Forensic Mental Health Nursing
Current Approaches

Edited by

Chris Chaloner
Michael Coffey

**Blackwell
Science**

© 2000 by
Blackwell Science Ltd
Editorial Offices:
Osney Mead, Oxford OX2 0EL
25 John Street, London WC1N 2BL
23 Ainslie Place, Edinburgh EH3 6AJ
350 Main Street, Malden
    MA 02148 5018, USA
54 University Street, Carlton
    Victoria 3053, Australia
10, rue Casimir Delavigne
    75006 Paris, France

Other Editorial Offices:

Blackwell Wissenschafts-Verlag GmbH
Kurfürstendamm 57
10707 Berlin, Germany

Blackwell Science KK
MG Kodenmacho Building
7–10 Kodenmacho Nihombashi
Chuo-ku, Tokyo 104, Japan

The right of the Author to be identified as the
Author of this Work has been asserted in
accordance with the Copyright, Designs and
Patents Act 1988

First published 2000

Set in 10/12.5pt Sabon
by Aarontype Limited, Easton, Bristol
Printed and bound in Great Britain by
MPG Books Ltd, Bodmin, Cornwall

The Blackwell Science logo is a
trade mark of Blackwell Science Ltd,
registered at the United Kingdom
Trade Marks Registry

DISTRIBUTORS

Marston Book Services Ltd
PO Box 269
Abingdon
Oxon OX14 4YN
(*Orders*: Tel: 01235 465500
              Fax: 01235 465555)

USA
Blackwell Science, Inc.
Commerce Place
350 Main Street
Malden, MA 02148 5018
(*Orders*: Tel: 800 759 6102
                    781 388 8250
              Fax: 781 388 8255)

Canada
Login Brothers Book Company
324 Saulteaux Crescent
Winnipeg, Manitoba R3J 3T2
(*Orders*: Tel: 204 837 2987
              Fax: 204 837 3116)

Australia
Blackwell Science Pty Ltd
54 University Street
Carlton, Victoria 3053
(*Orders*: Tel: 03 9347 0300
              Fax: 03 9347 5001)

A catalogue record for this title
is available from the British Library

ISBN 0-632-05031-4

Library of Congress
Cataloging-in-Publication Data

Forensic mental health nursing : current
    approaches / edited by Chris Chaloner,
    Michael Coffey.
        p. cm.
    Includes bibliographical references and
    index.
    ISBN 0-632-05031-4 (pbk.)
    1. Psychiatric nursing. 2. Forensic
    psychiatric nursing.
    I. Chaloner, Chris. II. Coffey, Michael.
    [DNLM: 1. Psychiatric Nursing.
    2. Forensic Psychiatry. WY 160
    F715 1999]
    RC440.F55 1999
    610.73'68–dc21
    DNLM/DLC
    for Library of Congress   99-34311
                                           CIP

For further information on Blackwell Science,
visit our website:
www.blackwell-science.com

This book is dedicated to our parents and
to Cathy, Pauline and Ruth

Contents

Preface

Forensic mental health nurses are principally concerned with the care, treatment and management of mentally disordered offenders within a variety of clinical settings. For many, the nursing care of such individuals still conjures up images of oppressive regimes and physical control within locked, isolated institutions surrounded by high walls and fences.

The purpose of this book is to explore and explain some of the diverse areas of clinical practice in which forensic nurses now work and, in so doing, demonstrate the evolution of the nurse's role from its in-patient, secure services origins to the diverse sub-specialism of mental health nursing that exists today.

The development of the forensic mental health nurse's role has gone largely unnoticed. Attention is most frequently drawn towards forensic services at times of crises in patient management when nurses and nursing practice are frequently a focus for public criticism. The many and varied positive ways in which nursing effectively contributes to the care of a potentially difficult patient group receives little acknowledgement and, for many forensic nurses, an acceptance of negative public and, in some cases, professional perceptions of their role is an unfortunate necessity.

Our initial decision to write a book about forensic mental health nursing was largely motivated by a desire to respond to the dearth of dedicated texts available to nurses working in forensic mental health care. The various books written about forensic mental health practice tend not to focus on the nursing contribution. However, it is clear that there is an increasing requirement for nursing skills and knowledge within this specialist area, further highlighted by the high levels of public and professional scrutiny to which forensic mental health services are subjected.

We subsequently recognised that not only were there no books specifically written *for* forensic nurses but that there were also no books *about* the forensic nurse's role. We therefore decided to write this book so that it would be accessible to both nurses and members of the many other professional groups who have contact with, or are interested in the care of, mentally disordered offenders. This is a book about what forensic nurses are currently doing: it is not a 'how to do it' style book but describes 'approaches' to forensic mental health practice.

We approached nurses with a variety of experiences of forensic mental health practice both within and beyond secure environments. We invited nurses working within various areas of practice and/or education to contribute. In drawing together aspects of current thinking and clinical approaches, we encouraged these contributors to explore the variety of roles, skills and knowledge which forensic mental health nurses have developed in recent years. These authors have adopted individual approaches to the completion of their chapters. This was felt to be an essential aspect of such a clinically diverse text and reflective of the disparate nature of forensic mental health nursing practice.

We have not attempted to present a definitive account of what forensic mental health nursing *is* although a number of authors infer some degree of definition within their individual accounts. Rather we have sought, through delineation and analysis of practice issues, to present an overview of what those who adopt the professional title 'forensic mental health nurse' have achieved, are currently achieving and may potentially achieve in the future.

The emphasis throughout the book is on the exploration of relevant aspects of nursing both within and beyond secure clinical environments, drawing on current research and clinical issues. Each chapter aims to explore current thinking on a particular topic area and present evidence from the literature to establish a basis for developing practice. We hope that the focus on an evidence base for practice will prompt further exploration and inquiry into the forensic nurse's role.

Many of the chapter authors have included case studies in order to illustrate 'real-life' issues. All such scenarios are compositions produced solely for the purposes of this book and do not refer to any patient with whom the individual author has had clinical contact.

It is important to note that not all the areas in which forensic mental health nurses practise are covered within this book. It was never our intention to address every care scenario, and we acknowledge the contribution that nurses working in important clinical areas such as high security hospitals and prison health care services have made, and continue to make, to the development of the forensic nursing specialism.

We have produced a multi-authored text which addresses many issues relevant to the nursing care and management of mentally disordered offenders and examines some of the disparate roles which forensic mental health nurses undertake. We believe that it represents an important contribution to the knowledge base of forensic mental health nursing. We hope that you will find this an informative book and one which you find enjoyable and challenging to read.

Chris Chaloner
Michael Coffey

Acknowledgements

In compiling this book we were fortunate to find a group of individuals, experienced in their field, who were willing to apply themselves to the task of writing about their work. We would like to extend our thanks to them for their efforts. Our thanks also go to Nicola Horton for helping us to set the ball rolling and to Julia Houston for her helpful comments when reviewing a early draft of the Working with Sex Offenders chapter. Finally, we thank the anonymous reviewers and referees of this text for their encouragement and helpful advice.

Contributors

Anne Aiyegbusi RMN, MSc   Forensic Nurse Consultant, The Ashworth Centre, Ashworth Hospital Authority, Liverpool

Chris Chaloner RMN, RGN, MSc, PgDip Health Care Ethics, PgDip Social Research Methods, FETC   Senior Lecturer, School of Health, The University of Greenwich, London

Jenifer Clarke RMN, ENB 770, Dip Forensic Psych, MSc   Clinical Nurse Specialist, South Wales Forensic Psychiatric Service, Caswell Clinic, Bridgend

Michael Coffey RMN, RGN, BSc (Hons), MSc   Lecturer in Community Mental Health Nursing, School of Health Science, University of Wales, Swansea

Carol Davies RNMH, RMN, MSc, CertEd, DipMDO, ENB 870   Ward Manager, Rampton Hospital Authority, Nottinghamshire

Mike Doyle RMN, DipN, BSc (Hons), MSc   Risk Management Coordinator and Forensic Community Mental Health Nurse, Mental Health Services, Salford NHS Trust

Nicola Evans RMN, BSc (Hons), CertEd, Cert Family Therapy   Forensic Community Mental Health Nurse, South Wales Forensic Psychiatric Service, Caswell Clinic, Bridgend

Geoff Haines RMN, RGN, MEd, BEd, RNT   Lecturer/Practitioner, John Howard Centre, Hackney, London

Gina Hillis RMN, RGN, MSc, Cert CPN   Community Forensic Psychiatric Nurse, formerly Reaside Clinic, Birmingham

Stephan D. Kirby RMN, MSc, DipMDO   Lecturer/Practitioner, Tees and North East Yorkshire NHS Trust

Ged McCann RMN, DPSN (Thorn), BPhil, MPH   County Development Officer for Mentally Disordered Offenders and Lecturer, North Yorkshire Health Authority and University of York

Tim McDougall RMN, Dip Nursing (MH), Dip Psychotherapy, BSc, ENB 603   Community Nurse Specialist, Child Mental Health Services, St Helens, Merseyside

Doug MacInnes PhD, BSc (Hons), RMN, PgDip ARM   Research Fellow, Centre for Nursing Research and Practice Development, Canterbury Christ Church University College, Kent

Mick McKeown RMN, RGN, DPSN (Thorn), BA (Hons)   Lecturer/ Practitioner, University of Liverpool and North Mersey Community NHS Trust

Allison Tennant RNMH, RMN, CertEd, RNT, BSc (Hons)   Lecturer/ Practitioner, Rampton Hospital Authority, Nottinghamshire

Ian Tennant RNMH, RMN, Adv. Dip Counselling, ENB 870   Clinical Nurse Manager, Rampton Hospital Authority, Nottinghamshire

Arthur Turnbull RNMH, BA, DipCPN   Community Nurse (Forensic Learning Disabilities), Tees and North East Yorkshire NHS Trust

Chapter 1
Characteristics, Skills, Knowledge and Inquiry

Chris Chaloner

INTRODUCTION

The primary purpose of this book is to contribute to the knowledge base of an emerging specialism and to demonstrate the range of roles and disparate areas of practice into which forensic mental health nursing has developed in recent years. Chapter authors have been encouraged to illustrate the boundaries of contemporary practice and to demonstrate nursing's ability to articulate its purpose and contribution to forensic mental health care.

The role of the forensic mental health nurse has expanded and there is a growing number and range of practice areas to which 'forensic' nurses make an active contribution. Many nurses (working within dedicated forensic mental health teams) undertake increasingly autonomous roles which extend the boundaries and perceptions of their specialism and show that 'forensic' is no longer the exclusive attribute of those working within secure clinical environments.

The expansion of the role has naturally extended the range of skills required by forensic mental health nurses and contributed to an increasing knowledge base relating to the diverse requirements of practice. The creation of specialist educational programmes, plus the diverse range of publications generated by forensic nurses, have contributed to the recognition of this specialism and enabled a nursing 'voice' to be heard within the varied and complex debates relating to the treatment, care and management of mentally disordered offenders.

However, for perhaps the majority of mental health professionals a clear conceptualisation of forensic mental health nursing remains uncertain. Associations with custody and control are a significant feature of many people's perception of 'forensic nurses' and, even within the specialism itself, the identification of a discrete body of skills and knowledge is incomplete.

This chapter will endeavour to illustrate the characteristics of forensic mental health nursing and explore the skills and knowledge required for effective practice. The nurse's role as a participant in academic develop-ments and research inquiry within forensic mental health care will be addressed.

THE CHARACTERISTICS OF FORENSIC MENTAL HEALTH NURSING

In recent years, the term 'forensic' has been applied to mental health care within a range of clinical areas. From being the exclusive property of those working in secure services, 'forensic' has been adopted by many mental health professionals whose role involves contact with mentally disordered offenders within or beyond in-patient services. The development of forensic mental health nursing has seen the concomitant emergence of forensic psychologists, forensic social workers, forensic occupational therapists and, of course, forensic psychiatrists.

'The term "forensic nurse" is a recent addition to the descriptions of nursing roles in mental health care and confusion remains over what the term in fact means and whether such a nurse really does exist.' (Whyte, 1997, p. 46).

The development of forensic mental health nursing as a discrete sub-specialism of mental health care has been affected by its perceived relationship to custodial and punitive responses to mentally disordered behaviour and traditional perceptions of the role of the 'mental nurse' in the management of 'mad' and potentially dangerous individuals. The application of the term 'forensic' (with its legal connotations) to an area of nursing practice (generally associated with caring and compassionate behaviour) is a basic source of confusion. Whyte (1997, p. 47) states:

'There is little in the current literature to endorse the existence of such a person as a forensic nurse, or the sub-speciality of forensic nursing, in the UK. However, what does appear to be happening is that the work of all mental health nurses is being influenced increasingly by the forensic aspect of mental health care as the relationship between healthcare services and criminal activity takes on a more explicit focus.'

The basis for such a dissenting view of the use of the title 'forensic nurse' by UK practitioners may relate to its failure to correlate with other con-ceptions of forensic nursing. For example, the United States 'forensic nurse' has an affirmed academic and professional base but direct comparisons with the role of the forensic mental health nurse are inappropriate. An overview of the US forensic nurse role states that:

'Forensic nurses apply the nursing process to public or legal proceedings; they engage in the scientific investigation of trauma, involving both living and deceased individuals. They are concerned with the impact of victimisation, offender motivations, crime scene analysis, self-destructive behaviour, and the exploitation of the vulnerable.' (Lynch, 1995, p. 6).

The US role is defined by its associations with the care of victims of offences rather than perpetrators and is thus not mirrored by the work of the majority of UK forensic mental health nurses. Although forensic services are increasing their clinical commitment to 'victims' (Huckle, 1995; Hilton & Mezey, 1996), the majority of nursing activities are directed towards the care and management of mentally disordered offenders. Aspects of 'forensic nursing' in some other countries, notably Canada and some parts of Australia, may possibly be more aligned with the goals of UK practice. When considering the UK role it is perhaps advisable to adhere to the descriptive (if not succinct) terminology of 'forensic mental health nurse'.

Conceptions of forensic mental health nursing are also handicapped by misunderstandings regarding the function and purpose of forensic mental health services. These services provide care, treatment and safe management for what are collectively, if somewhat erroneously, referred to as 'mentally disordered offenders'. The term is perhaps misleading as not all individuals who come into contact with these services will have committed offences (Coid in Murphy *et al.*, 1997). The majority of forensic mental health services are located within or attached to secure mental health establishments although recent developments in the size and nature of forensic provision have led to the development of many community-based forensic mental health teams. A frequently highlighted aspect of the role of all forensic mental health professionals is a responsibility to both patients and society. Indeed, both 'protecting the public' and 'needing continually to balance security and risk with therapy and patient needs' have been identified as primary aspects of the forensic mental health nurse's role (Kirby & McGuire, 1997, p. 408).

A definition of forensic psychiatry and a consideration of the general interests of forensic psychiatrists assist in the identification of the function of forensic mental health nursing. In its most fundamental interpretation, the forensic psychiatrist's role is concerned with the provision of treatment for the mentally abnormal offender and the preparation of psychiatric reports for the court on the mental state of offenders suspected of having a mental abnormality (Faulk, 1994).

Forensic psychiatry, although of comparatively recent origin – 'The speciality barely existed before the 1970s' (Chiswick, 1995, p. 2) – has developed and maintained an important academic profile and guided the expansion of services for mentally disordered offenders. The psychiatrist's role and range of clinical contacts and responsibilities (Bluglass & Bowden, 1990; Gunn & Taylor, 1993) provide evidence of the aims, expectations and associations of forensic mental health practice within which nurses participate as members of multi-professional and multi-agency teams.

Nurses have benefited from psychiatry-led advances and started to undertake activities reflecting a nurse-orientated forensic mental health role, for example with regard to community mental health practice (Chaloner & Kinsella, 1992; Evans, 1996), the needs of patients' relatives (McCann *et al.* 1995) and the emerging nursing advisory role (Friel & Chaloner, 1996). Nurses have also acknowledged the particular demands of forensic practice, the need for 'job satisfaction' (Kinsella & Friel, 1995; Morrison *et al.*, 1996) and the contribution of constructive self-awareness and 'appropriate attitudes' (Kinsella & Chaloner, 1995).

Traditional perceptions of forensic mental health care relate to detention and management within secure clinical environments. For many years this has been sufficient to determine the boundaries of the nurse's role, and such a view remains, for some, one of its defining characteristics (Box 1.1). An emerging reality (of which this book provides evidence) is that the nurse's role is increasingly diverse, and many 'forensic' nurses practise well beyond the confines of the locked clinical setting.

Box 1.1   The function of forensic mental health nursing

'The overall function could be described as providing health care for people with a recognised mental disorder under conditions of special security (high, medium and low) required to protect the public from their dangerous, violent and criminal propensities. While this view is somewhat simplistic, it captures the essence of the (nurse's) function.' (Kirby & McGuire, 1997, p. 396)

Burrow (1993a) addressed 'an inclusive forensic nursing speciality which has evolved out of general psychiatric competencies and has adapted specialist nursing skills but is progressing towards a more discrete forensic focus'. He proceeded to present a case for the existence of the specialism (Box 1.2).

Box 1.2   The case for forensic nursing (Burrow, 1993a, p. 903)

(1) The client category consists overwhelmingly of offenders with psychiatric pathology.
(2) Nurses contribute towards the therapeutic targeting of any mental disorder or offending behaviour related to psychiatric morbidity.

Contd.

(3) These care strategies are largely incorporated within institutional control and custody of patients.

(4) The configuration of patient pathology, criminal activity, therapeutic interventions and competencies, court/legal issues, and custodial care creates the need for a formidable and accelerating knowledge base.

(5) The advocacy role is different from that in other nursing specialities, embracing both the destigmatisation and decriminalisation of the patient group.

(6) Clients' potentials for future dangerousness require the formulation of risk assessment strategies.

The need to combine the promotion of individual well-being with obligations towards the wider society remains a contentious aspect of forensic mental health practice and may cause a degree of role confusion for nurses – particularly among those who regard their professional purpose to be the provision of individual patient care. The dual nature of the role and its effect on defining the nature of practice provides one of the determining aspects of the specialism. Burrow (1993b, p. 20) describes the 'double-barrelled conflict' which nurses face in attempting to align their roles as clinicians and guardians of public safety.

Perhaps, when one considers the joint role to which all health care professionals subscribe – i.e. to their patients and to society – the clash of obligations within forensic mental health practice has prominence due to the specialism's potentially 'sensational' connotations. Role conflict is not unique to forensic mental health care.

When examining the nature and attributes of forensic mental health nursing, one is inevitably tempted to produce a definitive list delineating its purpose and characteristics. Although such a task lies beyond the aspirations of this chapter, I would propose that some of the defining characteristics of forensic mental health nursing are:

(1) Nursing contact with mentally disordered offenders (not exclusively within secure services).

(2) Working as part of (or in close collaboration with) a dedicated forensic mental health service.

(3) Development of and participation in nurse-specific activities intended to contribute to the care and management of mentally disordered offenders.

(4) The ability to differentiate between the social and therapeutic aspects of the forensic mental health nursing role and to practise effectively with regard to both.

(5) An understanding and acknowledgement of the contribution which personal values and attitudes make to forensic mental health care.

Of course, it may be that some rather than all of these characteristics apply to nurses working within specific areas of practice. This attempt to define the characteristics of the specialism is intentionally limited to five items; the potential for deliberation and revision is almost endless and this list is simply a contribution to a much wider debate.

THE SKILLS AND KNOWLEDGE BASE

The Reed Report (Volume 3) recommended 'the speedy introduction of more flexible arrangements for, and content of, post-basic education and training in subjects related to forensic nursing, including greater opportunities for open learning and better links with further and higher education' (Department of Health/Home Office, 1992a).

Since the publication of this major review of services for mentally disordered offenders there has been a marked increase in the number of educational establishments offering dedicated 'forensic nursing' courses, and the majority of forensic mental health services have well developed academic links with higher education providers.

The knowledge base for all areas of forensic mental health care continues to develop. However, the provision of, in 'Reed' terms, 'training in subjects related to forensic nursing' raises questions relating to the identification of such 'subjects' and to the interpretation of the word 'training'. If 'training' implies instruction and/or skills development, a clear identification of these skills has yet to be achieved.

SKILLS

The majority of forensic mental health nurses practise within in-patient secure services and it is within such areas that the skills base of forensic mental health nursing has its origins.

Traditionally, the primary focus of such skills was on the maintenance of security and safety – possibly at the expense of acquiring a more therapeutic focus for the nursing role: '... in effect this means that while other health disciplines (psychiatrists, psychologists, social workers and occupational therapists) can afford the luxury of a more or less unadulterated 'therapeutic' role, the custodial role *per se* becomes the overriding responsibility of the nursing staff irrespective of any therapeutic activity in which they might be involved' (Burrow, 1993b, p. 21).

A need to deliver care and safely manage individuals within secure environments enabled nurses working within such areas to develop and maintain a considerable skills base relating to the traditional aspects of the role, i.e. physical control, detention, risk management and the management of aggressive and violent behaviour.

Nurses working within high secure services were the first health-care professionals to incorporate nationally approved methods of physical restraint into their practice. 'Control and restraint' techniques began to be practised within the special hospitals in the early 1980s. Nurses have been instrumental in developing and refining these techniques and in providing training and expert advice regarding methods of physical control to colleagues in many areas of health care and social services (Carton & Larkin, 1991; McDougal, 1996; Wynn, 1996).

In recent years nurses working in secure areas have made significant professional advances and demonstrated that effective practice in secure environments may demand, and offer, a great deal more than previously expected (McMurran & Thomas, 1991; Rogers & Hughes, 1994; Hall, 1995; Noblett & Ikin, 1997).

As nursing expanded beyond the locked environment, the range of skills required broadened, although a number of the 'specialist' skills in which some forensic mental health nurses have become accomplished demonstrate an extension of previously developed (if not formally acknowledged) in-patient expertise. For example, the formalisation of 'risk management' traditionally practised by nurses within secure areas has contributed to the identification of the key factors involved in the assessment and management of risk and dangerousness (Doyle, 1998; Fox, 1998).

The evolution of forensic mental health services has led to the creation of various community-based services involving, for example, the diversion of people with mental health problems from the criminal justice system (James *et al.*, 1997) and the treatment of sex offenders (Taylor, 1991). Such expansion has seen nurses adopt prominent roles within multi-professional and multi-agency teams whilst furthering the skills base of the specialism.

Working within forensic mental health teams, nursing has extended into specialist aspects of practice such as adolescent forensic nursing and working with personality disordered individuals. Nurses have also started to identify specific skills relating to the diagnostic and behavioural characteristics of their patients. Examples of specialised practice can be found within the chapters of this book.

In 1997, the key competencies of the 'forensic nurse' were defined as (Royal College of Nursing, 1997):

(1) Assessment of offending behaviour
(2) Assessment of dangerousness
(3) Management of dangerousness
(4) Management of personality disorders with associated offending behaviour
(5) Risk assessment
(6) Understanding associated ethical issues in the management of the mentally disordered offender

The Royal College's report proceeded to define 'advanced interventions' practised by forensic nurses, such as:

- Behavioural therapies
- Anger management
- Loss and bereavement counselling

The particular nature of these skills, competencies and advanced interventions and the means by which they are, or should be, acquired remain a source of debate within educational and training arenas.

KNOWLEDGE

It is generally acknowledged that a clearly defined evidence base is a significant contributory factor to effective nursing practice (Hunt, 1997). The evidence base of forensic mental health nursing has emerged primarily from the established body of generic mental health nursing knowledge developed over many years of in-patient and community care. As the distinctive aspects of forensic mental health practice become increasingly evident, nurses have established and continually supplement a dedicated knowledge base related to many aspects of their role.

Informed opinion and inquiry have furnished the knowledge base of forensic mental health nursing as a discrete specialism (Mason & Mercer, 1998) and in relation to specific areas of practice such as: community care (Hillis, 1993; Evans, 1996); risk management (Doyle, 1998); seclusion (Mason, 1993; Morrison & Lehane, 1995; Mason et al., 1996) and quality care (Robinson, 1995).

In addition to a knowledge base relating to clinical approaches, working effectively with mentally disordered offenders obviously demands knowledge of legal frameworks.

The legislative components of the forensic mental health process may occasionally appear less important to nurses than the acquisition (and demonstration) of clinical knowledge – particularly when practitioners are required to demonstrate their therapeutic priorities in response to critical inspection (a public inquiry, for example). At such times a thorough comprehension of relevant mental health law may be thought acceptable evidence of a nurse's 'legal knowledge'. However, it is important that forensic mental health nurses have a heightened awareness of many other aspects of the legislative process – not simply the workings of the Mental Health Act, for example the criminal justice system, the function of the courts, litigation procedures, relevant case law and non-mental health statutes such as the Access to Health Records Act 1990 and the Crime (Sentences) Act 1997.

ACQUIRING SKILLS AND KNOWLEDGE

Traditionally, the essential skills and knowledge acquired by nurses caring for mentally disordered offenders were passed on from experienced nurses to their junior colleagues over lengthy apprenticeship periods during which nurses were also required to gain the respect and peer acknowledgement essential to 'fitting in' to the isolated culture of secure institutions. Practice was, to a great extent, based upon received wisdom regarding established approaches to the care and safe management of potentially 'difficult' and dangerous individuals, largely based on medically authorised interventions. Emphasis was not placed on the specialist nature of the nurse's role or on the establishment of a theoretical base for practice. There was little specific education or training available to nurses seeking to develop their role or widen their knowledge base.

The development of the generic mental health nurse's role and, in 1923, the first acknowledgement of the registered mental nurse's status (Nolan, 1993) offered opportunities for nurses to explore the foundations of their practice although at that time the theoretical basis for their role was primarily focused on the acquisition of knowledge of psychiatry and medical approaches to treatment.

In more recent times, forensic mental health nurses have begun to investigate the specialist nature of their role and to identify those aspects which distinguish their practice from other areas of mental health nursing. The development of a discrete skills and knowledge base has occurred as nurses have identified a need for relevant education, training and professional development opportunities which assist them to effectively work *with*, rather than under the direction of, their medical colleagues.

It seems reasonable to expect the acquisition of 'forensic' skills and knowledge to commence during pre-registration nurse training and education. It is unfortunate that forensic mental health experience, although possibly offered as an elective placement for some student nurses, maintains a low profile within many pre-registration mental health nursing programmes. The focus on the acquisition of generic skills and knowledge within a limited time frame possibly diverts attention from the more specialist areas of practice. Recommendations for changes to current pre-registration programmes – for example, a proposal in favour of a discrete three-year mental health nursing programme (The Sainsbury Centre for Mental Health, 1997) – may reflect an acknowledgement of student nurses' need for the acquisition of specialist skills and knowledge.

Future development of forensic mental health services, particularly with regard to the provision of long-term medium secure beds, suggests that the establishment of a dedicated pre-registration forensic mental health nursing programme may not be inconceivable. An approved 'Registered Forensic Mental Health Nurse' qualification may be a possible means of responding to the need for an increase in both the numbers and 'quality' of nursing personnel.

Following registration, the diversification of forensic mental health nursing roles may affect the design and delivery of meaningful educational, training and development programmes. It would be difficult to design and deliver a programme to meet the requirements of all forensic mental health nurses as they are now such a disparate group of practitioners. This is a particular problem for those course providers who attempt to include skills development and assessment of practice within their curriculum. The identification of measurable 'forensic nursing skills' remains in its infancy, and the skills-based aspect of many courses relates strongly to an assessment of either in-patient or community-based generic mental health nursing competencies.

There are many formal educational opportunities available to nurses, and the breadth of issues covered is extensive. However, it may be claimed that too much emphasis is placed on the acquisition of formal higher education qualifications which are gained at the possible expense of meaningful education and training acquired within less formal, but well resourced, service-based settings. Although a diploma and/or degree qualification has become an apparently essential item on the professional development agenda of many nurses, the pursuit of higher education courses may not always be the most appropriate way of gaining the relevant 'forensic' skills and knowledge required for practice. Many of the fundamental needs of nurses' post-registration education, training and development may be met within comprehensive in-house training and development programmes.

THE PROVISION OF FORMAL EDUCATION, TRAINING AND DEVELOPMENT OPPORTUNITIES

'They are coached for their examination in a special schoolroom on the premises by a regular male tutor. At the beginning of their career student nurses can be as ignorant about Broadmoor as they are about nursing. One delighted his instructor by exclaiming "Everything seems to be done for the patients here. One would think the bloody place was built for them".' (Partridge, 1953, p. 154)

This illuminating insight into the training of 'forensic' nurses nearly 50 years ago suggests that some progress has been made with regard to educating nurses, but to what extent have the developments in forensic mental health nurse education, training and development met the needs of both the individual and the clinical service?

The provision of designated education and training courses for nurses working with mentally disordered offenders was, until recent years, an unfortunate deficiency in the provision of forensic mental health services. Volume 4 of the Reed Report noted that 'As long ago as 1974, the Glancy report suggested that there should be a formal qualification in forensic psychiatric nursing but this has not happened' (Department of Health/Home Office, 1992b).

The first dedicated educational programmes for nurses working with mentally disordered offenders were established in the late 1970s and early 1980s. The English National Board for Nursing, Midwifery and Health Visiting (ENB) courses 960, 'Nursing in Secure Environments', and 955, 'The Prevention and Management of Violence', were a means by which nurses could gain a level of relevant post-registration education and training. The emphasis on 'violence' and working in secure areas was perhaps reasonable as the 'forensic' role at that time was exclusive to secure establishments and its primary purpose was the maintenance of locked clinical areas in which patients could be safely treated and managed.

In the early 1990s a number of centres, in liaison with the three English Special Hospitals – Broadmoor, Rampton and Ashworth – established a new ENB course which generated a significant increase in the awareness, skills and knowledge of nurses. The ENB 770 'Nursing in Controlled Environments' course offered a wider range of educational opportunities than had been provided by the 960 and 955 courses. Nurses from various clinical locations undertook an educational programme which, in addition to relating and assessing knowledge, required that they conducted some form of investigative work of their own in the form of a short 'research study'. Although many of the studies undertaken for this purpose were purely of local (or even personal) relevance, a number of more generalisable findings were published (Burnard & Morrison, 1992). The fact that forensic mental health nurses were encouraged to formally explore issues pertaining to their practice was a major advance for both nursing and forensic services.

Although it represented a significant progression from what had been previously available, the ENB 770 course, in its initial conception at least, retained a focus on nursing practice within secure clinical areas. In recent years, as forensic mental health nursing has advanced, it has been necessary for educational programmes to acknowledge these developments and provide an appropriate range of opportunities for nurses working in different areas of the specialism. The ENB A71 course, 'Care of the Mentally Disordered Offender: Principles and Practice', was a subsequent attempt to provide a wider focus for nurses' education and training.

In the 1990s, changes in the provision of pre-registration nurse education and the development of links with higher education led to the establishment of a minimum diploma-level pre-registration programme for all nurses. Post-registration courses were subsequently adapted to fit in with the requirements of higher education providers. Courses such as the ENB 770 and A71 became modularised within educational 'pathways' leading towards diploma and degree qualifications. The theoretical aspects of courses were revised in line with these changes and assessment criteria modified in accordance with academic standards.

There are now a variety of short courses, modules and units, academically validated at diploma or degree level, specifically designed to meet the needs of forensic mental health nurses and others involved in the care management of mentally disordered offenders. Indeed, it is now possible for nurses to acquire a 'forensic nursing' degree (most commonly as part of a BSc in Higher Education award). Examples of the theoretical content of a diploma/degree level programme are illustrated in Box 1.3.

Box 1.3 Examples from the theoretical contents of a diploma/degree course in forensic mental health nursing (City University & St. Bartholomew School of Nursing and Midwifery, London, 1997/8)

- Forensic mental health theory: the history and aims of forensic mental health care
- Assessing and managing risk and danger
- Models of interdisciplinary and inter-agency care
- Managing patients in the community
- Dual diagnosis in forensic settings – issues for staff and managers
- Issues of power and control: the 'unpopular' patient
- Dealing with and supporting victims
- Providing 'expert' advice to 'non-forensic' colleagues
- Ethics and forensic mental health practice
- Ideological factors in the design of forensic mental health care settings
- Concepts of professional and therapeutic relationships
- The future of forensic mental health nursing
- Rehabilitation needs of forensic patients

THE PROVISION OF INFORMAL EDUCATION, TRAINING AND DEVELOPMENT OPPORTUNITIES

Many forensic facilities, in addition to fulfilling their clinical responsibilities, act as administrative, teaching and research centres for regional forensic services (Cordess, 1995). Many are extremely well resourced in terms of both equipment and available expertise. The majority of forensic services combine some form of academic programme into their regular activities and many have their own dedicated training and educational facilities.

Unfortunately, there may be differences between nurses' experience of in-house training and that of their non-nursing colleagues. There may be two reasons for this. First, forensic mental health nursing has yet to establish the academic purpose and credibility of its longer established and more 'academically confident' professional colleagues. Therefore the contribution of nurses and nursing to multi-professional learning opportunities may be impaired. However willing other disciplines may be to bring a nursing perspective to their education and training activities, many nurses are perhaps not ready or able to effectively participate.

Second, nurses may believe that in-house training activities lack the educational credibility or value of external courses or feel that they do not relate to the daily realities of their clinical practice (the establishment of the academic basis for practice is still, after all, in its infancy). They may feel threatened by their apparently more learned colleagues and opt for the comparative 'safety' of clinical work ('We're too busy to attend the lecture/seminar etc.'; 'We can't spare the time and/or staff to participate', etc.). Obviously the clinical workload of nurses is a contributory factor to the amount of time that they can devote to in-house activities – the majority of clinically based nurses do not enjoy the luxury of an appointments diary – but excuses for not wishing to be involved in the wider academic opportunities available in house may conceal a deeper fear of exposure to the wider multi-professional learning environment.

MULTI-DISCIPLINARY/MULTI-AGENCY TRAINING AND EDUCATION

'...despite the fact that they often have the greatest experience of the patient: they (nurses) may feel that they are not empowered with the same professional and coded language to achieve their aims of shared professional participation' (Killian & Clarke, 1998, pp. 104–5).

Unfortunately, multi-professional roles within some forensic mental health teams remain entrenched in 'traditional' disciplinary hierarchies; interdisciplinary divisions relating to perceived clinical effectiveness and contribution to care may also persist, thus minimising opportunities for the narrowing of knowledge gaps and promotion of cohesive working practices. It makes little sense that such a situation should endure at a time when the complex nature of forensic mental health practice demands a multi-skilled and effective professional workforce.

Fortunately, the late 1990s have seen an encouraging development in multi-disciplinary and multi-agency education initiatives. A number of multi-professional 'forensic' educational programmes have been established in which nurses, psychiatrists, psychologists, social workers, etc. participate on equal terms in the learning environment. Many nurses now undertake meaningful educational courses at diploma, first degree and higher degree levels alongside their non-nursing colleagues. Multi-professional programmes offer equivalent input and assessment criteria for all forensic mental health professionals. They do not have the negative connotations that 'forensic nursing' courses maintain for some members of the multi-disciplinary team (including, of course, many nurses), for whom such courses may be considered to have limited academic credibility.

Courses offered by, for example, St. George's Medical School, London; the University of Liverpool; and the University of Birmingham have pioneered meaningful multi-professional forensic mental health education (see Box 1.4).

Box 1.4   Contents of a multi-disciplinary diploma in forensic mental health care (St. George's Hospital Medical School, 1998)

Module 1: Violence and Dangerousness

Topics include:

- Mental disorder and crime
- Domestic violence
- Gender and deliberate self-harm
- Organic disorders and violence

Module 2: Ethics and Forensic Mental Health Care

Topics include:

- Ethical issues within secure environments
- Exploration of coercive practice
- Issues of confidentiality
- Mental health care and human rights

Module 3: Forensic Psychotherapy

Topics include:

- Key concepts within forensic psychotherapy
- An understanding of psychotic and borderline clinical problems
- Unmanageable affects (anger, shame and guilt in the genesis of violent behaviour)
- Personality problems

Contd.

Module 4: Law and The Mentally Disordered Offender

Topics include:

- Court processes and mentally disordered offenders
- Homicide and legal defences
- Child protection law
- Legal understandings of responsibility

Module 5: Social Policy

Topics include:

- History of secure institutions
- Interface between the criminal justice system and health and social care
- Institutions and their perils
- Media interest and coverage of 'forensic' individuals

NURSING AND RESEARCH INQUIRY

Forensic mental health nursing is rapidly establishing an identifiable research base and the number of important studies generated by nurses is increasing. Individuals from both clinical and academic backgrounds have examined a variety of practice-based and context-related topics. The methods employed are varied and many of the studies provide insight into the realities of practice, the identification of relevant aspects of service provision and indicators for education and practice development. The National Forensic Nurses Research and Development Group and the Royal College of Nursing's Forum for Forensic Nursing contribute to the academic base of forensic mental health nursing.

There are approximately 30 times as many nurses as there are doctors working within mental health care (Muijen, 1997). It would appear illogical if such a large workforce were unable, or unwilling, to adopt a prominent role in the investigation of all aspects of mental health practice.

Methodological issues are, perhaps, one of the important determining factors in the conduct of inquiry within forensic mental health settings. The nature of clinical locations has possibly led to an over-reliance on quantitative methods. The survey is an extremely useful source of knowledge and has many benefits in the exploration of numerous aspects of practice (e.g. Kinsella & Chaloner, 1995). However, its comparative ease of application may deter nurses from participating in more 'demanding' forms of inquiry. It is perhaps a less daunting task to distribute and analyse questionnaires from the comparative comfort of one's workplace (or home) than to physically enter the field of study to undertake a labour-intensive qualitative or mixed-strategy inquiry.

Nurses have exclusively close contact with patients, other members of the multi-professional/multi-agency clinical team and many of the other important, if more peripheral, sections of forensic mental health services. They are in a prime position to undertake non-numerical studies within clinical settings. Forensic mental health areas would undoubtedly benefit from the implementation of ethnographic methodology. An obvious limitation to this type of inquiry is that the researcher must pay particularly close attention to the unique nature of research location in addition to demonstrating respect for individual autonomy and the patients' potential role as participants in the study (Latvala *et al.*, 1998).

Within in-patient settings, particularly those sensitive to any form of inquiry, covert participation, although a valuable means of data collection (Clarke, 1996), is not perhaps the most acceptable method of obtaining information. But the requirement for a 'public' approach by the qualitative investigator should not necessarily dissuade nurses from considering this methodology within their wider research strategy.

The use of the single case study method would appear to have much to offer a forensic mental health researcher and may have valuable implications for specific aspects of practice (Duff, 1996).

Investigations into the patients' experiences as recipients of forensic mental health services, for example Skelly (1994a, b) and Morrison *et al.* (1996), seem to be an obvious focus for nursing research activity and evaluative studies (Chanpakkee & Whyte, 1996), and literature reviews (McDougal, 1996) can also be useful methods for nurses to examine the evidence base for their role.

In addition to exploring the varied aspects of practice discussed within this book, there are many areas on which nurses could (and hopefully will!) focus future research activities, to the benefit of clinical practice, skills training and professional knowledge. The scope for academic activity is vast. It is an extremely attractive and exciting aspect of the specialism that there remains a great deal of innovative academic activity to be undertaken.

A major initiative being undertaken as this book goes to press is the 'Nursing in secure environments project' conducted by The University of Central Lancashire. Utilising a range of research methods, this study aims to provide a comprehensive overview of the educational, occupational and professional practice expectations placed on forensic mental health nurses working in secure environments.

INPUT INTO THE WIDER ACADEMIC WORLD

Forensic mental health services generate and contribute to an abundance of knowledge pertaining to mental health care; the prevention and amelioration of mental disorder; social and criminological responses to offending behaviour and the development of national and international frameworks for the management of mentally disordered offenders.

Much of this activity is psychiatry-led but nurses are beginning to develop a greater participatory role in the wider academic world of forensic mental health practice and there has been an increase in publications by nurses within peer-reviewed, predominantly medico-legal journals (e.g. Brett, 1992; Mason, 1993; Kirby, 1997)

Nurses have also contributed to the dissemination of knowledge and critical thinking through international publications and conference presentations across the world (e.g. Chaloner, 1995; Mason & Mercer, 1996).

CONCLUSION

The forensic mental health nurse's unique role demands that suitably knowledgeable, experienced and skilled individuals participate in the undertaking and development of practice. Undoubtedly, there are particular requirements for effective forensic mental health nursing – the possession of common sense and a willingness to participate in the development of the specialism being perhaps the most essential! Obviously, the nursing role should develop within a realistic framework which relates to both the specialist requirements of forensic services and the wider needs of health care and society.

As all aspects of the specialism develop and the number of nurses prepared to undertake a participatory role in multi-professional academic work increases, the foundations of forensic mental health nursing will continue to solidify and prove increasingly meaningful and attractive to potential recruits. It has to be seen as a viable specialism into which registered nurses would wish to gain entry and progress their careers. Without an appropriately skilled and qualified nursing workforce it is difficult to envisage significant progress being made with regard to the care, treatment and management of mentally disordered offenders. It is particularly important that nurses develop and maintain the professional confidence and authority required to work effectively with their multi-disciplinary and multi-agency colleagues.

The demands of clinical practice must be met by the identification of the skills and knowledge base which forensic mental health nursing requires. In developing a coherent skills and knowledge base, nurses may confirm their specific contribution to multi-professional forensic mental health care. Although there is still some way to go before an all-encompassing skills and knowledge base is created or even fully defined, and this has obvious implications for any claim nurses may wish to make with regard to the status of their specialism, the evidence contained within this book demonstrates that forensic mental health nurses and nursing are progressing towards the confirmation of an important contributory role to both mental health care and society.

REFERENCES

Bluglass, R. & Bowden, P. (eds) (1990) *Principles and Practice of Forensic Psychiatry*. Churchill Livingstone, Edinburgh.

Brett, T. (1992) The Woodstock approach: one ward in Broadmoor Hospital for the treatment of personality disorder. *Criminal Behaviour and Mental Health* **2**, 152–8.

Burnard, P. & Morrison, P. (eds) (1992) *Aspects of Forensic Psychiatric Nursing*. Avebury Press, Aldershot.

Burrow, S. (1993a) An outline of the forensic nursing role. *British Journal of Nursing* **2**(18), 899–904.

Burrow, S. (1993b) The role conflict of the forensic nurse. *Senior Nurse* **13**(5), 20–5.

Carton, G. & Larkin, E. (1991) Reducing the violence in a special hospital. *Nursing Standard* **5**(17), 29–31.

Chaloner, C. (1995) The ethics of forensic mental health nursing. Presented at 'Celebrating a New Era', International Conference on Mental Health Nursing, Canberra, Australia, 29 September 1995.

Chaloner, C. & Kinsella, C. (1992) Care with conviction. *Nursing Times* **88**(17), 50–2.

Chanpakkee, J. & Whyte, L (1996) Evaluating primary nursing in a secure environment. *Psychiatric Care* **3**(5), 188–93.

Chiswick, D. (1995) Introduction. In *Seminars in Practical Forensic Psychiatry* (Chiswick, D. & Cope, R., eds), Chapter 1. Royal College of Psychiatrists, London.

City University & St. Bartholomew School of Nursing and Midwifery, London (1997/8) 'Forensic Mental Health Nursing' (ENB 770) and 'Care of Mentally Disordered Offenders' (ENB A71).

Clarke, L. (1996) Covert participation in a secure forensic unit. *Nursing Times* **92**(48), 37–40.

Cordess, C. (1995) Facilities and treatment. In *Practical Forensic Psychiatry* (Chiswick, D. & Cope, R., eds), Chapter 7. Gaskell, London.

Department of Health/Home Office (1992a) *Review of Health and Social Services for Mentally Disordered Offenders and Others Requiring Similar Services. Vol. 3: Finance, staffing and training*. HMSO, London.

Department of Health/Home Office (1992b) *Review of Health and Social Services for Mentally Disordered Offenders and Others Requiring Similar Services. Vol. 4: The academic and research base*. HMSO, London.

Doyle, M. (1998) Clinical risk assessment for mental health nurses. *Nursing Times* **94**(17), 47–9.

Duff, A. (1996) Case study of a female client on a regional secure unit. *Journal of Advanced Nursing* **23**(4), 771–5.

Evans, N. (1996) Defining the role of the forensic community mental health nurse. *Nursing Standard* 10(49), 35–7.

Faulk, M. (1994) *Basic Forensic Psychiatry* (2nd edn). Blackwell Science, Oxford.

Friel, C. & Chaloner, C. (1996) The developing role of the forensic community mental health nurse. *Nursing Times* 92(29), 33–5.

Fox, G. (1998) Risk assessment: A systematic approach to violence. *Nursing Standard* 12(32), 44–7.

Gunn, J. & Taylor, P. (1993) *Forensic Psychiatry: Clinical, Legal and Ethical Issues.* Butterworth-Heinemann, London.

Hall, G. (1995) Using group work to understand arsonists. *Nursing Standard* 9(23), 25–8.

Hillis, G. (1993) Mentally disordered offenders. Diverting tactics. *Nursing Times* 89(1), 24–7.

Hilton, M. & Mezey, G. (1996) Victims and perpetrators of child sexual abuse. *British Journal of Psychiatry* 169(4), 408–15.

Huckle, P. L. (1995) Male rape victims referred to a forensic psychiatric service. *Medicine, Science and the Law* 35(3), 187–92.

Hunt, J. (1997) Towards evidence based practice. *Nursing Management* 4(2), 14–17.

James, D., Cripps, J., Guilluley, P. & Harlow, P. (1997) A court focused model of forensic psychiatry provision to central London: abolishing remands to prison. *Journal of Forensic Psychiatry* 8(2), 390–405.

Killian, M. & Clarke, N. (1998) The nurse. In *Forensic Psychotherapy: Crime, Psychodynamics and the Offender Patient* (Cordess, C. & Cox, M., eds). Jessica Kingsley, London.

Kinsella, C. & Chaloner, C. (1995) Attitude to treatment and direction of interest of forensic mental health nurses: a comparison with nurses working in other specialties. *Journal of Psychiatric and Mental Health Nursing* 2(6), 351–7.

Kinsella, C. & Friel, C. (1995) Job satisfaction in a medium secure unit: a comparative study of male and female secure unit nurses. *Psychiatric Care* 2(1), 2–16.

Kirby, S. (1997) Ward atmosphere on a medium secure long-stay ward. *Journal of Forensic Psychiatry* 8(2), 336–47.

Kirby, S. & McGuire, N. (1997) Forensic psychiatric nursing. In *Stuart and Sundeen's Mental Health Nursing: Principles and Practice.* (Thomas, B., Hardy, S. & Cutting, P., eds), Chapter 26. Mosby, London.

Latvala, E., Janhonen, S. & Moring, J. (1998) Ethical dilemmas in a psychiatric nursing study. *Nursing Ethics* 5(1), 27–35.

Lynch, V. A. (1995) Forensic nursing: what's new? *Journal of Psychosocial Nursing and Mental Health Services* 33(9), 6–8.

McCann, G., McKeown, M. & Porter, I. (1995) Understanding the needs of relatives of patients within a special hospital for mentally disordered offenders: a basis for improved services. *Journal of Advanced Nursing* 23(2), 346–52.

McDougal, T. (1996) Physical restraint: A review of the literature. *Psychiatric Care* 3(4), 132–8.

McMurran, M. & Thomas, G. (1991) An intervention for alcohol-related offending. *Senior Nurse* 11(3), 33–6.

Mason, T. (1993) Seclusion theory reviewed – a benevolent or malevolent intervention? *Medicine, Science and the Law* 33(2), 95–102.

Mason, T. & Mercer, D. (1996) Forensic psychiatric nursing: visions of social control. *Australia and New Zealand Journal of Mental Health Nursing* 5(4), 153–62.

Mason, T. & Mercer, D. (eds) (1998) *Critical Perspectives in Forensic Care: Inside Out*. Macmillan, London.

Mason T., Henighan, M., Chandley, M. & Johnson, D. (1996) Decompression from long-term seclusion. *Psychiatric Care* 3(6), 217–25.

Morrison, P. & Lehane, M. (1995) Staffing levels and seclusion use. *Journal of Advanced Nursing* 22, 1193–1202.

Morrison, P., Phillips, C. & Burnard, P. (1996) Staff and patient satisfaction in a forensic unit. *Journal of Psychiatric and Mental Health Nursing* 3(1), 67–9.

Muijen, M. (1997) The future of training. *Journal of Mental Health* 6(6), 535–8.

Murphy, E., Coid, J. & Boa, W. (1997) Security cheques. *Health Service Journal* 107(5535), 28–9.

Noblett, S. P. & Ikin, P. T. (1997) Hostage incidents: first on the scene training for healthcare professionals. *Psychiatric Care* 4(6), 279–82.

Nolan, P. (1993) *A History of Mental Health Nursing*. Chapman & Hall, London.

Partridge, R. (1953) *Broadmoor. A History of Criminal Lunacy and its Problems*. Chatto & Windus, London.

Robinson, D. (1995) Developing clinical quality indicators in psychiatric nursing. *Journal of Psychiatric and Mental Health Nursing* 2(2), 111–12.

Rogers, P. & Hughes, A. (1994) Assessment and treatment of a suicidal patient. *Nursing Times* 90(34), 37–9

Royal College of Nursing (1997) *Buying Forensic Mental Health Nursing: an RCN Guide for Purchasers*. Royal College of Nursing, London.

Skelly, C. (1994a) The experiences of special hospital patients in regional secure units. *Journal of Psychiatric and Mental Health Nursing* 1(3), 171–7.

Skelly, C. (1994b) From special hospital to regional secure unit: A qualitative study of the problems experienced by patients. *Journal of Advanced Nursing* 20(6), 1056–63.

St. George's Hospital Medical School, University of London (1998/99) Multi-Disciplinary Diploma/MSc in Forensic Mental Health.

Taylor, P. (1991) Psychiatry for sex offenders: is anyone motivated? (editorial). *Criminal Behaviour and Mental Health* 1(2), iii–vii.

The Sainsbury Centre for Mental Health (1997) *Pulling Together: The Future Roles and Training of Mental Health Staff*. The Sainsbury Centre for Mental Health, London.

Whyte, L. (1997) Forensic nursing: a review of concepts and definitions. *Nursing Standard* 11(26), 46–7.

Wynn, R. (1996) Controlled Aggression. *Nursing Times* 92(2), 18–19.

Chapter 2
Working with Adolescent Patients

Tim McDougall

INTRODUCTION

Specialist mental health services for children and adolescents are frequently cited government priorities (Health Advisory Service (HAS), 1987, 1995). In any one year, up to 1 in 5 children and young people may experience mental health problems serious enough to require professional help (Royal College of Psychiatrists 1995; Rutter & Smith, 1995). Such needs may disturb psychological and social development, affect relations with family and friends and disrupt education and employment opportunities.

Many psychiatric disorders and mental health needs originate in childhood. Disorders of mood such as manic depression, severe psychotic disorders such as schizophrenia, and conduct and personality problems may persist into adulthood. There are increasing numbers of young people with psychological, emotional or behavioural difficulties who require care and treatment within a secure environment. Adolescent forensic mental health nursing is a unique and rapidly expanding area of practice. Nurses working within this challenging area are required to meet the complex needs of young people who present with dangerous, challenging or high-risk behaviours.

(In accordance with the Children Act 1989, the descriptions of 'young person', 'child' and 'adolescent' throughout the text refer to people under the age of 18 years old.)

SECURE PROVISION FOR CHILDREN AND YOUNG PEOPLE

Secure and related specialised services for children and adolescents were recommended by the Reed Committee (Department of Health/Home Office, 1992). Low, medium and high security placements for young people are provided by local authorities, the health service and the Home Office. These constitute young offender institutions, secure training centres and local authority secure care units.

An Adolescent Forensic Service provides in-patient assessment and treatment for young people aged 10–18 years within conditions of medium security. The Gardener Unit in Manchester is staffed by a multi-disciplinary team, many of whom have had training in both child and adolescent and forensic mental health care. The Forensic Adolescent Community Treatment Service (FACTS) provides a court diversion scheme, a psychiatric clinic in the Youth Court and a community-based assessment, treatment and liaison service. Outreach work is provided to secure care units, child and adolescent mental health services and the new multi-agency Young Offending Teams. Young people are referred to the Adolescent Forensic Service from both health and childcare services and the Criminal Justice System. Such referrals are taken from district child and adolescent mental health services, social services and the penal system. In addition, young people may come to the attention of the Adolescent Forensic Service through the intervention of court diversion schemes, youth justice and the probation service.

THE LITERATURE

Medical, psychology and social work texts have been published widely about mentally disordered young offenders (Farrington, 1995; Lyon, 1996). Research has addressed secure provision for adolescents (Bullock *et al.*, 1990; Bailey *et al.*, 1994) and, more specifically, young people who kill (Grant *et al.*, 1989; Bailey, 1996; Cavadino, 1996; Hardwick & Rowton-Lee, 1996); adolescent fire-setters (Kolko & Kazdin, 1994; Swaffer & Hollin, 1995); and young people who sexually abuse others (Becker, 1988; Epps, 1994; Vizard *et al.*, 1996). A small number of publications specifically explore adolescent forensic mental health nursing (McDougall, 1997, 1998a).

YOUNG OFFENDERS

In Britain, children and young people account for an estimated 7 million crimes a year (Health Advisory Service, 1995). The age of criminal responsibility in the United Kingdom is unusually low by European standards. In England, Wales and Northern Ireland it is 10 years, and in Scotland young people are held to be criminally responsible at 8 years (Bainham, 1993). In most other European countries children under 14 years do not appear before the criminal courts and are instead dealt with by youth authorities and family proceedings courts. Here, the emphasis is on the need for compulsory measures of care and rehabilitation rather than incarceration, retribution and punishment.

YOUNG PEOPLE, MENTAL HEALTH AND THE LAW

Young people who require in-patient assessment or treatment within conditions of security must be detained under provisions of the Mental Health Act 1983, the Children Act 1989 or the Children and Young Persons Act 1933. Children and adolescents cannot be informally assessed or treated within a secure environment.

There is no minimum age of admission to hospital under the Mental Health Act, and children and young people can be detained if they present a risk of danger to themselves or others. Young people can also be detained if they refuse voluntary admission, assessment or treatment. Similarly, Section 25 of the Children Act allows for a young person to be detained in hospital if they are deemed to be at significant risk of harm due to absconding and/or present a significant risk towards others. Adolescents detained under the Mental Health Act are exempt from Section 25 of the Children Act as lawful provision for their detention already exists.

The Children and Young Persons Act makes special provision for young people convicted on indictment for murder or other serious offences. Section 53[1] provides that a young person aged 10–17 convicted of murder can be detained during Her Majesty's Pleasure for an indeterminate period of time. Section 53[2] provides that a young person convicted of an offence for which an adult may be sentenced for 14 years' imprisonment or more can be detained. The period of detention (which may be for life) must be specified in the sentence and must not exceed the maximum period of imprisonment with which the offence would be punishable in the case of an adult (Criminal Justice Act 1991). Placement for young people detained within Section 53 is determined by the Home Secretary and can include secure psychiatric care.

RESTRICTING THE LIBERTY OF YOUNG PEOPLE

It is only in recent years that concern about the restriction of children's liberty has led to legislative safeguards (Gulbenkian Foundation, 1993). Until 1983 there was no statutory provision to limit the period of time a young person spent in secure care. Children and adolescents could be detained in secure units for indeterminate periods of time and with no statutory right of appeal. Such practice, clearly in breach of the European Convention on Human Rights, was highlighted in reports commissioned by the Department of Health and Social Security and in campaigns by the Children's Legal Centre and other organisations lobbying for children's rights (Children's Legal Centre, 1991). The United Nations Convention on the Rights of the Child, which the United Kingdom ratified in 1991, set standard minimum rules for the administration of juvenile justice (the Beijing Rules), the United Nations Guidelines for the Prevention of Juvenile Delinquency (the Riyadh Guidelines), and the United Nations Rules for the Protection of Juveniles Deprived of their Liberty (Gulbenkian Foundation, 1995).

Adolescent forensic mental health nurses work within a professional framework laid down by the United Kingdom Central Council (UKCC, 1992a, b), the Code of Practice for the Mental Health Act 1983, and the Children (Secure Accommodation) Regulations 1991 guidance for the Children Act 1989. This applies to any restriction of liberty of young people who are 'accommodated' by a local authority or NHS Trust in England and Wales. In addition to legislation, adolescent forensic mental health nurses are required to examine aspects of their practice which further restrict the liberty of young people in their care. This has been explored within the context of seclusion (Goren, 1991; Sampson, 1993), physical restraint (Mayton, 1991; McDougall, 1996) and enforced medication (Antoinette *et al.*, 1990). The 'pindown scandal' (Levy & Kahan, 1991) followed a catalogue of punitive childcare practice and explored restriction of liberty issues. Guidance for staff on permissible forms of control in children's residential care was developed (Department of Health, 1993) and close attention was paid to the use of locked doors, segregation and methods of physical restraint. Adolescent forensic mental health nurses are required to maintain a balance between young people's rights, restriction of liberty and the duty-to-care ethic. This interface relates to coercive interventions such as locking doors, searching and segregating adolescents, physical holding and the administration of medication against a young person's will.

ETHICAL ISSUES AND CONSENT TO TREATMENT

The right of young people to be involved in decisions about their mental health treatment is provided in common law, the Children Act 1989, the Mental Health Act 1983 and, for young offenders, criminal justice legislation (Criminal Justice Act 1991). The UN Convention on the Rights of the Child set minimum standards against which to base law, policy and practice as it affects children and young people (Gulbenkian Foundation, 1995). Adolescent forensic mental health nurses increasingly work within health authorities and trusts committed to the principles and standards of the Convention. The issue of consent to treatment by children and young people is complex and concerned with a balance of legal autonomy, empowerment and protection.

Consent refers to the ability of a young person to make an informed and knowledgeable decision (Bainham, 1993). The Family Law Reform Act 1969 first introduced the age of 16 years as the age at which young people could consent to or refuse their own treatment. Below the age of 16 years parental consent was necessary. However, in what became known as Gillick Competency, the House of Lords ruled that parental responsibility for children under 16 years is absolved 'if and when the child reaches a sufficient understanding and intelligence to make up their own mind on the matter requiring decision' (Bainham, 1993). In order for consent to be informed, the young person must be deemed competent and must understand the issues involved. Consent based on an informed decision must also be free from coercion, extrinsic pressure and secondary gain.

Medical treatment for adolescents can encompass both detention within secure accommodation under the Children Act and psychiatric treatment for mental disorder within the Mental Health Act. In general terms, children and adolescents have the same rights as adults, and consent is required before treatment can be given. However, in emergency circumstances or if statute provides that the consent of the adolescent is not required, treatment can be given against the young person's will. Here, consent is provided by those with parental responsibility. The Children Act dictates that a young person who is of sufficient understanding and intelligence can refuse psychiatric examination, assessment and treatment. However, the Act also states that the court can override the right of the young person who lacks the capacity to consent not to be assessed or treated.

STATUTORY SAFEGUARDS

Children and adolescents who are detained in hospital have a statutory right to complain about their care and treatment. Furthermore, young people have a statutory right to have their concerns and complaints fairly and impartially investigated. Adolescent forensic mental health nurses are required to ensure that children and adolescents with mental health needs have easy access to advice and support, advocacy and the procedure for making complaints. Furthermore, adolescent forensic mental health nurses must strive to create a culture of support that encourages young people to activate the complaints procedure. It is important to recognise that although a young person may feel that their care and treatment are unfair, unlawful or inappropriate, they may not feel able to use a well publicised and easily accessible formal complaints procedure. For these reasons nurses must ensure that children and adolescents know how to contact independent adults who will listen to their concerns or complaints.

The rights of children and adolescents who are compulsorily admitted to hospital under the Mental Health Act are protected by a number of safeguards. The Mental Health Act Commission (MHAC) monitors the care and treatment of young people, investigates complaints and externally reviews issues such as continued detention and consent to treatment. Young people have the right to appeal to the Mental Health Review Tribunal (MHRT) and to be legally represented at the Tribunal hearing.

Unlike the Mental Health Act, the Children Act does not allow for a young person's medical treatment decision to be overridden. An exception to this is where a young person is subject to a Secure Accommodation Order (Section 25) of the Children Act. Young people who are detained in secure accommodation within the Children Act are appointed a guardian *ad litem* by the court to investigate and represent their best interests. For children and adolescents who are detained within security the application for detention is externally audited and reviewed in a court setting. In addition, the young person may obtain assistance from a solicitor or independent visitor. Guidance on the role of the independent visitor issued by the Children Act suggests that they are not expected to act as advocates. The Independent Representative Service (A Voice for the Child in Care) is used by most secure units in England and Wales and combines aspects of the role of independent visitor and advocate.

SPECIALIST SKILLS

Children and adolescents detained within a secure environment have complex and unique needs. Adolescent forensic mental health nurses have a variety of skills and interventions to meet such needs. Specific interventions include anger management training, social and life-skills building and family work. The nature of the intervention and the type and length of treatment depend on the complexity or severity of the young person's mental health and developmental needs, legal requirements and the impact of any high-risk or offending behaviour. Specific interventions carried out by forensic nurses are related to patterns of offending or particular dangerous behaviours. Assessment and treatment interventions address mental health needs associated with fire-setting, sexually abusive behaviour and serious psychotic disorders.

All planned interventions should be culturally sensitive and appropriate to assessment and treatment requirements, involving evaluation by the young person themselves, and should be informed by current research and good practice initiatives. In addition to clinical skills, adolescent forensic nurses are required to meet the emotional, developmental and psychosocial needs of children and young people in their care. Many children and adolescents in secure mental health provision have experienced extremely dysfunctional and abusive family environments, as well as disruptive and numerous care placements. Young people in residential care need to be listened to, understood and cared for. In the absence of parents or carers, nurses may fulfil the role of *loco parentis* or substitute parent, a position clarified by the Children Act for those with parental responsibility.

RISK ASSESSMENT AND DANGEROUSNESS

Although formal and comprehensive risk assessment tools for young people have not yet been fully developed, the assessment of risk is a central and ongoing feature of the adolescent forensic mental health role. A detailed biography, predisposing stress factors and the propensity towards violence and dangerousness all inform systematic risk assessment. Cognitive, emotional and situational variables which might predispose a young person to act violently or dangerously are carefully considered. It is also vital to collect information from third-party sources. Deposition statements, witness statements, pre-sentence and probation reports, and information from family or carers all inform thorough risk assessment and analysis. Specific areas of risk related to particular patterns of offending or high-risk behaviours are measured using tools such as the Child Behaviour Checklist (Achenbach, 1986).

It has been suggested that one cannot empower another to reach their optimum mental health within a regime that is incapable of allowing therapeutic risk taking (Tarbuck, 1994). Consequently, adolescent forensic mental health nurses structure interventions based on what young people are able to do rather than focusing on what they cannot, must not or will not do. Whilst there may be legal restrictions on a young person's liberty and freedom, children and adolescents who are detained within security gradually move through levels of dependence and independence into conditions of lesser security and the community. Tarbuck (1994) believes that security can be invested in a therapeutic, needs-led and individualised way. He suggests that all human needs, including mental health needs, are based on the fundamental need for safety and security. This is pertinent for adolescent forensic mental health nurses who are required to consider the young person holistically, objectively and not just in the context of their high-risk or offending behaviour.

YOUNG PEOPLE WITH SERIOUS PSYCHOTIC DISORDERS

Whilst serious mental illness during adolescence is comparatively rare (Cornell *et al.*, 1987), a retrospective study of detained young people showed that over a third of those admitted with psychosis had committed violent offences (Bailey *et al.*, 1994). Similarly, in a series of nine young people who subsequently committed murder, all had experienced at least one psychotic symptom (Lewis *et al.*, 1988).

Assessment and treatment of young people with serious psychotic disorders is both psychological and pharmacological. A cognitive-behavioural model based on research by Bentall *et al.*, (1994) is used to assess individual symptoms such as auditory hallucinations, delusions and paranoia. Psychological interventions with young people involve a combination of distraction from persistent voices, focusing on auditory hallucinations and techniques where the primary aim of intervention is anxiety reduction. Psychological interventions for adolescents with severe psychotic illness comprise interviews, questionnaires and self-rating scales. The Cognitive Assessment Schedule (CAS: Chadwick & Birchwood, 1994) is used to assess the nature of auditory hallucinations, the evidence young people give for their beliefs, and emotional and behavioural responses to delusions, voices and paranoia. Similarly, the Beliefs About Voices Questionnaire (BAVQ) (Chadwick & Birchwood, 1995) is a psychometrically validated measure of key beliefs about auditory hallucinations. This measures the malevolence, benevolence or benignity of voices, and dimensions of coping, namely resistance and engagement. In addition, an adapted Topography of Voices Rating Scale (Hustig & Hafner, 1990) is used to measure the frequency, audibility and intrusiveness of young people's voices.

The primary aim of cognitive-behavioural interventions for psychotic symptoms is to allow the young person to cope with their symptoms, reappraise their meaning and make them less distressing. Positive psychotic symptoms such as command auditory hallucinations can be assessed within a cognitive framework. Close attention is paid to the voices themselves, the meaning a young person attaches to their voices and how they then feel and behave as a consequence. Coping strategy enhancement (CSE) is formulated from the work of Yusupoff & Tarrier (1996) and involves ways of empowering young people to cope with symptoms which may be upsetting or distressing. Alternative ways of thinking and behaving as a consequence are explored. Another psychological approach is focusing. Cognitive-behavioural interventions of focusing are based on the work of Haddock *et al.* (1993) and enable young people to recognise their experiences as internal and private.

Specific areas of assessment and treatment include examination of:

- Activating events prior to psychotic symptoms
- Levels of conviction, control and distress associated with psychotic symptoms
- Malevolence or benevolence associated with psychotic symptoms
- Dysfunctional assumptions, beliefs about others and psychological function of psychotic symptoms

- Adaptive and maladaptive coping strategies
- Concurrent risk of violence to self or others and compulsion to act on psychotic symptoms

CASE STUDY

Chantelle, 14 years old, is detained under Section 3 of the Mental Health Act 1983 following attempts to abduct a baby from outside a shop. Chantelle is an only child whose earlier life was affected by several house moves, the purpose of which were never explained to her. Chantelle never settled at school and had no close friends of her own age. She is described by her teacher as quiet and caring of others.

Chantelle had told both her teacher and her mother that she intended to steal a baby boy. When she was interviewed in police custody she stated that the baby was special and belonged to her. Chantelle believed that the child's mother was about to sacrifice him and so attempted to take him to save his life. Chantelle was assessed by a police surgeon, transferred from police custody without charge and later admitted to the Adolescent Forensic Service for an assessment of mental state and risk.

On admission it was evident that Chantelle was floridly psychotic. She described an elaborate delusional system, command hallucinations and a belief that nursing staff could place 'wishes' in her head. During the initial stages of assessment Chantelle was guarded, reticent and difficult to engage. With close support from her primary nurse and with involvement with her mother Chantelle was later able to complete the Beliefs About Voices Questionnaire (BAVQ) and a self-rating scale (SRS) which measured conviction, control and distress associated with her beliefs about command hallucinations.

During a five-month period of treatment Chantelle was diagnosed as having schizophrenia and stabilised on Risperidone (anti-psychotic medication). Whilst Chantelle's delusional system remained intact, her voices were less frequent and easier to control. Psychological interventions were cognitive and enabled Chantelle to recognise that her auditory hallucinations were triggered by strong feelings of loneliness and sadness. Associated levels of distress were low and Chantelle developed skills to cope by reappraising the meaning of her voices or distracting herself if they were upsetting or persistent.

Close attention was paid to beliefs and associated risks. Chantelle developed her education, completed a programme of social skills building and successfully returned home under the care and regular review of a support worker and child-and-adolescent psychiatrist. Chantelle now has fortnightly sessions with a mental health worker, attends a child-and-family unit for education and remains stable at home in the community.

In addition to pharmacological and psychological interventions for psychotic symptoms, treatment approaches focus on coping with associated emotions such as anger, distress and despair. Dynamic issues related to low self-esteem, worthlessness and hopelessness are addressed during individual session work.

YOUNG PEOPLE WHO SEXUALLY ABUSE OTHERS

Therapeutic interventions with young people who sexually abuse others occur either in the community or within secure environments dependent on legal restriction or level of risk posed. The underlying philosophy behind therapeutic work with young people who sexually abuse others is adapted from the work of O'Callaghan & Print (1994). They believe that sexually abusive behaviour and the cognitive distortions that maintain such behaviour arise from negative childhood experiences. The young person develops a need for control, power and acceptance that is enacted through a cycle of aggressive and sexually abusive behaviour. Despite a paucity of reliable evidence, it is clear that the majority of children who are sexually abused do not become abusers. Moreover, research indicates that around half of young people who sexually abuse others have not themselves been victims of sexual abuse (Ryan *et al.*, 1990; Bentovim & Williams, 1998).

In addition to causative factors that contribute towards sexually abusive behaviour in young people a model which illustrates reinforcement and maintenance is offered by Ryan & Lane (1991). Compulsive sexually abusive behaviour is explained in terms of thoughts, feelings and behaviour. Ryan & Lane developed a cyclical model that demonstrates the process of motivation, repetition and reoffending. Whilst the sexual abuse cycle differs for each young person, the more entrenched the cycle and the faster it is repeated, the more habitual the sexually abusive behaviour becomes (see Fig. 2.1).

The cycle shows that sexually abusive behaviour is rarely an impulsive act. Rather, it indicates that it is a result of thoughts, appraisals, feelings and action. The cycle represents the cognitive and behavioural patterns that occur before and after an assault and demonstrates the grounding of assaultive behaviour in a young person's poor self-image and low self-esteem.

For example, a child or adolescent expects to be disliked and rejected, and therefore avoids getting close to others and situations where intimate social contact may occur. The young person cannot respond assertively to the difficult or stressful situations that invariably arise and so becomes socially isolated, withdrawn and self-pitying. The child or adolescent who sexually abuses others often blames others for their discomfort and is angry towards them. The young person then fantasises about ways to become

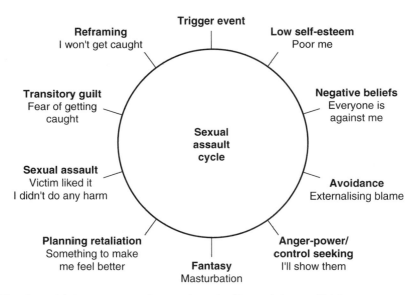

Fig. 2.1　Adolescent sexual assault cycle (Ryan & Lane, 1991).

powerful, make themselves feel better and increase their self-worth. By masturbating to such fantasies they are reinforced and eventually planned and acted out. The sexually abusive act is usually followed by a period of transitory guilt that is a combination of moral concern and fear of getting caught. If indeed the young person is not caught, such fears are gradually suppressed and cognitive distortions and self-serving biases are used in their place.

Whilst the primary aim of therapeutic work is the protection of others from sexual abuse, a secondary aim is to break the cycle of sexually abusive behaviour and promote cognitive and behavioural change within the adolescent perpetrator. Through anger management, social skills work and self-esteem building, young people are helped to recognise, understand and accept responsibility for their sexually abusive actions. This involves working through cognitive processes of denial and distortion, abusive sexual fantasies and victim empathy. The purpose of assessment with young people who sexually abuse others is to identify whether mental health intervention is appropriate, to evaluate level of risk and dangerousness and to predict recidivism. Collaborative assessment requires input from the young person, their carers and support networks, and any other professionals and agencies who are involved in their care.

There is a lack of research that addresses recidivism and dangerousness in young people who sexually abuse others. Risk assessment tools in use with adults are not generally transferable for use with young people (Vizard *et al.*, 1995). Assessment of future risk and relapse prevention are central to all therapeutic interventions. Risk assessment is an important consideration both in terms of public safety and in the interests of child protection. The nature of risk is dependent on situational factors, offence characteristics and the young person's attitudes, thoughts and feelings about sexual behaviour.

Support and supervision are essential for nurses working with young people who sexually abuse others. Entering into a therapeutic relationship where many of the core conditions are difficult to apply can be challenging. It may be difficult for nurses to remain non-judgemental because of the nature of the offending behaviour, the young person may not be the primary focus of concern, and the confidentiality ethic is shadowed by legal issues and child protection responsibilities.

Whilst the Children Act urges staff to consider the 'wishes and feelings' of the young person, this becomes ethically contentious when the young person may have 'wishes and feelings' about sexually abusing others. Nurses are required to pay close attention to their attitudes, beliefs and values when working closely with young people who sexually abuse others. The therapeutic relationship may produce personal issues about sexuality, identification with the young person and rejection or collusion. Strong emotional reactions such as anger and fear must be contained, processed during clinical supervision and used for the promotion of therapeutic activity.

YOUNG FIRE-SETTERS

It has been suggested that most children develop a fascination with fire at an early stage in their development (Kafry, 1980). For some, this fascination grows and becomes stronger as the child gets older (Hall, 1995). Whilst it has been noted that the majority of young people who set fires are not mentally disordered, a small minority exhibit features of mental illness (Rice & Harris, 1991; Jackson, 1994) and a large proportion are conduct disordered (Bailey *et al.*, 1991). It is generally agreed that a constellation of psychosocial variables contribute to fire-setting in young people. Low educational achievement (Showers & Pickrell, 1987), family dysfunction (Kolko & Kazdin, 1994) and experiences of failure, rejection or frustration (Kolko, 1989) are factors which appear throughout the literature. Whilst motivation is generally agreed to be multi-factorial and complex, various specific reasons to explain why young people set fires have been offered. These include revenge (Stewart, 1993; Swaffer & Hollin, 1995), excitement (Cox-Jones *et al.*, 1990), curiosity (Showers & Pickrell, 1987; Kolko & Kazdin, 1994) and issues surrounding low self-esteem (Kolko, 1989). Whilst sexual gratification has been attributed to adult fire-setters (Bourget & Bradford, 1987), no such link has been established with young people.

Whilst the underlying principles behind interventions with young people who set fires are psychodynamic in origin, the interventions themselves are cognitive behavioural and based on the work of Harris & Rice (1984). A working principle is that historical life events predispose a young person to act in antisocial and destructive ways. Environmental influences further teach, reinforce and encourage such behaviours.

During the assessment period young people who set fires are helped to identify precipitating events. These may include factors such as abuse, low self-esteem and poor family dynamics. Close attention is paid to any feelings a young person might have before, during and after lighting fires. Experiences of anxiety, guilt and anger are commonly described by adolescents.

Fire-setting appears to provide young people with an effective means to influence a situation which may feel out of control. By lighting a fire, the young person may relieve tension, avoid stress and achieve a sense of power and mastery. The process of assessment also involves looking at patterns of reinforcement and behaviour maintenance in young people who set fires. A thorough assessment informs risk assessment, fire-related dangerousness and suitability for treatment interventions. Other areas of assessment include:

- Detailed history of fire-setting
- Relationship between fire-setting and overall psychopathology
- Identification of internal and external triggers to fire-setting
- Thoughts, feelings and behaviour experienced before, during and after fire-setting
- Risk analysis, associated dangerousness and treatability

Treatment interventions occur in the community or within secure accommodation depending on the level of risk and recidivism. Through a behavioural model and cognitive interventions young arsonists are helped to dynamically understand, control and avoid their fire-setting behaviour. Treatment interventions focus on the dangers of fire, safety issues and the impact on others of lighting fires. Cognitive interventions explore personal beliefs, constructs and general coping strategies. Adolescents who set fires generally have a lack of problem-solving skills and experience low self-confidence. Providing young people with the skills to be assertive and solve problems helps them avoid situations that might produce conflict, stress and a subsequent increase in the risk of fire-setting.

Risk indicators for young people who set fires

- Low self-esteem
- History of physical, emotional or sexual abuse

- History of aggression and violence
- High expressed emotion and poor conflict resolution within family
- Fire-setting due to boredom, anger or perceived rejection
- Solitary fire-setting
- Ritualistic fire-setting
- Lack of insight into motives and fire-setting behaviour

VIOLENT AND AGGRESSIVE YOUNG PEOPLE

Whilst the majority of young people who are seriously aggressive or violent are not mentally ill, a minority have specific psychiatric needs or social development disorders (Lyon, 1996). Various studies have positively cor-related early traumatic experiences with violent and aggressive behaviour during adolescence (Boswell, 1995).

Factors such as family disruption, neglect and poor parental supervision are cited as important precursors to violent offending by young people (Farrington, 1995; Gulbenkian Foundation, 1995). The growing body of work on post-traumatic stress disorder (Pynoos & Eth, 1985) shows that children and young people may respond to unresolved abuse and trauma in an aggressive and violent manner. Adolescent forensic mental health services offer containment and security to young people who are aggressive or violent. Through positive role modelling and consistent limit setting, children and adolescents learn or develop adaptive ways to cope with anger and aggression.

In a retrospective analysis of aggression and violence within the Adolescent Forensic Service (McDougall, 1998b) it was shown that the large majority of violent incidents (91%) were generated by mentally disordered non-offenders. This group of young people had presented challenging, dangerous or high-risk behaviour to mainstream child and adolescent mental health services. By contrast, a small minority of violent incidents (9%) were generated by mentally disordered young offenders with a prior history of violent and assaultive behaviour including murder, attempted murder and manslaughter.

YOUNG PEOPLE WHO KILL

Children and adolescents who kill constitute a heterogeneous group. Whilst violent offending in young people has increased steadily over the past 30 years (Hardwick & Rowton-Lee, 1996), rates of adolescent homicide have not increased to any significant extent (Shepherd & Farrington, 1996).

Research indicates that a high proportion of young people who have committed homicidal acts have themselves been the victims of childhood trauma, abuse and loss (Boswell, 1995; Bailey, 1996; Hardwick & Rowton-Lee, 1996).

In a study of 40 murderers referred to the Adolescent Forensic Service, Dolan *et al.* (1996) recorded high levels of physical and sexual abuse, violent parenting and mental illness within the families of homicidal adolescents. Similarly, in a study of 38 violent young offenders, Smith (1997) highlights a history of emotional abuse (44%), physical abuse (23%) and sexual abuse (13%) in young people who committed murder, attempted murder and manslaughter.

Psychosocial characteristics of young people who commit murder include neuro-psychological abnormalities (Lewis *et al.*, 1988), alcohol abuse (Labelle *et al.*, 1991) and a history of violence towards others (Busch *et al.*, 1990).

The role of the adolescent forensic mental health nurse working with young people who kill is primarily supportive. The adolescent forensic psychiatrist frequently undertakes pre-trial psychiatric assessments. The court may ask for an expert opinion on criminal responsibility, whether the child or adolescent can distinguish right from seriously wrong, level of future risk and appropriate placement recommendations.

Post-conviction nursing interventions are psychotherapeutic in nature. Interventions which enhance and enable insight, catharsis and under-standing are used. Contrary to popular media belief, young people who have killed can, and do, show remorse for their crimes. Following a period of dissociation, children and adolescents who have killed usually move through a process similar in nature to grief (Hambridge, 1990). Whilst this may initially be self-serving and related to a loss of freedom, the young person is helped to work through the circumstances of their homicidal act and is later able to grieve about their victim (Bailey, 1996). Post-traumatic stress reactions frequently arise from participation in the homicidal act directly, from witnessing the actions of co-defendants or as a result of previous abusive experiences. Psychotherapeutic techniques are often central to treatment and can be used to assess empathy, self-reflection and the capacity to form emotional attachments.

Post-conviction therapeutic work can often raise painful childhood memories, and the nurse is required to help the young person face unresolved anger, distress and loss. Children and adolescents who have killed may internalise anguish through self-injury or externalise feelings of hatred, rage, terror and blame. Emotional distress is frequently acted out in a chaotic, destructive or disruptive manner. It is essential to offer a high level of care, containment and security. This positive nurturing experience, which may have previously been lacking, is consistent, non-abusive and delivered within a climate of therapy and rehabilitation.

DELIVERING BEST PRACTICE

It is vital that adolescent forensic mental health nurses have access to education and training in terms of mental health and childcare law, policy guidance and good practice initiatives. Providing young people with a safe, secure and caring environment requires an awareness of fundamental issues related to security, safety and control and how they impact on the delivery of quality nursing care. Important areas of consideration include:

- Awareness of developmental factors and how these impact on care and treatment
- Awareness of child protection procedures, good practice guidelines and duty-to-care responsibilities
- Understanding of permissible forms of control and restriction of liberty (Department of Health, 1993)
- Relevant aspects of childcare legislation, mental health law and both civil and criminal statutes
- Awareness of jurisdiction and process of youth court, family proceedings court, magistrates' and crown courts
- Awareness of religious and ethnic diversity, and the cultural and linguistic needs of young people

Although much progress has been made within both child and adolescent mental health and forensic nursing, there is a paucity of research relating to adolescent mentally disordered offenders. There is a pressing need for further research into the causes of childhood mental health and developmental disorders, their effects and long-term consequences, and the best methods of intervention and treatment. Although a number of agencies within youth treatment, childcare and mental health services are now conducting research with adolescent mentally disordered offenders, further development is required. Research and development is currently being undertaken with psychotic children and adolescents, young people who set fires, and female offenders. Areas of further development are required that will focus on the needs of young people with severe psychosis and coexistent conduct disorders, the role of intensive care within conditions of medium security, and the unmet mental health needs of young people in forensic mental health care.

CONCLUSION

Working alongside severely disturbed and dangerous young people is a complex and challenging task. Societal and political debate has blurred the distinction between treatment and punishment for mentally disordered young offenders. It has been over ten years since the Health Advisory Service report, *Bridges over Troubled Waters*, stated that the nursing profession needs to define the specialist contribution which nurses can make to the care and treatment of adolescents with specific psychiatric disorders (HAS, 1987). A decade on, the Health Advisory Service review of the commissioning, role and management of child and adolescent mental health services, *Together We Stand*, highlighted the need for specialist provision in which secure forensic services played a central role (HAS, 1995). The untreated mental health of young people increases the demand placed on the social services, education, youth justice and prison systems.

Whilst the focus of this chapter has been on the nursing care and treatment of adolescent mentally disordered offenders, the mental health needs of the young people described cannot be met by a single practice discipline or agency. Interdisciplinary team working, multi-agency liaison, comprehensive planning and collaborative after-care are essential. Commitment from a variety of agencies including social services, education and the criminal justice systems will help ensure that young people with complex, challenging and dangerous behaviour get the care and treatment they deserve. Adolescent forensic mental health nursing is a unique and rapidly expanding speciality. In order to meet the distinctive mental health needs of these young people, adolescent forensic mental health nurses must continue to create a specialist knowledge base, develop and create benchmarks for evidence-based interventions, and disseminate examples of good practice.

REFERENCES

Achenbach, T. (1986) *Manual for the Child Behavior Checklist and Revised Child Behavior Profile*. University of Vermont, Burlington.

Antoinette, T., Iyengar, S. & Puig-Antich, J. (1990) Is locked seclusion necessary for children under the age of 14? *American Journal of Psychiatry* **147**(10), 1283–9.

Bailey, S. (1996) Adolescents who murder. *Journal of Adolescence* **19**, 19–39.

Bailey, S., Stowell, B. & Garrett, H. (1991) Characteristics of adolescent sex offenders. Unpublished. Adolescent Forensic Service.

Bailey, S., Thornton, L. & Weaver, A. (1994) The first 100 admissions to an adolescent secure unit. *Journal of Adolescence* **17**, 207–220.

Bainham, A. (1993) Children, parents and the law: non-intervention and judicial paternalisation. In *The Frontiers of Liability* (Birks, P., ed.). Oxford University Press, London.

Becker, J. (1988) Adolescent sex offenders. *Behaviour Therapist* **11**, 185–7.

Bentall, R., Haddock, G. & Slade, P. (1994) Psychological treatment for auditory hallucinations: from theory to therapy. *Behavior Therapy* **25**, 51–6.

Bentovim, A. & Williams, B. (1998) Children and adolescents: victims who become perpetrators. *Advances in Psychiatric Treatment* **4**, 101–7.

Boswell, G. (1995) *Violent Victims: the Prevalence of Abuse and Loss in the Lives of Section 53 Offenders*. The Prince's Trust, London.

Bourget, D. & Bradford, J. (1987) Fire fetishism, diagnostic and clinical implications: a review of two cases. *Canadian Journal of Psychiatry* **32**(6), 459–62.

Bullock, R., Hosie, K., Little, M. & Millham, S. (1990) Secure accommodation for very difficult adolescents: some recent research findings. *Journal of Adolescence* **13**, 205–16.

Busch, K., Zagar, R., Hughes, J., Arbit, J. & Bussell, R. (1990) Adolescents who kill. *Journal of Clinical Psychology* **46**, 472–85.

Cavadino, P. (1996) Children who kill. *Young Minds* **27**, 12–13.

Chadwick, P. & Birchwood, M. (1994) The omnipotence of voices: a cognitive approach to auditory hallucinations. *British Journal of Psychiatry* **164**, 190–201.

Chadwick, P. & Birchwood, M. (1995) The omnipotence of voices, Part 2: The Beliefs About Voices Questionnaire (BAVQ). *British Journal of Psychiatry* **166**, 773–6.

Children's Legal Centre (1991) *Mental Health Handbook: Young People, Mental Health and the Law: a Handbook for Parents and Advisors*. The Children's Legal Centre, London.

Cornell, D., Benedek, E. & Benedek, D. (1987)   Characteristics of adolescents charged with homicide: review of 72 cases. *Behavioural Sciences and the Law* **5**(1), 11–23.

Cox-Jones, C., Lubetsky, M., Fultz, S. & Kolko, D. (1990) Inpatient treatment of a young recidivist firesetter. *American Academy of Child and Adolescent Psychiatry* **29**(1), 936–41.

Department of Health (1993) *Permissible Forms of Control in Children's Residential Care*. HMSO, London.

Department of Health/Home Office (1992) *Review of Health and Social Services for Mentally Disordered Offenders and Others Requiring Similar Services*. HMSO, London.

Dolan, M., Holloway, J., Bailey, S. & Kroll, L. (1996) The psychosocial characteristics of juvenile sex offenders. *Medicine, Science and the Law* **36**(4), 343–52.

Epps, K. (1994) Treating adolescent sex offenders in secure conditions: the experience at Glenthorne Centre. *Journal of Adolescence* **17**(2), 105–22.

Farrington, D. (1995) The development of offending and antisocial behaviour from childhood: key findings from the Cambridge Study in Delinquent Development. *Journal of Child Psychology and Psychiatry* **6**, 560.

Goren, S. (1991) What are the considerations of the use of seclusion and restraint with children and adolescents? *Journal of Psychosocial Nursing* **29**(3), 32–3.

Grant, C., Burgess, A. & Hartman, C. (1989) Juveniles who murder. *Journal of Psychosocial Nursing* **27**(12), 4–11.

Gulbenkian Foundation (1993) One scandal too many: the case for comprehensive protection for children in all settings. *Report of a Working Group Convened by the Gulbenkian Foundation*. Calouste Gulbenkian Foundation, London.

Gulbenkian Foundation (1995) Children and Violence. *Report of the Commission on Children and Violence Convened by the Gulbenkian Foundation*. Calouste Gulbenkian Foundation. London.

Haddock, G., Bentall, R. & Slade, P. (1993) Psychological treatment of auditory hallucinations: two case studies. *Behavioural and Cognitive Psychotherapy* **21**, 335–46.

Hall, G. (1995) Using group work to understand arsonists. *Nursing Standard* 9(23), 25–8.

Hambridge, J. (1990) The grief process in those admitted to Regional Secure Units following homicide. *Journal of Forensic Sciences* 35(5), 1149–54.

Hardwick, P. & Rowton-Lee, M. (1996) Adolescent homicide: towards assessment of risk. *Journal of Adolescence* 19(3), 263–76.

Harris, G. & Rice, M. (1984) Mentally disordered firesetters: psychodynamic versus empirical approaches. *International Journal of Law and Psychiatry* 7(1), 19–34.

Health Advisory Service (1987) *Bridges Over Troubled Waters: a Report on Services for Disturbed Adolescents*. HMSO, London.

Health Advisory Service (1995) *Together We Stand: The Commissioning, Role and Management of Child and Adolescent Mental Health Services in England and Wales*. HMSO, London.

Hustig, H. & Hafner, R. (1990) Persistent auditory hallucinations and their relationship to delusions and mood. *Journal of Nervous and Mental Disease* 178, 264–7.

Jackson, H. (1994) Assessment of firesetters. In *The Assessment of Criminal Behaviours of Clients in Secure Settings* (McMurran, M. & Hodge, J., eds). Kingsley Publishers, London.

Kafry, D. (1980) Playing with matches: children and fire. In *Fires and Human Behaviour* (Canter, D., ed.). Wiley, Chichester.

Kolko, D. (1989) Firesetting and pyromania. In *Handbook of Child Psychiatric Diagnosis*, pp. 443–459 (Last, C. & Hersen, M., eds). Wiley, New York.

Kolko, D. & Kazdin, A. (1994) Children's descriptions of their firesetting incidents: characteristics and relationship to recidivism. *Journal of the American Academy of Child and Adolescent Psychiatry* 33, 114–22.

Labelle, A., Bradford, J., Bourget, D., Jones, B. & Carmichael, M. (1991) Adolescent murderers. *Canadian Journal of Psychiatry* 36, 583–7.

Levy, A. & Kahan, B. (1991) The pindown experience and the protection of children: the report of the Staffordshire Child Care Inquiry. Staffordshire County Council, Stafford.

Lewis, D., Lovely, R., Yeager, C. & Ferguson, G. (1988) Intrinsic and environmental characteristics of juvenile murderers. *Journal of the American Academy of Child and Adolescent Psychiatry* 27, 582–7.

Lyon, J. (1996) Adolescents who offend. *Journal of Adolescence* 19, 1–4.

McDougall, T. (1996) Physical restraint: a review of the literature. *Psychiatric Care* 3(4), 132–8.

McDougall, T. (1997) Adolescent forensic mental health nursing. *Mental Health Practice* 1(4), 13–16.

McDougall, T. (1998a) Children who kill – protection not revenge. *Nursing Times* 94(21), 14.

McDougall, T. (1998b) Violent incidents on a secure adolescent unit: a retrospective analysis. Unpublished. Adolescent Forensic Service.

Mayton, K. (1991) What are the considerations of the use of seclusion and restraint with children and adolescents? *Journal of Psychosocial Nursing* 29(3), 33–6.

O'Callaghan, D. & Print, B. (1994) Adolescent sexual abusers: research, assessment and treatment. In *Sexual Offending Against Children: Assessment and Treatment of Male Abusers*, pp. 146–77 (Morrison, T., Erooga, M. & Beckett, R., eds). Routledge, London.

Pynoos, R. & Eth, S. (1985) Children traumatised by witnessing acts of personal violence: homicide, rape or suicide behaviour. In *Post Traumatic Disorder in Children* (Eth, S. & Pynoos, R., eds). American Psychiatric Association, Washington, DC.

Rice, M. & Harris, G. (1991) Firesetters admitted to a maximum security psychiatric institution: offenders and offenses. *Journal of Interpersonal Violence* 6(4), 461–75.

Royal College of Psychiatrists (1995) Severe and chronic mental disorder in children and young people: Factsheet. RCP, London.

Rutter, M. & Smith, D. (1995) *Psychosocial Disorders in Young People*. Wiley, Chichester.

Ryan, G. & Lane, S. (1991) *Juvenile Sexual Offenders: Causes, Consequences and Corrections*. Lexington Books, Massachusetts.

Ryan, G., Metzner, G. & Krugman, R. (1990) When the abuser is a child: the assessment and treatment of the juvenile sex offender. In *Understanding and Managing Child Sexual Abuse* (Oates, K., ed.). Harcourt Brace Jovanovich, Sydney.

Sampson, K. (1993) Acting with restraint. *Nursing Times* 89(38), 40–3.

Shepherd, J. & Farrington, D. (1996) The prevention of delinquency with particular reference to violent crime. *Medicine, Science and the Law* 36, 331–6.

Showers, J. & Pickrell, E. (1987) Child firesetters: a study of three populations. *Hospital and Community Psychiatry* 38(5), 495–501.

Smith, C. (1997) The psychosocial characteristics of violent offenders. Unpublished. Adolescent Forensic Service.

Stewart, L. (1993) Profile of female firesetters: implications for treatment. *British Journal of Psychiatry* 163, 248–56.

Swaffer, T. & Hollin, C. (1995) Adolescent firesetting: why do they say they do it? *Journal of Adolescence* 18(5), 619–23.

Tarbuck, P. (1994) The therapeutic use of security: a model for forensic psychiatric nursing. In *Mental Health and Disorder*, 2nd edn (Thompson, A. & Mathias, P., eds). Baillière Tindall, London.

UKCC (1992a) *The Scope of Professional Practice*. UKCC, London.

UKCC (1992b) *The Code of Professional Conduct for the Nurse, Midwife and Health Visitor*. UKCC, London.

Vizard, E., Monck, E. & Misch, P. (1995) Child and adolescent sexual abuse perpetrators: a review of the research literature. *Journal of Child Psychology and Psychiatry* 36, 731–56.

Vizard, E., Wynick, S., Hawkes, C., Woods, J. & Jenkins, J. (1996) Juvenile sex offenders. Assessment issues. *British Journal of Psychiatry* 168, 259–62.

Yusupoff, L. & Tarrier, N. (1996) Coping strategy enhancement for persistent hallucinations and delusions. In *Cognitive Behavioural Interventions with Psychotic Disorders* (Haddock, G. & Slade, P., eds). Routledge, London.

Chapter 3
Working with Sex Offenders

Michael Coffey

INTRODUCTION

Sexual offences can be committed by both male and female offenders on both male and female victims of any age. Within this chapter offenders will commonly be referred to in the male gender as they present the majority of referrals for assessment and treatment. Sexual offending is defined here as a criminal act involving a sexual behaviour to which one party has not given or is incapable of giving informed consent. This includes offences where the power differential between the persons involved is such that the victim is unable to make a free decision, such as sexual offences against children. Although much of this chapter refers to child sex offenders, the broad concepts and interventions described can be more generally applied to other sexual offences.

The very concept of offering treatment to sex offenders is anathema to many mental health nurses as well as to the public in general. The abhorrent nature of the offences committed by sex offenders may make the prospect of developing therapeutic relationships with them unthinkable.

Allocating limited treatment resources to individuals whom many members of the public may wish to see castrated and locked away forever can also present a dilemma for health professionals. The ingrained recidivistic behaviour of many sex offenders raises the question of whether this behaviour can be treated at all. Indeed Furby *et al.* (1989) concluded that there was no evidence that treatment reduces the risk of reoffending in sex offenders in general. This study did, however, find some evidence to suggest that, in certain types of sex offenders, recidivism rates were different, implying that treatment works differently for different types of offender.

A more optimistic series of studies suggests positive results for cognitive-behavioural treatments of child sex abusers and exhibitionists but not for rapists (Marshall *et al.*, 1991). In Britain it has been recent government policy to provide multi-disciplinary management of sex offenders as highlighted in the Reed Report (Department of Health/Home Office, 1992). Reconciling these expectations with the feelings about such work can be a difficult process. The one constant which runs through the literature in this area is the firmly held belief that the best way to protect potential victims of this damaging crime is by helping the abusers to change their behaviour. O'Connell *et al.* (1990, p. 8) go further and state that methods of 'evaluating and controlling' offenders assume central importance in the provision of services to this group. Assisting offenders to control and not cure their behaviour is the prime goal of sex offender treatment programmes (Prins, 1991).

Whilst a variety of treatment strategies have been used to provide treatment to sex offenders, including behavioural, psychoanalytical and even biological, efficacy of such treatment modalities remains unproven. Demonstrating efficacy remains a peculiarly difficult problem with this group. Their behaviour often is surreptitious and remains undetected for long periods of time. Offenders' motivation for treatment may be questionable and their honesty in wanting to truly change their behaviour may be doubtful.

Among therapists offering treatment to this group there remains a notable ambivalence as to whether treatment is indicated or if long-term vigilance and supervision are a more realistic goal (Taylor, 1991). Kaul (1993) suggests that psychiatry with its traditions of long-term management and supervision of people with serious mental illness is best placed to offer this continuing care.

Treatment strategies used with sex offenders have varied over the years. They range from the starkly physical and popular public choice of physical castration (Sturup, 1972) and chemical castration (Berlin & Meinecke, 1981) through to the less emotive but ethically questionable behavioural approach of aversion therapy (Quinsey *et al.*, 1976). As mentioned above, however, the current emphasis is now on cognitive-behavioural approaches with most forensic and prison services adopting this approach in their treatment programmes (Thornton & Hogue, 1993).

VICTIMOLOGY

Before further exploring sexual offenders and treatment approaches it is worth considering the victims of these offences and the traumatic effects of such abuse. Finkelhor & Browne (1985) suggest that the effects on victims be considered under the categories of traumatic sexualisation, stigmatisation, betrayal and powerlessness.

Traumatic sexualisation

This is often recognisable in children who develop inappropriate sexuality for their age. There may be evidence of precocious sexual development such as sexual elements (beyond the normal childhood curiosity) in their play with other children. Alternatively the victim may develop negative phobic feelings surrounding intimacy and in children this may be seen with enforced isolation in an attempt to avoid being touched. The abuse disrupts the child's normal sexual development and the child confuses love and caring with sexual contact. The child may develop inappropriate sexual behaviour and learn to use this as a way of seeking approval.

Stigmatisation

Victims of child sexual abuse often have feelings of guilt, shame and worthlessness. The offender often asks or forces them to keep the abuse secret with frequent pressure being applied in the form of threats such as 'It will kill your mother if she ever finds out' or 'You will be taken into a home'. The fear of worse things to come and enforced separation from siblings or parents, even when one of the parents is the abuser, serves to reinforce these feelings. The victim has a sense of being a bad person, different from other people and may even feel like 'spoilt goods'. These feelings become part of their self-image. Self-harming or reckless behaviour such as acting-out may be seen in some children. Future sexual development and forming of adult relationships can become difficult and fraught with crises.

Betrayal

Frequently, victims have experienced betrayal either as a result of someone important to them such as a parent abusing them or by the fact that those whom they look to for protection have failed to prevent the abuse occurring. A sense of abandonment may be felt by the victim, leading them into indiscriminate and often desperate attachment to others.

Powerlessness

The victim, as a result of being unable to prevent their body being violated, experiences a strong sense of powerlessness. Some offenders will often cite the child's lack of resistance as mitigation or evidence that the child must have enjoyed or wanted the sexual contact. This, however, should be seen for what it is. The offender will always seek to justify his actions. The child in such a position is unable to prevent the offence occurring and so adopts survival behaviour. The offender chooses to ignore the resistance and uses the presumed co-operation as justification. The repetition of the abuse reinforces the sense of powerlessness the victim experiences and may persist into adulthood and can be replicated in other areas of life.

Mullen *et al.* (1993) identified sexual abuse in childhood as a contributing factor in adult psychopathology with the severity of abuse related to the degree of psychopathology. The authors were, however, unable to declare a direct causal link with childhood sexual abuse and mental ill health in later life due to the complex range of social disadvantage from which many of those studied had arisen. Certain factors appear to predict poorer outcome for victims. Finkelhor (1979) suggests that abuse by a father or stepfather as opposed to a stranger, for instance, can have a worse effect on the victim. Sexual assaults involving violence (Russell, 1986) or penetrative acts (Bagley & Ramsay, 1986) also have a more deleterious effect on the victim.

CLASSIFICATION

Sex offenders are not a homogeneous group. This makes dividing them into categories that meaningfully describe them difficult. In terms of the criminal justice system, sex offenders are defined in terms of the nature of their offences, e.g. rape, indecent exposure. While these terms are generally understood, they do not provide the depth of description which can enable treatment approaches to be formulated.

Within the field of psychiatry some texts have based descriptions on attempts to develop clinically valid categories to enable targeting of treatments (American Psychiatric Association, 1987). The argument for this medicalised or psychiatrised approach, as Mercer (1998) has termed it, has been that effective treatment outcomes will remain an unattainable goal until such time as the individual characteristics of sexual offending are defined (Grubin & Kennedy, 1991). Whatever arguments exist about the purpose or otherwise of the description of offender characteristics, there remains the view that changing these behaviours is imperative. Classification of the offending behaviours may assist the development of interventions which help some offenders to change these behaviours. Identifying those offenders whose behaviour is not amenable to change and who are at increased risk of reoffending then becomes possible.

Grubin & Kennedy (1991, p. 124) suggest that for a classification scheme to be useful it must contain three criteria:

(1) It must first be reliable, that is, when different people use it they must get the same results.
(2) It must be easy and straightforward to use so that it will be widely applied.
(3) It must be valid for its purpose.

Many classification systems do not meet any of these criteria. Describing sex offenders in terms of their offences does not satisfactorily define the behaviour. Rapists for instance are not in themselves a homogeneous grouping. Those clinicians who work with child sex abusers will recognise the distinct differences between some offenders whilst acknowledging that many share the same characteristics. Developing a classification system which is therefore meaningful for all sex offenders is fraught with difficulties.

It may be that separate systems of categorisation will be required for different types of behaviour. It is important at this stage, however, not to be lulled into the trap often set by offenders themselves in therapy, that is, one of hierarchies. Whatever the sexual offence, it is devastating for the victim and involves well documented approach behaviours from the offender, some of which are described below.

PRESENTING CHARACTERISTICS OF SEX OFFENDERS

Sex offenders display some common characteristics on presentation which create unique problems for therapeutic work. These will briefly be described here.

Emotional congruence

The child sex offender often appears to have an emotional congruence with children. In other words the offender feels better able to relate to children and is more emotionally attracted to children than adults. For offenders who have been abused themselves as children it is believed that repetition and identification with the aggressor may be an important factor. The possibility of attraction to deviant stimuli as a conditioned response in offenders who have been abused has also been raised (Fisher, 1994, p. 21). The difficulty with this theory, as Fisher (1994) recognises, is that it does not explain why those who have not been abused sexually offend nor indeed why many people who have been abused never sexually offend.

Targeting

The offender will often choose their victim carefully. This indicates a level of planning which many sex offenders will initially deny. Child sex abusers will often choose female partners with young children. They may occupy respected positions within the community, which enable them to have access to children. The friendly neighbour who volunteers his services for childminding or babysitting is a frequent ploy.

Grooming

Sex offenders commonly make preparation for their offences. Classically in the case of child sex offenders, this involves breaking down the resistance of the child with gifts, the introduction of sexualised conversation and the gradual introduction of physical and sexualised play. The offender will often groom the environment by ensuring he will not be interrupted, for instance. Grooming may even take place with adults responsible for a child by persuading them to leave that child in the offender's care on a regular basis.

Lack of victim empathy

Sex offenders often have a marked absence of empathy for the person they have abused. Marshall *et al.* (1997) have found that when compared with non-offenders, child sex offenders were deficient in empathy. The result of this lack of empathy is that they appear unable to understand the harm they are doing to the person, or justify their behaviour as 'educational'. One aspect of treatment aims to develop victim empathy, the theory being that this will act as an internal control or inhibitor for future offending.

Denials of behaviour

Kennedy & Grubin (1992) describe patterns of denial in sex offenders and have identified four groups: those who admitted offending but denied harming the victim; externalisers who blamed the victim or others; internalisers who admitted and accepted harm to the victim; and those exhibiting absolute denial. While many treatment programmes have found that offenders with absolute denial are not amenable to therapy, there is now emerging evidence that such offenders can be engaged in treatment (Schlank & Shaw, 1996).

Minimising

The offender minimises his behaviour to make it seem less abhorrent or less socially unacceptable, for example admitting to a less serious offence or suggesting that the victim was less harmed than was in fact the case. There is also now some suggestion in the personal construct literature that sex offenders may construe themselves and others in ways which attempt to avoid deviant self-identity (Houston, 1998).

Cognitive distortions or thinking errors

These include convincing themselves that the victim wanted to have sex, that children enjoy sex, that children are sexually provocative and therefore know what they are doing, or that the child must have enjoyed the abuse otherwise they would have told someone sooner. Child sex abusers often convince themselves that the sexual contact is educational for the child.

Other problems with which offenders present is their questionable motivation to change and their propensity to be dishonest. Sex offenders have frequently committed many more offences than they have been arrested or charged for (Abel *et al.*, 1987). It can often be the case that an offender will learn the jargon of treatment but not have internalised the learning. He may appear to therapists to have made shifts in his thinking but will still hold the attitudes and beliefs that allow him to offend. Assessment of motivation to change is a prime factor in deciding to offer treatment to sex offenders. The offender may say he wants to change but either lacks the ability to change his attitudes or does not want to change them. He may successfully disguise his attitudes, his motivation being primarily to avoid prison or removal by social services.

Finkelhor (1984) places many of the above factors together in a model of aetiology of sex offending and the process by which it occurs:

(1) Motivation to sexually abuse. Put simply, for an offence to occur the offender has to want it to occur. Factors that contribute to motivation include, for example, sexual arousal and emotional congruence.

(2) Overcoming internal inhibitions. Many people may find deviant sexual thoughts arousing but never progress to offending. For instance, rape fantasies are thought to be prevalent among many 'normal' men but only a small proportion progress to committing an offence. Overcoming internal inhibitors may be facilitated by the development of cognitive distortions. Alcohol or drugs may be used to further facilitate disinhibition and then conveniently blamed for the offence.

(3) Overcoming external inhibitions. This is similar to the planning and grooming stage of the offending cycle. Getting access to victims, preparing the environment for offending or engineering opportunities to offend are part of this process.

(4) Overcoming the resistance of the victim. The offender will go to great lengths to prepare the victim for the offence. Bribery, gifts, conditional affection, and threats invoking fear of violence to the victim or their relatives and siblings are often used.

ASSESSMENT AND TREATMENT APPROACHES

While early behaviour therapy programmes conceptualised sexual offending solely in terms of sexual motivation, more recently researchers have favoured a broader, more comprehensive approach. This has incorporated cognitive components, social skills training and relapse prevention techniques.

Eldridge (1992) notes that thoughts, feelings and behaviours contribute to offending. Therefore all these areas require addressing in treatment. It is for this reason that cognitive-behavioural approaches have gained prominence in the treatment of sex offenders. Perkins (1991) states that treatment for sex offenders is broadly divided into two types:

(1)   treatment which concerns itself with helping the offender gain insight into his offending
(2)   treatment that helps him to control or remove those influences which maintain offending

Given the complex nature of sex-offending behaviour, Perkins advocates the use of both avenues of treatment. The emphasis will change depending on where the client is in terms of changing behaviour. In the early stages treatment is concerned with facilitating insight and accepting responsibility for offending behaviour. Later the emphasis switches to relapse prevention and maintaining new learning.

Initial treatment programmes are often centred on a group treatment approach. The development of insight into the behaviour and challenging of cognitive distortions and minimisations are more readily facilitated within such an environment. Offenders within the group may be at varying stages in their understanding of their offences and are encouraged to challenge other group members when they display distorted cognition. Offenders themselves may more readily accept challenges from other offenders and feel less able to dissemble than if seeing a lone therapist. Houston *et al.* (1995) describe such a group approach within a prison environment. The group members attended voluntarily and were encouraged to talk 'about their individual offence histories and cycles' to challenge 'their distorted ways of thinking about children and adults', to promote victim empathy, address issues of sexuality and assertion and accept peer feedback (Houston *et al.*, 1995, p. 361).

Group treatments using this cognitive-behavioural model are highly structured and time limited. A cycle of offending (for example see Fig. 3.1) is presented and explained to group members. This provides a loose cognitive structure around which the offender can begin to explore his offending and develop some understanding and insight into his behaviour. Group members are asked to complete a personal cycle of offending within the group and other members are asked to contribute or challenge as appropriate. While many groups are cognitive-behavioural in orientation, Houston *et al.* (1995) caution that it remains important to recognise dynamic processes occurring within such structured groups. Lewin *et al.* (1994) report on a community treatment programme for sex offenders which was not highly structured and used a psychodynamically orientated model. The group did seek to develop insight, victim empathy and 'new powers of control' (Lewin *et al.*, 1994 p. 306). No outcomes are given for this group other than that one infrequent attender had reoffended.

The use of relapse prevention techniques in working with sex offenders has been adapted from the field of addictive disorders. Relapse in this context refers to a failure in the person's attempt to change or remove the target behaviour. George & Marlatt (1989) describe relapse prevention as a

Pro-offending thinking

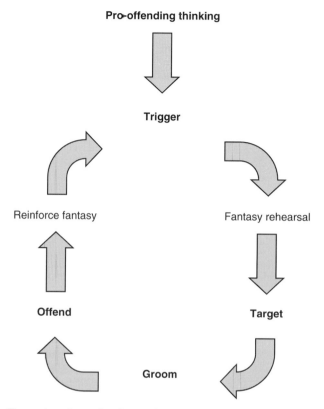

Fig. 3.1 Example of a simple cycle of offending used in sex offender treatment groups.

'self-control program designed to teach individuals who are trying to change their behaviour how to anticipate and cope with the problem of relapse'.

Relapse prevention is aimed at helping the offender to recognise and anticipate what are termed as high risk situations (Nelson & Jackson, 1989). These are situations that place the offender at greater risk of reoffending. It is critical that the offender exhibits some appreciable recognition of the need to change and some genuine intrinsic desire to seek change (George & Marlatt, 1989). The assumption of relapse prevention is that the offender has voluntarily chosen to adopt a new set of rules in regard to his behaviour.

CASE STUDY

The treatment strategy employed with the patient described here was primarily a cognitive-behavioural approach. This aims to challenge the client's distorted cognitions, develop insight into the motivations for his behaviour and encourage him to develop coping strategies.

Alan is a 49-year-old man referred by his probation officer following his conviction and sentencing for indecent assault on a 12-year-old boy. He has served four years of his prison term and has been released under the supervision of his probation officer. He has convictions for similar offences against young boys over a 20-year period. Alan has had treatment for his offending whilst in prison where he attended the Sex Offender Treatment programme in Prison (SOTP). Alan's offences have adopted a similar pattern in that he has used his position as a music teacher and later as a shopkeeper to target young boys and groom them to allow him to offend against them.

He has supervised access to his children whom it is believed he had not offended against. He has accepted responsibility for his offences and does not display open denial. He now recognises that he has a primary attraction to pre-pubescent males. His probation officer has requested that he be seen for relapse prevention work with the aim of assisting him to develop coping strategies to prevent further offending.

Session 1: Assessment

The assessment interview established that Alan was capable of following and understanding a line of reasoning. The components of this comprehensive assessment are outlined in Box 3.1. This information coupled with his education history indicated suitability for treatment (Box 3.2). Alan turned up on time for the assessment and co-operated throughout the process even when difficult and challenging questions were being asked. He appeared genuinely interested in changing his behaviour. Alan saw treatment as a way of 'finally sorting out' his behaviour. He stated that he accepted full responsibility for his offending but occasionally used the word 'relationship' to describe his contact with young boys. This appeared to be a minimisation on his behalf and was one area highlighted for future challenging. One of the benefits of a detailed assessment is that patterns of behaviour can be identified and used to form treatment goals. Experience of personal victimisation is used within treatment to challenge minimisations and develop victim empathy.

Box 3.1   Multi-modal analysis used for assessment purposes (Perkins, 1991)

(1)   Cognitive, i.e. what was going through the offender's mind before, during and after the offence

(2)   Emotional, i.e. how the offender was feeling at the time of his offence

---

Contd.

(3) Attitudinal, i.e. what attitudes the offender holds about offending and the victim

(4) Physical condition, i.e. the offender's physical state at the time of his offence

(5) Personal relationships, i.e. how the offender was relating to others at the time of the offence

(6) Sexual interests, i.e. the extent to which the offender is sexually aroused by fantasies of offending, pornographic material

(7) Behavioural, i.e. what the offender was doing at the time of his offence

Box 3.2   Some factors indicating suitability for treatment

(1) Motivation to attend for interview and treatment
(2) Open to challenges to denial, minimisations and distortions
(3) Displaying some understanding of victim's feelings
(4) Intellectual ability

It became clear from the assessment interview that Alan had not constructed any plan to avoid relapse into offending behaviour. He remained unaware of risky situations and had constructed no coping strategies to remove him from these situations when they arise. He was unable to see the part his mood may have to play in his offending.

Session 2: Aims, process and outcomes

The goals for this session were to clarify with Alan the number of sessions being offered and what the sessions would be used for. Perkins (1991) describes this as negotiating outcomes for treatment. This process involves clarifying what the therapist's responsibilities are and what responsibilities are those of the client. The emphasis is on self-management and Alan was seen as responsible for the problem solution (Brickman *et al.*, 1982). George & Marlatt (1989) suggest that the resultant sense of ownership over the process helps to create an internal control and lasting behaviour change. Perkins (1991) also suggests that the therapist should ensure that the offender attributes good therapeutic ideas to himself. This will make it more difficult for him to justify removing himself from treatment should he find it too difficult at a later stage. This was achieved with Alan by reinforcing good suggestions and by making him aware of the options available to him. This included the option of no treatment versus the types of treatment available. Reminding Alan of external reinforcers such as prison and loss of family contact was used to encourage him to remain in treatment. Alan was encouraged to view treatment as his choice, the theory being to capitalise on the principle of 'cognitive dissonance' (Festinger, 1957) in an effort to maximise attitude change.

The relapse prevention model used is essentially a self-maintenance model. The offender is responsible for monitoring his own behaviour and taking evasive action when placed in risky situations. Alan was responsible for attending appointments on time and contributing constructively to the process. He was also responsible for his honesty or lack of it during the sessions. He admitted during this interview that he was frequently dishonest within treatment: 'I tell them whatever they want to hear'. He also acknowledged that he regularly lied to himself about his behaviour.

The principal aim of the treatment being offered is to help Alan to complete a relapse prevention plan (RPP) and to encourage him to recognise the distorted cognitions he uses which place him at risk of reoffending. The model used for the relapse prevention plan is adapted from that suggested by Eldridge (1992) (see Fig. 3.2). It was agreed with Alan that he would be offered six sessions to complete a personal RPP. The first session was largely taken up with definitions and concepts of each element of the plan. As Alan had had previous treatment he was able to suggest many possible routes to relapse as outlined in the first stage of the plan.

While consideration was given to using some standardised measure for assessing change it is recognised that measuring behaviour change in such a short period as planned here is difficult. Alan was asked to complete a relapse prevention questionnaire as homework for the next session. This was designed to prompt Alan to think further about possible roads to relapse and how he acted previously and what he might do differently

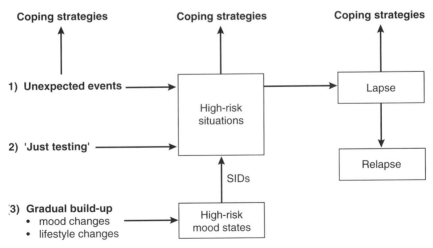

Fig. 3.2 Example of relapse prevention plan as suggested by Eldridge (1992). SIDs = Seemingly irrelevant decisions.

now. Homework is a useful method of consolidating work completed in the session and enables the offender to transfer his new repertoire to the real world.

The main outcome of the sessions being offered is that Alan will have completed a personal relapse prevention plan in the time offered. It is hoped he will remain offence-free during this period. It has to be recognised, however, that this cannot be evaluated with any objectivity.

Session 3: High-risk situations

Alan was able to recognise his routes to relapse with little prompting. It had become clear from the assessment interview, however, that he had little insight into possible risky situations and had no clear strategies for coping with these situations. The goals for this session therefore were to begin work on facilitating insight into and developing anticipation of high-risk situations. A high-risk situation is defined as any situation which poses a threat to perceived control and thereby increases the probability of a lapse or relapse (George & Marlatt, 1989).

The technique used to identify high-risk situations was that suggested by Nelson & Jackson (1989). Alan was asked to describe past situations which resulted in offences. He was then assisted to identify risk elements in these situations. Alan was readily able to identify obvious high-risk situations such as 'being alone with children' but had more difficulty with less obvious situations. For example he did not see as a high-risk situation the fact that he walked his dog on the common when children were leaving school. Children regularly approached him to pet his dog, which was a popular breed with children. It is not possible or even desirable to identify every possible high-risk situation for an offender. It is more practical to identify a range of situations the offender has experienced and some he can expect to experience. Coping strategies, which are developed as a result, can then be generalised to a broader range of situations.

In the case described here it remains too early in treatment to declare an outcome. Alan will have at least three more sessions. He has yet to see the value in having a support network of friends or family who will act as external controls and who will know his RPP. Future sessions will assist him to develop coping strategies for dealing with high-risk situations as well as instruction on positive lifestyle changes. There remains a great deal of work to complete with Alan. When the current sessions are completed, consideration will be given to what further treatment is required. It is possible that further work on victim empathy and problem-solving techniques will be required.

One of the difficulties in one-to-one sessions with sex offenders is that it is difficult to challenge them about their cognitive distortions. While the therapist may readily see the distortions, the offender can choose to disagree. For this reason future treatment options may include group work. Offenders find it more difficult to deny motivations and easier to accept challenges from other offenders who have similar experiences. The relapse prevention model is primarily a cognitive-behavioural approach. It is however difficult to assess any real behaviour change in sex offenders. Prolonged or even lifetime follow-up and monitoring may be the only real alternative to long-term incarceration.

DILEMMAS OF TREATMENT

Treating sex offenders brings with it increased legal and ethical concerns which present a number of challenges for many forensic mental health nurses working in this area. As with many such issues, in practice there is never one simple answer to these concerns. Underlying these concerns is a fundamental dilemma for nurses of providing care to those who have demonstrated an amazing lack of care or concern for others. However, providing care for such people is nothing new for nurses, and for forensic mental health nurses in particular many of our patients will have committed serious offences.

Some authors have eloquently questioned the rationale for treatment of sex offenders by health services (Mercer, 1998). This may be a reflection of the ambivalence nurses feel about treating these offenders. It also appears to challenge our concepts of nursing and deep-seated feelings about one of the last pariahs of our society.

Legal dilemmas

Sex offenders who were sentenced after September 1997 are now required under the Sex Offenders Act 1997 to notify and register with the police. Together with these requirements social services, probation officers and the police are forming what have become known as risk management panels. These panels are convened to discuss and communicate potential risk posed by sex offenders in local areas. The dilemma for health-care staff is that these panels often request information from clinicians on offenders in treatment. Balancing these requests with the confidentiality of the offender in treatment can be difficult. This is especially the case when offenders are not compelled to attend for treatment. They may see the involvement of the police and social services as threatening and either refuse treatment or contribute less of themselves to treatment. In practice it is important to frame the involvement of the risk management panels in the context of relapse prevention. Thus requests by the police and other agencies for information on risk status may be dealt with in terms of providing a comprehensive relapse prevention treatment package. The offender will also receive the message that the flow of information is in both directions and that health-care staff will not engage in collusion with the offender. This is important as there is now an obligation, often framed by locally agreed guidelines, for clinicians to report concerns about the welfare of children to the appropriate authorities. In terms of other possible sexual offences it should be made clear to offenders in treatment that, where an offence comes to light and where the victim is identifiable, clinicians have a responsibility to report such offences. To do otherwise would be to collude in the secretive world in which many child sex offenders thrive.

Ethical dilemmas

Other than issues of confidentiality, which legal and professional obligations present, it may be assumed that sex offenders in treatment are entitled to the same levels of confidentiality as any other patient in the care of a nurse. There may, however, be other instances where these issues are less clear, and access to appropriate professional supervision and advice is an absolute prerequisite in such situations.

For nurses there may also be difficulty in reconciling spending-limited health-care resources on what are commonly regarded as 'evil men' or social pariahs. This can often be starkly highlighted when considering the disparity in service provision for victims of these offences. While a large number of sex offenders are now being treated in prisons (Thornton & Hogue, 1993) many more are being treated in community programmes (Barker & Morgan, 1993). This may present a number of concerns for clinicians. It is clear that many sex offenders will have increased risk of offending when opportunities to offend are present. Clinicians are dependent upon the offender to remain offence-free while in community treatment. Coupled with risks that the offender may continue to offend while in treatment is the risk the offender may present to himself. For many offenders the process of accepting responsibility for offences and acknowledging the depth of deviant thinking may be so devastating that they take their own lives (Mezey, 1991). It is therefore incumbent upon mental health nurses treating offenders to consider the risk they present in broader terms.

Concepts of harm reduction and living with risk of further offending of offenders in treatment may also create difficulties for nurses. It is true that some offenders in treatment will go on to commit further offences. Exactly how many we do not as yet know. Forensic mental health nurses grapple with such concerns on an often daily basis. With mentally disordered offenders we may reconcile ourselves to the potential for further offending by acknowledging the part the illness has to play in the process. With sex offenders this is often a less obvious factor. Positive outcomes of treatment may be less tangible and re-conviction rates are a poor measure of re-offending (Furby *et al.*, 1989). It may be that clinicians working with these offenders will have to accept that even where positive outcomes are realised, the clinician may not bear witness to them. However, the development of more sophisticated methods of risk assessment and treatment may yet provide us with the information to decide on who will benefit most from different methods of treatment.

Personal dilemmas

The personal feelings and experiences of nurses working with sex offenders and the impact of working in close proximity to them is an important factor when providing these treatments. Hilton & Mezey (1996, p. 413) acknowledge that working with these offenders is likely to 'evoke strong emotions which may include fear, dread and disgust'. As such it may be difficult for the clinician to approach treatment with the same level of empathic understanding and respect that is integral to mental health nurses' professional functioning. Indeed, adopting punitive and overly confrontational techniques in an attempt to somehow make the offender 'pay' for the offence may more clearly reflect the content of such treatments where these fundamental components are missing. Associated with this are feelings of being manipulated or manoeuvred by people whom most of us would cross the street to avoid. Expert clinical supervision and professional support are absolute necessities in working with sex offenders, many of whom are skilled in the art of manipulating people and environments to their own ends.

OUTCOMES

There is some evidence that cognitive-behavioural programmes are useful in this type of work. Marshall *et al.* (1991) in a comprehensive review of treatment outcomes concluded that cognitive-behavioural programmes are likely to be more effective with child sex abusers than other treatments.

There remain difficulties in measuring change although a number of standardised measures are now appearing. Recidivism rates are a poor measure due to under-reporting of sexual offences (Furby *et al.*, 1989), while sex offenders themselves when allowed complete confidentiality have reported thousands more offences than they had been apprehended for (Abel *et al.*, 1987). Most studies appear to have insufficient follow-up periods to enable recidivism to be used as an evaluative measure. Burchard & Wood (1982) have demonstrated behaviour change in offenders while in institutional settings but were unable to show if this generalised to community settings.

CONCLUSIONS

Working with sex offenders may present a number of difficulties for forensic mental health nurses. This is not least because the acts which these offenders have committed are socially abhorrent. It presents a direct challenge to the humanistic principles on which much of mental health nursing is based. Maintaining therapeutic integrity and avoiding punitive styles of interaction demand much of clinicians engaged in this type of work. Therapist selection must therefore consider personal feelings, beliefs and attitudes towards these offenders.

Nurses engaged in this work must achieve the difficult balancing act of providing appropriate challenges and confrontation to sex offenders within treatment while resisting the urge to use treatment as another form of punishment. O'Connell *et al.* (1990) provide interesting reading on how to determine suitable therapist selection for sex offender treatment. It is, however, imperative, whatever the level of experience possessed by mental health nurses in assessment and group treatments, that they receive expert clinical supervision. This may take many forms. Psychodynamic interpretation of group processes may be useful in understanding the complexities of interactions when working with sex offenders. Individual supervision with experienced clinicians in this field will help develop the assessment and analytic skills required to make detailed judgements on suitability for treatment of offenders with limited motivation to change.

The development of a sound theoretical basis for assessment and treatment of sex offenders is also important. Mental health nurses will not have encountered such specialised work in their basic training. Formal training in this area is limited. There is, however, a wealth of research literature and regular national conferences which could usefully be accessed by mental health nurses. Given the high rates in clinical populations of childhood sexual abuse it may be worthwhile to develop specialist programmes to address this training deficit (Briere, 1988).

The development of research that seeks to demonstrate efficacy of treatment of nurse-led interventions in this field could provide interesting information. Research of this nature may then prompt development of specialist training programmes that could address current deficits in forensic mental health nurse training.

In terms of treatment responses there are now a number of validated approaches centring on cognitive-behavioural models of intervention. Relapse prevention is one useful method of managing risk once initial treatment has established for the offender where responsibility lies for the offence and he has gained some understanding of his behaviour

Sex offenders present with a range of behaviours which pose some unique challenges for therapists. The recidivistic nature of their offences, their limited motivation to change and their frank dishonesty might dissuade many mental health nurses from entering this field of work. However, there is now good evidence that these behaviours can be changed and as assessment and treatment protocols become more sophisticated there now exists an opportunity for forensic mental health nurses to expand their practice into this challenging area.

It is appropriate to conclude this chapter by recalling the purpose of sex offender assessment and treatment. If difficulties arise for forensic mental health nurses in reconciling the provision of limited treatment resources to these offenders, then possibly a recognition of the plight of their victims may sway the argument. Sex offender treatment may provide, by reducing the number of future victims, a possible solution to this damaging and ultimately self-destructive crime.

REFERENCES

Abel, G. G., Becker, J. V., Mittelman, M., Cunningham-Rathner, J., Rouleau, J. L. & Murphy, W. D. (1987) Self-reported sex crimes of non-incarcerated paraphiliacs. *Journal of Interpersonal Violence* **2**(1), 3–25.

American Psychiatric Association (1987) *Diagnostic and Statistical Manual of Mental Disorder*, 3rd edn, revised. APA, Washington, DC.

Bagley, C. & Ramsay, R. (1986) Sexual abuse in childhood: psychological outcomes and implications for social worker practices. *Journal of Social Work in Human Sexuality* **4**, 33–47.

Barker, M. & Morgan, R. (1993) *Sex Offenders: A Framework for the Evaluation of Community-based treatment*. A report for the Home Office. Faculty of Law, University of Bristol.

Berlin, F. S. & Meinecke, C. F. (1981) Treatment of sex offenders with antiandrogen medication. *American Journal of Psychiatry* **138**, 601–607.

Brickman, P., Rabinowitz, V. C., Karuza, J., Coates, D., Cohn, E. & Kidder, L. (1982) Models of helping and coping. *American Psychologist* **37**, 368–84.

Briere, J. (1988) The long term clinical correlates of childhood sexual victimisation. In *Human Sexual Aggression: Current Perspectives* (Prentky, R., ed.), pp. 327–34. Annals of the New York Academy of Sciences, New York.

Burchard, J. D. & Wood, T. W. (1982) Crime and delinquency. In *International Handbook of Behaviour Modification and Therapy* (Bellack, A. S., Hersen, M. & Kazdin Q.E., eds). Plenum, New York.

Department of Health/Home Office (1992) *Review of Health and Social Services for Mentally Disordered Offenders and Others Requiring Similar Services* (The Reed Report). HMSO, London.

Eldridge, H. (1992) Relapse prevention and its application to patterns of adult male sex offending – implications for assessment, intervention and maintenance. Paper presented at the National Offender Treatment Association Conference, Dundee University, September 1992.

Festinger, L. (1957) *A Theory of Cognitive Dissonance*. Harper & Row, New York.

Finkelhor, D. (1979) *Sexually Victimised Children*. Free Press, New York.

Finkelhor, D. (1984) *Child Sexual Abuse: New Theory and Research*. Free Press, New York.

Finkelhor, D. & Browne A. (1985) The traumatic impact of child sexual abuse: a conceptualization. *American Journal of Orthopsychiatry* **55**, 530–41.

Fisher, D. (1994) Adult sex offenders: Who are they? What and how do they do it? In *Sexual Offending against Children: Assessment and Treatment of Male Abusers* (Morrison, T., Erooga, M. & Beckett, R. C., eds). Routledge, London.

Furby, L., Weinrott, M. R. & Blackshaw, L. (1989) Sex offender recidivism: a review. *Psychological Bulletin* **105**(1), 3–30.

George, W. H. & Marlatt, G. A. (1989) Introduction. In *Relapse Prevention with Sex Offenders* (Laws, R. D., ed.). The Guildford Press, New York.

Grubin, D. H. & Kennedy, H. G. (1991) The classification of sexual offenders. *Criminal Behaviour and Mental Health* **1**, 123–9.

Hilton, M. R. & Mezey, G. C. (1996) Victims and perpetrators of child sexual abuse. *British Journal of Psychiatry* **169**, 408–15.

Houston, J. (1998) *Making Sense with Offenders: Personal Constructs, Therapy and Change*. Wiley, Chichester.

Houston, J., Wrench, M. & Hosking, N. (1995) Group processes in the treatment of child sex offenders. *Journal of Forensic Psychiatry* **6**(2), 359–68.

Kaul, A. (1993) Sex offenders – cure or management? *Medicine Science and Law* **33**(3), 207–12.

Kennedy, H. G. & Grubin D. H. (1992) Patterns of denial in sex offenders. *Psychological Medicine* **22**, 191–6.

Lewin, J., Beary, M., Toman, E., Skinner, G. & Sproul-Bolton, R. (1994) A community service for sex offenders. *Journal of Forensic Psychiatry* **5**(2), 297–310.

Marshall, W. L., Jones, R., Ward, T., Johnston, P. & Barbaree, H. (1991) Treatment outcome with sex offenders. *Clinical Psychology Review* **11**, 465–85.

Marshall, W. L., Champagne, F., Brown, C. & Miller, S. (1997) Empathy, intimacy, loneliness, and self-esteem in nonfamilial child molesters: a brief report. *Journal of Child Sexual Abuse* **6**(3), 87–98.

Mercer, D. (1998) The nature of the beast: sex offender treatment. In *Critical Perspectives in Forensic Care: Inside Out* (Mason, T. & Mercer, D., eds). Macmillan Press, London.

Mezey, G. (1991) Treatment in the community. *Criminal Behaviour and Mental Health* **1**, 169–72.

Mullen, P. E., Martin, J. L.., Anderson, J. C., Romans, S. E. & Herbison, G. P. (1993) Childhood sexual abuse and mental health in adult life. *British Journal of Psychiatry* **163**, 721–32.

Nelson, C. & Jackson, P. (1989) High risk recognition: the cognitive-behavioural chain. In *Relapse Prevention with Sex Offenders* (Laws, R. D., ed.). Guildford Press, New York.

O'Connell, M. A., Leberg, E. & Donaldson, C. R. (1990) *Working with Sex Offenders: Guidelines for Therapist Selection*. Sage Publications, Newbury Park, California.

Perkins, D. (1991) Treatment in hospital. *Criminal Behaviour and Mental Health* **1**, 152–68.

Prins, H. (1991) Some aspects of sex offending – cause and cures? *Medicine, Science and the Law* **31**(4), 329–37.

Quinsey, V. L., Bergensen, S. G. & Steinman, C. M. (1976) Changes in physiological and verbal responses of child molesters during aversion therapy. *Canadian Journal of Behavioral Science* **8**, 202–12.

Russell, D. E. H. (1986) *The Secret Trauma: Incest in the Lives of Girls and Women.* Basic Books, New York.

Schlank, A. M. & Shaw, T. (1996) Treating sexual offenders who deny their guilt: a pilot study. *Sexual Abuse: A Journal of Research and Treatment* **8**(1), 17–23.

Sturup, G. K. (1972) Castration: the total treatment. In *Sexual Behaviours* (Resnick, R. L. P. & Wolfgang, M. F., eds). Little, Brown, Boston.

Taylor, P. (1991) Psychiatry for sex offenders: is anyone motivated? (editorial). *Criminal Behaviour and Mental Health* **1**(2), iii–vii.

Thornton, D. & Hogue, T. (1993) Large-scale provision of programmes for imprisoned sex offenders. *Criminal Behaviour and Mental Health* **3**(4), 371–80.

Chapter 4
Working with the Offender Patient with Psychosis

Geoff Haines

INTRODUCTION

Although forensic mental health services cater for individuals with a variety of diagnostic characteristics, the majority of patients, particularly those detained within secure environments, suffer from some form of psychotic disorder. Such individuals provide the bulk of the forensic clientele and therefore the issues pertaining to psychosis and offending behaviour are central to the nurse's role.

The term psychosis is generally applied to psychiatric conditions in which contact with reality is lost or impaired; examples are schizophrenia and bipolar affective disorder. In this chapter the main focus will be on the care of offenders diagnosed as suffering from schizophrenia. The chapter will begin with a case study followed by a review of the relevant literature, and conclude with an examination of future directions for investigation.

CASE STUDY

Paul is a 20-year-old man who has been remanded in prison following allegations of sexual abuse of his eight-year-old female cousin.

Paul was the second of three brothers and also had a younger sister. His father died when Paul was three and is reported to have sexually abused him. Paul's mother had experienced difficulties bringing up the family on her own in their flat. Paul was often aggressive towards his mother and siblings. His mother retaliated by hitting Paul or by locking him in his bedroom, sometimes for days.

Paul lived in a number of care homes until he was 16. He also attended a number of schools where he was described as aggressive and having reading and writing difficulties. He was reported to have become involved in 'inappropriate sexual activities' with other children. On two occasions unsuccessful attempts were made to place Paul with foster parents but both ended when Paul became violent and abusive.

When he was 16, Paul's local council placed him in a flat. After several months, according to Paul, he met his first girlfriend, who later died suddenly. He also gained employment as a labourer and enrolled at a local college. By the age of 19, however, he began drinking large quantities of alcohol and using cannabis and heroin. He lost his place at college and was cautioned by the police for fighting. He regularly visited his doctor complaining of a variety of ailments such as breathlessness and chest pains. On several occasions he was admitted to hospital for observations but no abnormalities were detected.

Paul resumed contact with one of his aunts and began looking after her nine-year-old daughter whilst his aunt was at work. The child later complained that Paul had interfered with her sexually. Paul appeared in court and was placed on a six-month probation order. He tried to hide his sentence from his family. Two months later Paul began to visit a second aunt who also allowed Paul to look after her eight-year-old daughter. This child also complained that Paul was sexually interfering with her. Paul was eventually charged with indecent assault and with breaching his previous probation order and was remanded in custody.

Since being remanded his behaviour has become increasingly bizarre. Initially he isolated himself in his cell and began shouting in different voices for no apparent reason. Paul told the prison staff that 'the master' was speaking through him in tongues and that he, Paul, could control other inmates through telepathy. Eventually, Paul began attacking other inmates and staff and was transferred to the prison medical centre. On two occasions Paul accepted oral neuroleptic medication and became more settled. Eventually, however, he began to refuse medication saying that 'the master' had forbidden him to accept any more, and he carried out two further unprovoked attacks on inmates and prison staff.

Paul continued to isolate himself, refused oral medication and started shouting again for no apparent reason. When interviewed by the prison doctor he said that he thought that other inmates and members of staff were plotting to kill him. A referral was made to the local forensic psychiatry service with a view to transferring Paul to a local medium secure unit.

After interviewing Paul it was agreed that he was suffering from mental illness and he was transferred on Section 38 of the Mental Health Act 1983 to the local medium secure unit.

REVIEW OF THE LITERATURE

Tidmarsh (1990) argues that schizophrenia can be defined either broadly or narrowly and can mean different things to different people. Jablensky

(1993) adds that schizophrenia is a hypothetical disease which lacks validated disease markers. Its diagnosis thus depends on the investigator's analysis of subjective and phenomenological data. The type of phenomena usually associated with schizophrenia include social impairment, thought disorder, hallucinations and delusions (Jamerson, 1985). Moreover White (1987) emphasises the socially produced nature of schizophrenia and how the person is objectified as a 'schizophrenic'.

Der *et al.* (1990) produced evidence that hospital admissions for schizophrenia in the United Kingdom had fallen by 50% in the last two decades. Harrison *et al.* (1991), however, found that the rate of first-onset schizophrenia in Nottingham had remained stable. They attributed this trend to an increase in the diagnosis of the condition in local migrant groups and in the children of such groups, and argued that it might also exist in similar urban areas of the UK. Harrison *et al.* (1991) suggest that the reason for the overall decline in the administrative incidence of schizophrenia is the availability of improved diagnostic techniques and the development of community services.

Norman & Malla (1993) argue that there is considerable genetic and neurophysiological evidence to support the biological basis of schizo-phrenia. From a nursing perspective Gournay (1996) supports this view and proposes that nursing practice accommodates the detection of brain and dopamine abnormalities and genetics. Dawson (1997), however, after examining the research, argues that there is little evidence that people with schizophrenia have larger brain ventricles than others in the population (Chua & McKenna, 1995); a consistent pattern of elevated dopamine levels (Carlson, 1990); or a genetic loading which will ultimately develop into schizophrenia regardless of environmental factors (Suddath *et al.*, 1990).

Zubin & Spring (1977) argue that those with schizophrenia develop varying levels of vulnerability to the condition which can be triggered by environmental, social, developmental, psychological and biological factors. They note that a schizophrenic episode often follows a period of acute stress which may be prevented through prior therapeutic intervention. The individual facing an episode is liable to experience a reduction in coping effort, an inability to perceive the discrepancy between their stressed and optimum states, and a loss of social competence (French & Stewart, 1976). Zubin & Spring's (1977) theory of vulnerability may explain the many anomalies surrounding the course of a schizophrenic episode. It is, how-ever, a difficult concept to measure due to the overlapping characteristics of the various subtle phenomena presented.

Some emphasise the effects of external stimuli whilst others highlight the individual's internal response to stress. Zarski (1984) describes how reactions to stress are recorded behaviourally, phenomenologically and biologically, and adds that it is often difficult to record corresponding measures even in the same domain (Steptoe *et al.*, 1990). People relapsing into schizophrenia often record higher levels of stress on biological indicators (Grillon *et al.*, 1990). It is unclear, however, if such changes are caused by symptoms strengthening reactions to external events or solely by external stimuli. People with schizophrenia are also considered to have fewer internal recourses for coping with stress and experience higher levels when confronted by situations which are effectively negotiated by other members of the population (Nicholson & Newfeld, 1989). Norman & Malla (1993) conclude that the stress that people with schizophrenia experience involves daily life encounters and concerns about the future rather than actual major life events.

Boyle (1997) acknowledges a possible biological basis for some people's disturbing experiences but doubts the existence of a scientifically testable category of mental illness called schizophrenia. The diagnosis, nevertheless, can have a drastic effect on people's lives. She produces evidence that acknowledgement of hallucinations is discouraged in this culture but cites studies which indicate that up to 50% of the population experience such phenomena (Bentall & Slade, 1985), either hypnotically (Barber & Calverley, 1964) or as a result of stress (Slade, 1976). Boyle also argues that the label of schizophrenia is more likely to be applied to bizarre behaviour if the individual's social functioning is considered inadequate or not corresponding to social norms (Littlewood & Lipsedge, 1982). She further argues that there are no specific criteria to differentiate schizophrenic hallucinations from normal imagery (Al-Issa, 1977) and that hallucinations may be under individual control and used as a response (or guide) to action in aversive situations (Slade, 1976).

Boyle (1997) criticises Clare's (1980) claim that delusions are false, preoccupying beliefs held with absolute conviction which are not amenable to reason or culturally shared. She argues that there is no evidence that schizophrenic beliefs are held with any greater conviction or preoccupation than beliefs not labelled as symptoms. Boyle considers there is little evidence that schizophrenic delusions are not amenable to reason or that the beliefs of 'ordinary' people are routinely changed by 'rational' persuasion (Anderson *et al.*, 1980). Moreover, Milton *et al.* (1978), using interventions derived from work on attitude change, demonstrated a decrease in the stated level of conviction, of people with schizophrenia, to their delusional beliefs.

Boyle (1997) contests the medical implication that radically different beliefs cannot arise within a culture except under the influence of mental disorder. She argues that psychiatrists appear to know little about the interrelationship between environmental and personality factors in the development of beliefs, and that patients are rarely diagnosed within the context of their home environment. Psychiatrists also appear not to acknowledge that the extent to which someone can convince another of the value of their beliefs will vary in relation to time and place, and in relation to the attributes of the 'believer'. She concludes that a belief therefore becomes a delusion when a psychiatrist decides others no longer want to hear it and the patient will not modify their belief in relation to what is socially valued.

MENTAL ILLNESS, OFFENDING AND CRIME

Many questions concerning the relationship between mental illness and crime are raised by the case of Paul. Can Paul be said to be suffering from 'mental illness' or more specifically 'schizophrenia'? Did Paul's condition develop at, or before, the time of his offence or did he commit the offence as an indirect result of tension related to his 'illness', and was Paul driven to commit the offence as a result of disordered thoughts and perceptions or did he develop the disorder at a later date due to his imprisonment?

Tidmarsh (1990) argues that the personality of the patient who develops schizophrenia may be of a schizoid type (i.e. lacking in empathy, detached, rigid and suspicious) which has developed before the onset of the disorder (Wolf & Cull, 1986) and may lead the patient into crime and have an underlying influence over their illness. Zitrin *et al.* (1976) identified that patients with schizophrenia had higher than average arrest rates in the two years prior to admission.

Tidmarsh (1990) considers that schizophrenic patients often show less emotion than might be expected when one considers the degree of threat they perceive they are under. If, however, the patient is convinced of their delusions and feels jealous and angry (Hafner & Boker, 1982), then even a mildly abrasive statement from another might increase the possibility of violence. This relates to the work of Leff *et al.* (1982) which indicates that those suffering from schizophrenia are prone to develop more pronounced symptoms in families with high levels of expressed emotion.

Yesavage (1982) suggests that assaults by in-patients diminish when they are treated with anti-psychotic medication and that serious assaults, if committed in hospital, often go unprosecuted. Hughson (1981) argues that such patients, after being transferred to high security hospitals, are often more disturbed than those admitted via the courts.

Coid (1988a), in his study of remand prisoners in Winchester Prison, estimated that 2.5% were suffering psychosis. Many of this group had committed burglary and theft to obtain food, or criminal damage and minor assaults to provoke arrest.

Taylor & Gunn (1984a, b) provided evidence of a higher than average level of criminal behaviour in remand prisoners diagnosed with schizophrenia. The figures, however, only represent a small percentage of the total number of people diagnosed nationally with the condition. Their evidence may have been distorted by the greater likelihood of people with schizophrenia being remanded (Faulk, 1994). Nevertheless, Humphreys *et al.* (1992), from their study of people recently diagnosed with the condition, concluded that 20% had exhibited life-threatening behaviour to others. Only a small percentage were arrested or admitted to hospital. It remains to be concluded if similar results would be found in a comparable national study.

Taylor (1985), in a study of prisoners with schizophrenia, found a direct relationship, in 80% of those studied, between their positive symptoms and their offences. Faulk (1994) doubts these findings and argues that patients sometimes rationalise or hide their 'true' motives.

In relation to Paul, Power (1976) concludes that, although a high proportion of people with schizophrenia report fluctuations in sex drive and difficulties with their sexual identity, such people are rarely charged or convicted with sexual offences including rape. However, Tidmarsh (1990) points to the increased level of risk posed by the rare insightless person with schizophrenia who is sexually disinhibited as a result of command hallucinations. In Paul's case it is to be hoped that he will be offered treatment for his alleged sexual offending (and use of illicit drugs) after his psychosis has resolved.

THE APPROPRIATE CLINICAL ENVIRONMENT

Bowden (1978), Taylor & Gunn (1984b) and Coid (1988a) found that a high number of offenders with schizophrenia were considered socially incompetent, had previous hospital admissions and experienced florid symptoms, yet were often rejected by the NHS and given custodial sentences. Coid (1988b) also found disparities between health regions' acceptance or rejection of chronically disturbed prisoners with schizophrenia. Tidmarsh (1990) suggests, however, that not all defendants with schizophrenia allow evidence of their illness to be presented in court, and a proportion, rather than being admitted to hospital, prefer to remain in prison where they will rarely have to undergo rehabilitation or comply with medication. He adds that there are a number of often chronically ill prisoners who, due to their compliance, are rarely seen by mental health professionals.

It is, nevertheless, considered that low, medium and high security mental health services provide a more appropriate environment for the care of mentally disordered offenders than prison. As Faulk (1994) indicates, prison health centres are not recognised as hospitals within the meaning of the Mental Health Act 1983 and are unable, except in emergencies, to treat patients against their will. Floridly psychotic patients, therefore, if they are refusing medication, only receive treatment if their condition deteriorates into an emergency or when they are transferred to a hospital setting.

In England there are approximately 1590 patients in high security hospitals, 75% of whom are diagnosed as suffering from schizophrenia

(Faulk, 1994). In such settings there is an emphasis on preventing potentially dangerous patients from absconding because, on admission, they were usually considered a grave and immediate risk to others. There is anecdotal evidence that patients suffering from schizophrenia are liable to be admitted to high security settings if they are persistently suffering from delusions and hallucinations linked to past violent attacks; are unpredictable and don't respond to medication; have killed another person; incorporate those close to them into their delusional system; pose a continual risk to other patients, staff or members of the public; and have an increasing history of violence predicting future harm.

Although it is estimated that a high proportion of patients within such settings could be cared for at a lower level of security, it is difficult to predict which patients would be in this group (Acres, 1975). Patients often stay for longer periods in high security hospitals due to their conditions being more difficult to treat and due to anxieties related to their level of risk. Some patients, however, relapse, possibly due to anxieties related to transfer or because they lose hope that they will ever move to a lower level of security.

Medium secure units (MSUs) are erratically distributed and vary considerably in size and level of security. They admit patients who are difficult to manage at lower levels of security yet are not deemed to require care in a high security setting. MSUs usually have the capacity to prevent patients absconding but also focus therapeutic programmes linked to external community resources.

A number of hospitals have locked intensive care wards, which often experience higher levels of disturbance, especially in inner city areas, than other secure settings. They treat short periods of disturbance. Such patients may have a history of aggression and violence against persons or property but their level of risk is not considered sufficient to warrant admission to medium security.

Finding the most appropriate clinical environment is usually determined by the legal system, the resources available and the forensic mental health team. Nurses are usually involved in the assessment of patients moving between varying levels of security. This provides continuity between clinical environments and hopefully helps to reduce the stress of transfer (Ritter, 1989).

AGGRESSION AND VIOLENCE

Taylor (1982), in a review of schizophrenia and violence, came to the following tentative conclusions:

- Violence often accompanies the illness especially if the illness remains untreated.

- It is more common in patients with recurrent exacerbations than in those who are continuously ill.
- The offence often arises from a loss of 'insight' after the patient has conducted investigations in an attempt to validate their delusions and hallucinations.
- Such violence is rarely of a bizarre nature except when inflicted on themselves.
- Violence may arise more as a result of pressure from the patient's environment rather than as a direct result of their mental state.

Taylor (1993), in a later study of violent offenders in Brixton Prison, produced evidence that psychotic men are less likely to engage in violence against others than non-psychotic men and that non-psychotic men commit more serious violence. Taylor also demonstrated that psychotic offenders were more likely to become socially isolated and unemployed, that 46% acted on their delusions at the time of their offence, that 10% drank alcohol prior to the offence, that strangers were rarely assaulted, that police officers were often assaulted, that victims were just as likely to be males as females, and that they were slightly more likely to know their victim than non-psychotic prisoners. Both psychotic and non-psychotic prisoners were found to have suffered from substantial periods of maternal and paternal loss through childhood and a substantial minority had spent some time in institutional care before the age of 16. Taylor (1993) concludes that most violence committed by psychotic people should be predictable and preventable through treatment, and adds that material resources, sensitive supervision and peer group support should all be taken into account when providing care and treatment.

There is little comparative work concerning what levels and types of violence may exist within low, medium and high security settings in urban, suburban and rural areas. It is also unclear what proportion of people with schizophrenia, in such settings, are involved in violent incidents and if the type of behaviour they exhibit is different from that of other groups. Violence may arise due to breakdowns in communication between staff and patients (Brailsford & Stevenson, 1973). Philips (1977), however, considered that a core of incidents are unpreventable. Considerable work has therefore been carried out in analysing the signs of impending violence and devising strategies to manage it effectively (Moran, 1984).

REHABILITATION

Therapeutic interventions associated with the rehabilitation of patients suffering from schizophrenia in forensic mental health settings may be identified by the use of the Care Programme Approach (Department of

Health, 1990) and are intertwined with the ongoing evaluation of the level of risk linked to the level of security required to manage that risk.

Tarbuck (1994) in his model of forensic mental health nursing advocated a patient-centred rather than a custodial approach to care linked to the individual patient's security needs. Tarbuck proceeded to identify minimum values for the care of people within forensic mental health settings which reflect human rights, are open to external scrutiny and work where possible towards the patient's returning to the community. Tarbuck considered that a large part of the forensic nurse's role involves risk assessment and advocated a multi-disciplinary and problem-solving approach to care which is regularly evaluated and delivered within a framework of specified standards. However, his model did not acknowledge fundamental problems associated with the diagnosis of mental illness, and lacked a community focus encompassing collaborative working between statutory, voluntary, user groups and independent agencies.

Patients suffering from schizophrenia are often caught up in distorted forms of communication which may exacerbate their problems (Lemert, 1968). The Clunis Report (Ritchie *et al.*, 1994) and a number of other inquiry reports indicate the tragic consequences which can arise when there is a breakdown in communication between professions. To reduce the possibility of such breakdowns occurring within and between forensic settings and generic services, it is essential that nurses work towards perfecting their systems of communication. It is also important that the model of care chosen is not framed in esoteric language and does not appear inaccessible to nurses and representatives from other disciplines and agencies.

Macdonald (1992) argues that the main features of rehabilitation are to limit the cause of the disability and help the individual develop their talents and self-esteem in successfully accomplishing social roles. Wing (1983) argues that reduced motivation, of some patients, is a secondary disablement brought on by environmental factors such as institutionalisation. Morgan (1980), however, argues that it is a negative symptom of the illness occurring independently of environmental factors. Shepherd (1985) advises that goals for such patients often need to be small, realistic and negotiated.

Rogers (1997) considers social skills training as an important intervention for patients with schizophrenia in secure settings to enhance their general functioning and prevent the onset of institutionalisation. Smith *et al.* (1996), in a review of the literature on social skills training with patients with schizophrenia, found strong evidence that skills are acquired and maintained as long as the patient has at least two sessions a week and that the sessions last for at least six months. Wing & Brown (1970) point out that patients are often resistant to staying in psychiatric services when they are first admitted but eventually do not wish to leave. Deterioration in patients is attributed to loss of contact with friends and relatives, their illness, institutionalisation and a lack of privacy and to the low priority given to interactions (Altschul, 1972). Wing & Brown (1970) suggest that staff with the most optimistic attitudes gravitate to employment in the least restrictive environments.

To combat institutionalisation Barton (1966) suggested a 'step approach' to rehabilitation where patients are encouraged to have contact with the outside world, to maintain their own possessions and to be involved in acknowledging personal events. He added that the ward atmosphere should be homely and permissive and that patients should be involved in planning and making decisions. Halek (1993) advocates nurses establishing strategies to attempt to engage relatives and friends. Pilling (1991), however, warns against constantly putting pressure on patients to develop ever higher levels of independence, and advises teams to acknowledge and learn to cope with setbacks. Many staff involved in the rehabilitation of mentally disordered offenders are working towards ideals of rehabilitation despite the many deficits which exist in the provision of community care facilities for this group.

Lyttle (1990) argued that patients suffering from schizophrenia often retreat into their own fantasy world where they can become neglected by staff to a point where their bizarre behaviour is tolerated as long as it does not directly impose on others. Ritter (1992) points out the importance of patients having some structure to their day so that, even if their inner world is chaotic, they are given an opportunity to feel contained by some social boundaries. It is, however, important that patients like Paul are helped to structure their time in relation to their own needs rather than the needs of the institution. Part of the nurse's role, therefore, is involved in establishing plans of care to help patients structure their time. A number of dilemmas can arise, however, if patients do not have a structure to their day. For example, the patient's sleep pattern can alter so that they sleep more during the day than at night, they can retreat or avoid interpersonal difficulties rather than learn strategies to overcome them, they can lose contact with morning therapeutic activities, they can become more isolated within their rooms and may ultimately prejudice their move into the community.

It might reasonably be argued that the patient has been placed in a hospital setting and thus staying in bed is part of the sick role and that lack of motivation could be related to prescribed medication. Therefore, the argument may proceed, patients should not have work-related time boundaries imposed on them, especially if they are liable to be unemployed when they are discharged and if there are not sufficient activities relating to their background for them to be involved in.

It can be a skilled process to gradually induct a patient from medium security, who may have initially come from a high security setting, into a hostel or back to their families. As well as the amount of time it takes to obtain a hostel place which suits the particular patient's needs, it also often takes time to work with the anxieties of hostel staff. Many patients are apprehensive about leaving their friends and the predictable environment of a secure setting. For these reasons patients are gradually discharged into the community beginning with visiting the hostel, attending for short periods during the day, possibly working from the unit, staying for periods of overnight leave and then eventually being discharged.

Some patients, usually because their symptoms have not abated and they still pose a significant level of risk, need long-term care within a secure setting. The Reed Report (Department of Health/Home Office, 1992) recommended increased funding for medium secure services beyond the 18 to 24-month limit generally applied to MSU patients.

Repper *et al.* (1994) from a community perspective provide evidence of the worth of developing trusting, long-term relationships with the patient experiencing enduring mental health problems, based on empathy and understanding. They add that it is also important to continually reassess and monitor the patient through the duration of the relationship, use a wide range of therapeutic and educational interventions to help meet their assessed needs, and be flexible enough to adapt to the patient's schedule. They futher add that it is important that such workers are given the opportunities, time and support to engage with this traditionally marginalised group.

ASSESSMENT AND MANAGEMENT

Escorts and leave

A significant aspect of the in-patient forensic nurse's role involves escorting patients either in hospital or in the community. The escorted activities Paul may experience could take a number of different forms such as providing security and support for him whilst he is having investigations or appearing in court, assessing his abilities to cope with the general public whilst on rehabilitation outings, or examining his relationship with members of his family whilst on home visits. This aspect of the nurse's role needs further investigation to establish how nurses are inducted into it and how outcomes are achieved.

Medication

Dixon *et al.* (1995), after reviewing four decades of research, concluded that there is overwhelming evidence of the efficacy of traditional anti-psychotic medication in the treatment and long-term maintenance of acute symptoms of patients diagnosed as suffering from schizophrenia. They consider, however, that physicians often prescribe in excess of the required levels and advise trials in low versus standard maintenance dose strategies. They add that little work has been carried out on non-clinical outcomes such as the patient's subjective feelings of well-being, family relations, anxiety and employment.

There is a general lack of long-term studies into the effects of such medication in relation to negative symptoms, compliance, monitoring practices and the integration of pharmacotherapy into other services. Evidence from such research could well affect the quality of Paul's subjective experience of the medication he is prescribed, and influence his long-term compliance.

Insight

Insight can have a number of different interpretations depending on which area of psychology or therapy is being analysed. In relation to the care of mentally disordered offenders the term is often associated with:

- the patient's recognition that they are or have been suffering from a mental disorder
- their understanding of the factors contributing to their disorder
- their own perceived need for after-care and/or supervision
- their understanding of the reasons for prescribed treatment
- their understanding of the nature of their offending and or disturbed behaviour plus the risk it has presented to themselves and/or others.

It may be difficult for Paul, after the positive symptoms of schizophrenia have subsided, to admit to his offending behaviour or that he has been through a period of mental illness. It may nevertheless be considered therapeutic for him to attempt to relieve himself of any guilt through discussing his past antisocial behaviour (Bateman, 1996). One reason for Paul's denial may be that he honestly believes that he has not been mentally ill or has carried out an antisocial act. Another may be the double social stigma associated with mental illness and offending (Pilgrim & Rogers, 1993).

FUTURE RESEARCH AND INVESTIGATION

From the work of Boyle (1997) and Jablensky (1993) a number of epistemological and ethical difficulties arise in relation to the term 'schizophrenia', some of which might be overcome by further, more generalised research and some of which may be unmeasurable and insurmountable.

More research is required into areas relating to the patient's pharmacological history. More general studies also need to be carried out to validate the various psychosocial and family interventions being adopted in the treatment of schizophrenia which might ultimately be of use in the care and treatment of patients like Paul.

Further analysis is required into the nurse's role in linking with staff in police stations, magistrates' courts and prison medical centres and carrying out assessments on potentially psychotic patients. Nurses involved in such assessments need a greater appreciation of how such institutions function so they can retrieve the required information to aid their colleagues in the hospital setting and develop a realistic picture of the potential patient. Sometimes only the disturbing aspects of the patient's history are given, with little information about how the patient occupies themselves on a day-to-day basis and what successful interventions have been used in the past to defuse outbursts. Nurses may therefore need to review their assessment tools to ensure that they are gathering information which might ultimately help divert patients like Paul away from prison settings and into mental health services. Such information can help in the development of the initial admission care plan rather than merely duplicating past medical findings.

To aid the rehabilitation process, joint staff–patient studies need to be promoted to examine how patients can become more involved in day-to-day decision making and planning for the service. Similarly, user representative groups and patients need to be involved in quality assurance initiatives.

More analysis is also required of the effectiveness of and the ethical issues surrounding physical restraint techniques. Investigations also need to be carried out into the long-term effects on staff of working in continually disturbed environments. There appears to be anecdotal evidence that nurses working in such areas are more effective in managing disturbed situations. The cost of this, however, may be that they resort to either dehumanising patients, due to burnout, or taking such stresses into their personal relationships to help cope with the intensely erratic emotions of the work environment.

A worrying trend amongst mental health professions is their current emphasis on attempting to find accurate measures of risk. Such approaches may be changing the emphasis of services from working with, and caring for, people with schizophrenia to one of assessing and monitoring risk factors, thus ensuring that individuals possessing such factors are contained in the correct environment (Castel, 1991). This may be due to the heightened yet unrealistic public fear of people with mental health problems perpetuated by wishes for an entirely safe predictable world. Such hopes and fears are accentuated by the media and reflected in, for example, the security concerns arising from public inquiries.

More work needs to be carried out on establishing what public attitudes are to mentally disordered offenders and how these attitudes might be modified if required. Another facet of the role of nurses working with offenders with schizophrenia is in developing a more educative role in their local communities to try to reduce the conceptual barriers and stigma surrounding patients detained in secure settings.

REFERENCES

Acres, D. I. (1975) The aftercare of special hospital patients. In *Home Office and DHSS Report of the Committee on Abnormal Offenders*. Appendix 30 Cmnd 6244. HMSO, London.

Al-Issa, I. (1977) Social and cultural aspects of hallucinations. *Psychological Bulletin* **84**, 570–87.

Altschul, A. T. (1972) *Patient Nurse Interactions: A Study of Interaction in Acute Psychiatric Wards*. Churchill Livingstone, Edinburgh.

Anderson, C. A., Lepper, M. A. & Ross, L. (1980) Perseverance of social theories: the role of explanations in the persistence of discredited information. *Journal of Personality and Social Psychology* **39**, 1037–49.

Barber, T. X. & Calverley, D. S. (1964) An experimental study of 'hypnotic' (auditory and visual) hallucinations. *Journal of Abnormal Social Psychology* **68**, 13–20.

Barton, R. (1966) *Institutional Neurosis*. Wright, Bristol.

Bateman, A. (1996) Defence mechanisms. In *Forensic Psychotherapy: Crime Psychodynamics and the Offender Patient* (Cordess, C. & Cox, M., eds). Jessica Kingsley Publishers, London.

Bentall, R. P. & Slade, P. D. (1985) Reliability of a scale measuring disposition towards hallucinations: a brief report. *Personality and Individual Differences* **6**, 527–9.

Bowden, P. (1978) Men remanded into custody for medical reports: the selection for treatment. *British Journal of Psychiatry* **132**, 320–31.

Boyle, M. (1997) *Schizophrenia: a Scientific Delusion?* Routledge, London.

Brailsford, D. S. & Stevenson, J. (1973) Factors relating to violent and unpredictable behaviour in psychiatric hospitals. *Nursing Times* **69**(3), 9–11.

Carlson, A. (1990) Early psychopharmacology and the rise of modern brain research. *Journal of Psychopharmacology* **4**, 120–6.

Castel, R. (1991) From dangerousness to risk. In *The Foucault Effect: Studies in Government* (Burchell, G., Gordon, C. & Miller, P., eds). Harvester Wheatsheaf, London.

Chua, S. E. & McKenna, P. J. (1995) Schizophrenia – a brain disease? A critical review of the structural and functional cerebral abnormality in the disorder. *British Journal of Psychiatry* **166**, 563–82.

Clare, A. (1980) *Psychiatry in Dissent: Controversial Issues in Thought and Practice*, 2nd edn. Tavistock, London.

Coid, J. W. (1988a) Mentally abnormal prisoners on remand: (i) Rejected or accepted by the NHS? *British Medical Journal* **296**, 1779–82.

Coid, J. W. (1 988b) Mentally abnormal prisoners on remand: (ii) Comparison of services provided by Oxford and Wessex Regions. *British Medical Journal* **296**, 1783–4.

Dawson, P. J. (1997) A reply to Gournay's 'Schizophrenia: a review of the contemporary literature and implications for mental health nursing theory, practice and education'. *Journal of Psychiatric and Mental Health Nursing* **4**, 1–7.

Department of Health (1990) Circular *Caring for people: The Care Programme Approach for People with Mental Illness*, H(C) 23, Department of Health, HMSO, London.

Department of Health/Home Office (1992) *Review of Health and Social Services for Mentally Disordered Offenders and Others Requiring Similar Services* (The Reed Report). HMSO, London.

Der, G., Gupta, S. & Murray, R. (1990) Is schizophrenia disappearing? *Lancet* 335, 513–16.

Dixon, L. B., Lehman, A. F. & Levine, J. (1995) Conventional antipsychotic medication for schizophrenia. *Schizophrenia Bulletin* 21(4), 567–77.

Faulk, M (1994) *Basic Forensic Psychiatry*, 2nd edn. Blackwell Science, London.

Gournay, K. (1996) Schizophrenia: a review of contemporary literature and implications for mental health nursing theory, practice and education. *Journal of Psychiatric and Mental Health Nursing* 3, 7–12.

Grillon, C., Courschesne, E. & Ameli, R. (1990) Increased distractability in schizophrenic patients: electrophysiologic and behavioural evidence. *Archives of General Psychiatry* 47, 177–88.

Hafner, H. & Boker, W. (1982) *Crimes of Violence by Mentally Abnormal Offenders*. New York, Cambridge University Press.

Halek, C. (1993) Nursing interventions: individual and family group systems. In *Mental Health Nursing* (Wright, H. & Giddey, M., eds). Chapman & Hall, London.

Harrison, G., Cooper, J. E. & Gancarczyk, R. (1991) Changes in the administrative incidence of schizophrenia. *British Journal of Psychiatry* 159, 811–16

Hughson, A. V. M. (1981) A comparison of 'offending' and 'non-offending' male patients admitted to the state hospital, Carstairs between 1966 and 1975. *British Journal of Psychiatry* 139, 431–5.

Humphreys, M. S., Johnstone, E. C., Macmillan, J. K. & Taylor, P. J. (1992) Dangerous behaviour preceding first admission schizophrenia. *British Journal of Psychiatry* 161, 501–5.

Jablensky, A. (1993) The epidemiology of schizophrenia. *Current Opinion in Psychiatry* 6, 43–52.

Jamerson, R. (1985) Personal view. *British Medical Journal* 291, 541.

Leff, J., Knipers, L., Berkowitz, R., Eberlein-Vriess, R. & Strugeon, D. (1982) A controlled trial of social interventions in the families of schizophrenic patients. *British Journal of Psychiatry* 141, 121–34.

Lemert, M. (1968) Paranoia and the dynamics of social exclusion. In *The Mental Patient: Studies in the Sociology of Deviance* (Spitzer, S. P. & Denzin, N. K., eds). McGraw-Hill, London.

Littlewood, R & Lipsedge, M. (1982) *Aliens and Alienists: Ethnic Minorities and Psychiatry*, 2nd edn. Unwin Hyman, London.

Lyttle, J. (1990) *Mental Disorder: its Care and Treatment*. Baillière Tindall, London.

Macdonald, H. (1992) Rehabilitation. In *A Textbook of Psychiatric and Mental Health Nursing* (Brooking, J. I., Ritter S. A. H. & Thomas, B. L., eds). Churchill Livingstone, Edinburgh.

Milton, F., Patwa, V. K. & Hafner, R. J. (1978) Confrontation versus belief modification in persistently deluded patients. *British Journal of Medical Psychology* 51, 127–30.

Moran, J. (1984) Response and responsibility. *Nursing Times* 80(14), 28–31.

Morgan, R. (1980) A regional rehabilitation unit. In *Handbook of Rehabilitation Practice* (Wing, J. K. & Morris, B., eds). Oxford Medical Publications, Oxford.

Nicholson, I. R. & Newfeld, R. W. J. (1989) Forms and mechanisms of susceptibility to stress in schizophrenia. In *Advances in the Investigation of Psychological Stress* (Neufeld, R. W. J., ed.). John Wiley, New York.

Norman, R. M. G. & Malla, A. K. (1993) Stressful life events and schizophrenia I: A review of the research. II: Conceptual and methodological issues. *British Journal of Psychiatry* **162**, 161–74.

Philips, M. (1977) Aggression control in psychiatric hospitals. *Dimensions in the Health Service* **54**(3), 39–41.

Pilgrim, D. & Rogers, A. (1993) *A Sociology of Mental Health and Illness*. Open University Press, Buckingham.

Pilling, S. (1991) *Rehabilitation and Community Care*. Routledge, London.

Power, D. J. (1976) Sexual deviation and crime. *Medicine, Science and the Law* **16**, 119–28.

Repper, J., Ford, R. & Cooke, A. (1994) How can nurses build trusting relationships with people who have severe and long-term mental health problems? Experience of case managers and their clients. *Journal of Advanced Nursing* **19**, 1096–104.

Ritchie, J., Dick, D. & Lingham, R. (1994) *The Report of the Inquiry into the Care and Treatment of Christopher Clunis*. HMSO, London.

Ritter, S. (1989) *Bethlem Royal and Maudsley Hospital Manual of Clinical Psychiatric Nursing Principles and Procedures*. Harper & Row, London.

Ritter, S. (1992) Schizophrenia. In *A Textbook of Psychiatric and Mental Health Nursing* (Brooking, J., Ritter, S. A. H., Thomas, B. L., eds). Churchill Livingstone, London.

Rogers, P. (1997) Behaviour nurse therapy in forensic mental health. *Mental Health Practice* **1**(4), 22–6.

Shepherd, G. (1985) Planning the rehabilitation of the individual. In *Theory and Practice of Psychiatric Rehabilitation* (Watts, F. N. & Bennett, D. H., eds). Wiley, Chichester.

Slade, P. D. (1976) Towards a theory of auditory hallucinations: outline of a hypothetical four-factor model. *British Journal of Social and Clinical Psychology* **15**, 415–24.

Smith, T. E., Bellack, A. S. & Liberman A. P. (1996) Social skills training for schizophrenia: review and future directions. *Clinical Psychology Review* **16**(7), 599–617.

Steptoe, A., Moses, J. & Edwards, S. (1990) Age related differences in cardiovascular reactions to mental stress tests in women. *Health Psychology* **9**, 18–34.

Suddath, R. L., Christison, G. W., Torrey, E. F., Casanova, M. F. & Weinberger, D. R. (1990) Anatomical abnormalities in the brains of monozygotic twins discordant for schizophrenia. *New England Journal of Medicine* **322**, 789–94.

Tarbuck, P. (1994) The therapeutic use of security: a model for forensic nursing. In *Lyttle's Mental Health and Disorder*, 2nd edn. Baillière Tindall, London.

Taylor, P. (1982) Schizophrenia and violence. In *Abnormal Offenders, Delinquency and the Criminal Justice System* (Gunn, J. & Farrington, D. P., eds). Wiley, New York.

Taylor, P. (1985) Motives for offending among violent and psychotic men. *British Journal of Psychiatry* **147**, 491–8.

Taylor, P. (1993) Schizophrenia and crime: distinctive patterns of association. In *Mental Disorder and Crime* (Hodgins, S., ed.). Sage, London.

Taylor, P. J. & Gunn, J. (1984a) Violence and psychosis I – risk of violence among psychotic men. *British Medical Journal* **288**, 1945–9.

Taylor, P. J. & Gunn, J. (1984b) Violence and psychosis II – effect of psychiatric diagnosis on conviction and sentencing of offenders. *British Medical Journal* **289**, 9–12.

Tidmarsh, D (1990) Schizophrenia. In *Principles and Practice of Forensic Psychiatry* (Bluglass, R. & Bowden, P., eds.). Churchill Livingstone, London.

White, M. (1987) Family therapy and schizophrenia: addressing the 'in the corner' life style. *Dulwich Centre News Letter*, Spring Edition, pp. 47–57.

Wing, J. K. (1983) Schizophrenia. In *Theory and Practice of Psychiatric Rehabilitation* (Watts, F. N. & Bennett, D. H., eds). Wiley, Chichester.

Wing J. K. & Brown, G. W. (1970) *Institutionalism and schizophrenia – A Comparative Study in Three Mental Hospitals.* Cambridge University Press, London.

Wolf, S. & Cull, A. (1986) 'Schizoid' personality and antisocial conduct: a retrospective case note study. *Psychological Medicine* **16**, 677–87.

Yesavage, J. A. (1982) Inpatient violence and the schizophrenic patient: an inverse correlation between danger related events and neuroleptic levels. *Biological Psychiatry* **17**, 1331–7.

Zarski, J. J. (1984) Hassles and health: a replication. *Health Psychology* **3**, 243–51.

Zitrin, A, Hardesty, A. S. & Burdock, E. L. (1976) Socially disruptive behaviour of ex mental Patients. *American Journal of Psychiatry* **133**, 142–6.

Zubin J. & Spring, B. (1977) Vulnerability: a new view of schizophrenia. *Journal of Abnormal Psychology* **86**, 103–26.

Chapter 5
Working with Learning Disabled Offenders

Arthur Turnbull

INTRODUCTION

In recent years, through the work of authors such as Day (1993), Craft (1984) and Murphy *et al.* (1995), issues relating to the care of learning disabled offenders have begun to be examined and acted upon and forensic mental health nursing within learning disability services has developed as a discrete speciality.

The increased focus on the needs of learning disabled offenders has high-lighted an area of deficit within the existing services for learning disabled people. The Mental Health Acts of 1959 and 1983 provided alternatives to prison for learning disabled offenders. However, the deinstitutionalisation or transcarceration hypothesis, as promoted by Fowles (1993), resulted in many learning disabled offenders being detained in penal establishments rather than in hospital environments.

This chapter aims to give an overview of some of the issues relating to the nursing care of learning disabled offenders. It will cover the provision of services for learning disabled offenders, their treatment needs and subsequent after-care provision.

ASSESSMENT, PREVALENCE AND LEGISLATION

'Mental impairment' has a number of definitions. Within the Mental Health Act 1983 it is divided into two areas. 'Severe mental impairment' is defined as 'a state of arrested or incomplete development of the mind which includes severe impairment of intelligence and social functioning when it is associated with abnormally aggressive or seriously irresponsible conduct on the part of the person concerned'. 'Mental impairment' is defined as 'the state of arrested or incomplete development of the mind which includes significant impairment of intelligence and social functioning and is associated with abnormally aggressive or seriously irresponsible conduct on the part of the person concerned'.

The ICD-10 (WHO, 1992) criteria define 'mental impairment' as: 'having an IQ of less than 70 and associated impairment in adaptive behaviour'. There are numerous assessment tools in use to measure the intelligence quotient (IQ) of an individual. The number of assessment tools themselves can cause difficulties in the identification of people with a mental impairment, due to the diversity of results given and their subsequent interpretation.

Some of these difficulties relate to the particular test used. For example, the WAIS-R (Psychological Corporation, 1986) measures verbal and performance levels, giving a measurement of each but also giving a joint score to provide a full-scale IQ. In contrast to this the National Adult Reading Test (NART) (Nelson, 1991) gives a measurement of the pre-moded level of intelligence and measures the verbal skills of the person. The Raven Matrices (Raven, 1986) gives a measurement of performance not verbal skills. The accuracy of these tests and determination of a person's intellectual ability have particular importance for the nursing care of learning disabled offenders.

The prevalence of learning disabled offenders within the penal system has been the subject of studies across the world. These studies offer a range of opinions. Murphy *et al.* (1995) found, in a study of 157 men, that 33 were reported to have an intellectual disability but following formal assessment none had an IQ of 70 or below. In America, Targan *et al.*, in a study carried out in 1973, estimated the prevalence of mental impairment in the general population to be between 0.2% and 2.4% (Targan *et al.*, 1979). However, various studies in the 1970s estimated that the percentage of mentally impaired offenders within the total offender population in the United States varied greatly but levels were all above 2.4% with a high of 39.6% in the state of Georgia (MacEachron, 1979).

MacEachron (1979) suggests a number of possible reasons for these differences in prevalence, amongst which are environmental and psychometric factors. The environmental factors described include the differences in state attitudes, parole regulations and the availability of community services for retarded persons (MacEachron, 1979).

The psychometric explanation described by MacEachron (1979) relates to the different intellectual tests carried out and how a standard deviation appears to have little influence on the results given and subsequent adjustments required to give accurate results.

When IQ testing is carried out, allowances should be made for cross-cultural differences (WHO, 1992). Therefore it would appear that, before any accurate figures can be identified for the prevalence of mental impairment, a standardised set of criteria or tests would need to be accepted by future studies. With developments in legislation and service development it is imperative that an accurate screening method is used to ensure that mentally impaired offenders are identified at an early stage in the criminal justice system.

Services for learning disabled offenders have changed and developed rapidly over the past 20 years. Prior to the publication of *Better Services for the Mentally Handicapped* (DHSS, 1971) and the move towards community care, the mentally impaired were largely detained in a long-stay institution. With the move to community care and the closure of hospitals, mentally impaired offenders are more likely to proceed through the criminal justice system or transcarceration (Fowles, 1993).

The Glancy Report (Glancy, 1974) suggested that mentally impaired offenders should share regional secure facilities with the mentally ill. However, the report by the Royal College of Psychiatrists (RCP, 1980) recommended that only mentally impaired offenders with a borderline IQ would benefit from sharing facilities with the mentally ill offender and that those offenders with a severe or profound impairment should have secure facilities provided within a mental handicap hospital.

The report 'Needs and Responses' (Department of Health, 1989) looked at a range of topics relating to mental impairment. Within the area of mentally impaired offending it commented on the lack of knowledge or information available to the police, courts or other agencies about services for people with mental impairment who offend. The report also suggests the setting up of a wide range of secure facilities to offer assessment and treatment for mentally impaired offenders, and the use, where possible, of the Mental Health Act 1983 to ensure that detention takes place in an environment which can offer assessment and treatment.

The Reed Report (Department of Health/Home Office, 1992) highlighted the need for mentally impaired offenders to be diverted from the criminal justice system as early as possible and treated in hospital rather than prisons, with the lowest appropriate level of security. The Mansell Report (Mansell, 1993), established to look at aspects which affect learning disabled people with challenging behaviour, advocated the use of existing services with the emphasis on appropriate staff numbers and training as a means of keeping the mentally impaired offender out of the penal system.

Implications for nurses caring for learning disabled offender patients relate to issues of professional practice and training. For example, the UKCC *Guidelines for Mental Health and Learning Disabilities Nursing* (UKCC, 1998) state that 'nurses have a professional responsibility to promote client independence and autonomy'.

Since the publication of *Better Services in Mental Handicap* (Department of Health and Social Secuerity, 1971) the move has been towards community living and normalisation.

SERVICE PROVISION

Learning disabled offenders require as wide a variety of disposals by the courts as any other offender group. The traditional disposal to long-stay mental handicap hospitals has been removed, to a degree, by the closure of these hospitals. Consequently service provision development has ranged from medium secure units to non-hospital-based therapeutic programmes.

It could be argued that, as part of the principles of normalisation, the learning disabled offender should serve a sentence in the penal establishment. However, Day (1993) points out that the learning disabled person in prison is less able to adjust to prison life and is either victimised or exploited by other prisoners or is more likely to demonstrate aggression or violence.

With the advent of Court Diversion teams following the Home Office Circular 66 (90) (Home Office, 1990), increasing numbers of learning disabled offenders are being identified at the pre-court or pre-sentencing stage of the criminal justice process, giving specialist services the opportunity to have a greater influence over ultimate disposal. For a community disposal to be effective, treatment requirements are important areas for consideration. Lindsay & Smith (1998), in a study of learning disabled offending men who have committed sex offences, highlighted the need for probation orders of at least two years' duration to allow for the consolidation of the treatment given.

Many studies have indicated the importance of social skills development, structured occupation and leisure to assist the learning disabled offender to develop the necessary skills to function in society and to assist in the promotion of self-esteem and worth (Craft, 1984; Day, 1988). Day (1993) points out that these services are seldom offered successfully by mainstream learning disability service providers, and suggests the need for a specialist service to meet this need.

An important factor associated with community-based disposal is the attitude of staff in the residential area in which these individuals are to live. Lyall *et al.* (1995) carried out a study into staff attitudes to offending behaviour. In hostels where some of the residents had had contact with the criminal justice system, they found that staff were more likely to consider offending behaviour as challenging. In some circumstances staff were less inclined to report some minor offences to the police. Only 23% of the establishments taking part in the study said they would always report a sexual assault or indecent exposure. In 9.9% of the establishments, staff said they would hesitate to inform the police if a resident were to rape a member of staff, another resident or a member of the public.

The importance of recognising and working with the attitudes of staff to offending behaviour needs addressing if learning disabled offenders are to be placed in non-specialised learning disability establishments. This is essential to ensure that the learning disabled offender receives appropriate help and support to discourage reoffending.

Needs and Responses (DHSS, 1989) identified the need for a range of services in learning disabilities. In recent years medium secure units providing services for learning disabled offenders have been created. Cumella & Sansom (1994) described the setting up of a medium secure unit with 12 beds for learning disabled offenders. In common with other in-patient facilities the focus is on assessment and treatment. As suggested by Day (1988) and Craft (1984) the provision of structured day activity and leisure time appears to be significant in supporting management and treatment programmes.

A common difficulty experienced by in-patient facilities is the issue of moving people on from secure accommodation once a period of treatment has been completed (Mayor *et al.*, 1990). This is exacerbated by the traditional placing of secure units within existing hospital sites, and suggests that priority should be given to the development of small, intensively supervised, residential units offering assessment, treatment and rehabilitation as well as intensive supervision.

Cumella & Sansom (1994) suggest a multi-disciplinary community team which could offer ongoing assessment treatment and support to learning disabled offenders. These authors also recognise the role that such a team can play in the identification of those at risk of offending, through liaison with school, police and other local services. Additionally, access to employment can make a valuable contribution to the care of the learning disabled offender. In all these areas the community nurse for the learning disabled offender can provide direct treatment as well as support or networks for service access.

The implementation of the Sex Offenders Act 1997 may make more difficult the process of possible rehabilitation of learning disabled offenders, especially sex offenders. The Sex Offenders Act 1997 allows police to inform significant people within the community, i.e. headmasters, about the presence of a sex offender in the local area. It is arguable that any disclosure of information can lead to leaks to the public which will increase public anxiety, therefore resulting in a situation of vigilantism or public demonstrations. The already sparse resources available to the learning disabled sex offender can be further limited by fears of adverse publicity and the potentially damaging effects of local reaction. This difficulty will undoubtedly present service providers with their next challenge and be an opportunity for research into public attitudes and perceptions on such an emotive issue.

OFFENDING BEHAVIOUR

Offences for which learning disabled offenders are convicted vary. Day (1993) suggested that sex offenders are over-represented in offenders with a learning disability. Supporting this opinion Gross (1984) found that, in a study of incarcerated learning disabled offenders, almost 50% had committed sexual offences. Swanson & Garwich (1990) suggest that this may be because initial sex offences are minimised with minor consequences, but if the offence continues tolerance is lost and punishment becomes severe. It has been suggested that this may be due to the policy of de-institutionalisation (Day, 1993). In the past, learning disabled offenders may originally have been placed in hospital after the first few offences, whereas now they are placed in the community which allows greater opportunity for such offences to take place and leads to a subsequent reduction in tolerance by the community.

Other offences commonly committed by learning disabled offenders include fire-setting and assault. An overview of the range of therapeutic interventions available for learning disabled sex offenders assists an exploration of treatment needs and availability – although these techniques can be used successfully with other learning disabled offender groups.

TREATMENT OF LEARNING DISABLED SEX OFFENDERS

Perkins (1993) describes traditional treatments as being broadly based on Freudian psychodynamic models which assist the offender to gain an insight into the offence and to subsequently develop self-control of their behaviour. There appears to be a considerable move away from the psychodynamic model of treatment, and various recent research findings indicate that a package of treatment using a variety of techniques gives greater success with learning disabled sex offenders.

Clare (1993) examined the use of a cognitive-behavioural approach to people with a learning disability who commit sex offences, and highlighted various issues which require addressing when engaged in this work. The issues included the simplification of treatment to facilitate intervention for those with poor verbal language and the necessity to give clear messages. The apparent reliance of adults with a learning disability upon external feedback suggests that they need to receive clear messages about the acceptability of behaviour.

Taylor (1996) suggests that factors such as self-esteem and cognitive processing capacity can be associated with the development of sex offending and that people with learning disability are vulnerable to low self-esteem.

Gardener *et al.* (1996) describe the setting up of a group for sex offenders with a learning disability. They suggest that because of the poor attention span of the client group, contact time should be limited to $1\frac{1}{2}$ hours and that treatment programmes need to be a long-term process, possibly two to three years. Prior to any treatment plan being carried out an assessment of cognition and problem behaviour has to be made. Models include multi-model analysis as described by Lazarus (1976), which is used to identify the behaviour and the thoughts of the offender at the time the offence took place.

Cullen (1993) describes using a behavioural approach incorporating functional analysis as described by Donnellan *et al.* (1988) originally designed for people who present with challenging behaviours. The techniques provide an added dimension to programmes and can assist with the development of comprehensive treatment programmes for offending behaviour. The approach encompasses ecological changes, positive programming and direct treatment. As a result of being in the unique situation of providing 24-hour care, nurses can ensure the consistency required so that a behavioural programme succeeds.

Various authors comment on the pharmacological interventions available for learning disabled offenders. Day (1993) discusses how the use of drugs that reduce aggression and control libido can be useful in controlling socialisation and rehabilitation. The use of pharmacological intervention is suggested by Swanson (1986) who describes its application in conjunction with psychotherapeutic intervention strategies.

Examples of complementary or diversionary treatment which can be used as part of a multi-model programme have been proved useful. Cullen (1993) describes the education of the person on the nature of anger, and the acquisition of skills to provide new ways of dealing with anger using different scenarios. Social skills training to enable the learning disabled offender to develop the skills required to develop appropriate relationships with others and the promotion of adaptive ways of spending their time is described by Lindsay and Smith (1998) in the context of structured occupation and weekend activity. Group work can be useful to examine the offender's attitudes and beliefs and is often a vehicle to facilitate development of positive attitudes through the challenges given by other offenders in the group.

It is also necessary to direct attention to relapse prevention. Laws (1990) suggests looking at social pressures which may lead to reoffending, such as alcohol and drug use, peer pressure, and negative emotions, which again can be affected by alcohol and drugs, and finally identifying high risk situations. Once an offender has identified these main areas he can then, with the help of a therapist, develop strategies to avoid them. Plans to reduce recidivism are important in the light of research carried out by Klimecki & Jenkinson (1994) who found that 30.8% of male learning disabled offenders who have committed sex offences will reoffend. The higher rate of recidivism within learning disabled sex offenders is also acknowledged by Day (1993).

CASE STUDY

Norman is a 45-year-old man who has a mild learning disability with an IQ of 68. He has an older brother who lives locally and a younger brother who is currently detained on the same in-patient unit as Norman. Norman is a Schedule 1 Offender as described by the Children and Young Persons Act 1933 due to the nature of his offences against children.

Norman experienced a rather traumatic childhood. At the age of eight years he was taken, with his brothers, into the care of the local authority due to severe parental neglect. During this time Norman alleged that he was sexually abused by a senior member of care staff. Norman's parents divorced during his teenage years following continuing conflict and dysfunction, but both still reside locally.

Whilst at secondary school, allegations were made against Norman that he sexually assaulted two girls. Norman was moved quickly to another school. He has held a number of work placements which have all broken down due to his inability to relate to other trainees and his poor attendance.

At the age of 16 Norman left the care of the local authority and returned home. After his parents divorced, Norman lived with his father until he gained the tenancy of his own flat. This unfortunately only lasted for six weeks and Norman returned to his immediate family to live with his cousins. It was at this time that he was arrested for indecently assaulting his younger cousins for whom he was babysitting at the time.

Norman has a history of depressive illness which responds well to medication. Whilst in a depressive state Norman has been known to self-injure. There has also been one attempt to hang himself whilst waiting to give evidence against a male perpetrator who abused him.

Past offences include drink-related offences, minor thefts, indecent assault against minors and his index offence, indecent assault against four children. For this he received a custodial sentence. He was later transferred to a mental handicap hospital many miles from his home.

Whilst in hospital Norman was considered very skilled and self-motivated and was well liked by his peers. He is reported to have experienced problems regarding his sexual identity and to have had relationships with both male and female partners. He received therapeutic input from psychologists, working on emotional awareness, index offences and relapse prevention, and was considered to be a 'low risk' patient.

In line with current trends Norman was eventually returned to a new in-patient hospital service nearer his home where he was treated by the Learning Disability Forensic Team. The holistic approach offered by the service ensured that Norman received input from all relevant agencies. Whilst on the new unit Norman attended a Sex Offender Group on a weekly basis, which examined his cycle of offending and relapse prevention.

After completion of all assessments the forensic team and Norman began the process of planning his rehabilitation into the community. The nature of Norman's offending behaviour clearly indicated that he required a well structured living environment and ongoing high levels of support and supervision. Once a suitable establishment was identified offering the structure, support and supervision required, the staff were given an insight into Norman's needs and offending history. Input was provided by nursing, social work and psychology professionals from within the Learning Disability Forensic Team.

Norman began to have escorted leave to the home, and unescorted hospital parole which progressed to unescorted visits to local shops. He then had unescorted leave to the home for a few hours at the weekend and subsequently for a full week. Norman was finally discharged under Section 17 of the Mental Health Act 1983.

Unfortunately after three months in his new environment local people found out that Norman was residing in the home and that he was a Schedule 1 offender. Local pressure made the placement untenable, resulting in a move to a local authority hostel in a different part of the area.

MANAGEMENT OF VIOLENCE AND AGGRESSION

The issues relating to the management of violence and aggression within the area of learning disabled offenders are very much the same as those for mental disordered offenders in general. However, some of the techniques used may have to be adapted to take into account cognitive or physical abilities.

A traditional response to violent and aggressive incidents is the use of physical restraint, seclusion and 'as required' (PRN) medication. There have been many comments on the realities of physical restraint including those of Stilling (1992) and Tarbuck (1992). However, McDougall (1995) points out that the literature on these issues tends to be narrow in its scope.

Recent research suggests that the traditional methods of management appear to be less popular in today's services, and the development of psychotherapeutic skills by nurses has prompted a move to preventative rather than reactive strategies for dealing with aggression.

The contribution of medication is acknowledged. As Swanson (1986) suggests, the correct medication can be used to facilitate psychotherapy, and McLaren et al. (1990) describe how PRN medication is still used for the management of violent behaviour. Kennedy et al. (1995) in a four-year study at a medium secure facility found that 36% of incidents that occurred resulted in physical restraint and 13% were treated with PRN medication. Therefore approximately half of the recorded incidents were dealt with by other means.

These other interventions were described as counselling and persuasion to move to a quieter area and the use of anger management and relaxation by the nursing staff. The development of relaxation and anger management skills and the apparent success of the interventions in dealing with violent incidents appear to support McDougall's (1995) observation that the focus of intervention should be moved away from reactive management to a more proactive method of controlling aggression and violent incidents.

The development of programmes based on a psychotherapeutic model such as the teaching of anger management and relaxation have been advocated by a number of authors. Deakin (1995) describes the setting up of a relaxation scheme in Rampton Hospital. He identified some of the key areas which need to be considered in the development of such a programme and indicated the need for prompts during sessions. Prompts could be physical or verbal but physical prompts should not be mistaken for restraint. Physical prompts are especially important to assist the person with a learning disability to relax as they may have difficulty understanding concepts on verbal prompts alone. Teaching people with a learning disability to practise anger management or relaxation is an advanced and developing area of nursing practice.

There has been an increase in nurse-led therapies used in various establishments. As more proactive management strategies develop, there are still numerous incidents in which physical restraint is used. There continue to be ethical questions as to the use of restraint (Hopton, 1995). The training of staff in physical restraint is provided on a basis of local policy. This has led to a wide variety of methods being taught, from the use of wrist locks in some establishments to the alternative, more dignified wrist holds in others.

Some of the complexities of seclusion surround its definition and purpose. Morrison & Lehane (1995) highlighted discrepancies in how the term 'seclusion' was used and noted that seclusion is often synonymous with the term 'time out' or even used in response to a patient's request. There have been some suggestions that the number of staff in the clinical area has an effect on the use of seclusion, a hypothesis that is supported by studies such as that of Higgins (1981).

Within the specialist service for learning disabled offenders an increasing trend is the use of behavioural management as a means of controlling violence and aggression. The theories of Donnellan *et al.* (1988) and subsequently Emerson (1995) have been incorporated to reduce the incidence of aggression. Use of functional analysis and positive programming allow for assessment of the function of the behaviour and the possible reason for its presentation. Through the use of functional analysis and identification of the cause of the behaviour it may be possible to change the underlying difficulty and remove the individual's need for aggression.

The successful use of other behavioural techniques such as token economy-based incentive schemes has been commented on by such authors as Mayor *et al.* (1990) and Day (1988). These studies both describe how incentive schemes have been a successful tool in an overall management structure. The flexibility of token economy schemes allows for them to be used for a variety of identified needs, and they can be adjusted to meet targets for an individual.

AFTER-CARE

Sheppard (1995), in a report collating recommendations of inquiries into deaths associated with the mentally ill, highlighted the apparent lack of after-care for many patients. It could be argued, however, that these enquiries represent only a very small percentage of the discharges taking place from hospital over that period of time. However, during the period of study of these reports the Department of Health established the Care Programme Approach (CPA) for people who have been accepted for treatment within psychiatric services (DoH, 1990).

The main focus for the development of CPA was psychiatric services but some learning disability services have acknowledged it as a means of standardising good practice. Although the Home Office directed trusts to have CPA in place by 1991, during a recent enquiry (Freeman & Brown, 1996) it was found that the CPA process had not been used effectively.

The team providing the services to the learning disabled offender may feel that a period of trial leave is required whereby the patient is given conditions to adhere to while on community leave to assess a level of compliance as part of the treatment programme. The Mental Health Act 1983 already provided Section 17 Leave of Absence which allows the patient to be returned to the hospital if the period of leave is unsuccessful.

There is also the Guardianship Order, Section 7 of the Act, which enables the establishment of an authoritarian framework for working with patients. The Guardianship Order allows for the Guardian to require the person to reside at a specified place and attend for medical treatment or occupational education. However, its success has been limited by the lack of power to force a person to abide by these requirements.

In 1996 the Mental Health (Patients in the Community) Act 1995 came into force. This allowed for supervised discharge to take place. The Act allows for restrictions to be placed on a person following discharge and if not complied with the key worker has the power to take and convey the patient to hospital. It may be argued that this Act is open to abuse in so far as a person may feel they must comply with restrictions or they will be 'sectioned'.

The importance of a good after-care service for learning disabled offenders is not only to reduce the risk of reoffending and subsequent enquiries but also to address the difficulties of moving people out of this level of supervision (Mayor *et al.*, 1990). Good after-care may assist in the identification of an appropriate place in the community and therefore help in rehabilitation of learning disabled offenders with structured support for the identified placement as well as the patient themselves.

Commencing with the official after-care process the community nurse for the learning disabled offender can provide the necessary supervision and support to identify and manage the risk of reoffending by the patient. The process of regularly revisiting the risk assessment carried out prior to discharge and regular meetings with all persons involved in the care of the learning disabled offender after discharge will assist identification of areas of concern before they can become problems. These strategies should also enable the patient to be aware of the external controls which are put in place to avoid the offending behaviour and to monitor general behaviour. These strategies will allow for rapid intervention should reoffending take place, to facilitate access to the appropriate services or in-patient facilities as identified.

APPROPRIATE ADULT

The rights of the learning disabled offender have been recognised by legislative authorities and provision made under the Code of Practice for the Police and Criminal Evidence Act (PACE) 1985. The PACE Code of Practice identifies the Appropriate Adult as someone who has experience of dealing with mentally handicapped people. The importance of the Appropriate Adult is further highlighted by research by Clare & Gudjonsson (1993) which shows that a learning disabled person is more vulnerable to acquiescence than those without a learning disability. Clare & Gudjonsson (1993) showed that a learning disabled person was relatively unconcerned about making false confessions and was more likely to believe they would return home, at least until the trial.

The Code of Practice for the Police and Criminal Evidence Act (PACE) 1985 notes that it is important to bear in mind that, although persons who are mentally ill or mentally handicapped are incapable of providing reliable evidence, they may without knowing provide information which is unreliable, misleading or self-incriminating. It is in cases such as the Confait case (Fisher, 1977) where a man with a learning disability and two other juveniles were convicted because of a confession later held to be unsound, that the Appropriate Adult, or more importantly the absence of the Appropriate Adult, is highlighted.

There are various schemes operating throughout Britain to provide Appropriate Adults at police stations. In practice, police officers often contact Social Services or health departments outside working hours to seek an Appropriate Adult, meaning that these schemes tend to operate on an out-of-hours basis. Because of this, these schemes are often voluntary in nature as cost can be considered to be an unacceptable expense to statutory organisations. The result is that the training of Appropriate Adults and availability of the people providing the service can vary greatly from area to area.

Until some form of national standards for Appropriate Adults can be set up, then it is destined to remain fragmented. It might be suggested that the role of the Appropriate Adult could become an extension of the services provided by nurses working with learning disabled offenders. They are already experienced in working with people with a learning disability and would require little extra training in the legislative aspect of the work.

DIVERSION FROM CUSTODY

With the development of Diversion Schemes following the Home Office Regulations HC66 (90) it is important to consider the number of schemes which have designated staff experienced in the recognition and identification of learning disabled people. Some areas now have psychologists as part of the teams providing these services. However, most diversion schemes are operated by community mental health nurses and psychiatrists. This can result in delay in psychometric testing for the identification of a learning disabled person. If a specialist learning disability nurse was available or formed part of this team, initial screening of persons suspected of having a learning disability would be possible. The secondment on an *ad hoc* basis of a learning disability nurse for this purpose would bring benefits for both sets of disciplines. For example, the in-depth knowledge of local learning disability facilities would facilitate a decision by the court on appropriate disposal.

FURTHER INVESTIGATIONS

This chapter has attempted to address some of the pertinent issues related to the nursing care and management of the learning disabled offender. There is a need for a variety of local services for these individuals. Although there are developments in some areas, provision remains patchy with many learning disabled offenders being cared for in facilities well away from their own locality. There is also a pressing need for increased, organised occupation and leisure services, both for people living in the community and for those within a hospital setting. The value of such services to treatment programmes and as a preventative measure with regard to reoffending suggests that nurses may be inclined to take a leading role in further research into this area.

The identification of learning disabled offenders at the stage of arrest and pre-court suggests that learning disability nurses could work as part of diversion teams. Studies into appropriate adult schemes throughout the country could possibly assist in the development of national standards for appropriate adult services to ensure that mentally disordered offenders receive assistance at a stage where they are at their most vulnerable.

Within clinical practice it is important to identify appropriate training needs to facilitate true therapeutic interventions with this client group. Nurses could usefully explore how to modify existing assessment and treatment programmes to meet the needs of learning disabled offenders.

For the nurse working within the learning disability forensic services there needs to be greater emphasis on the role of providing treatments and therapies as well as on the traditional role of care. This should begin at the stage of identification through to in-patient treatment, and continue into the after-care process.

REFERENCES

Clare, I. (1993) Issues in the assessment and treatment of male sex offenders with a mild learning disability. *Sexual and Marital Therapy* 8(2), 67–80.

Clare, I. C. & Gudjonsson, G. H. (1993) Interrogative suggestibility, confabulation, and acquiescence in people with mild learning disabilities (mental handicap): implications for reliability during police interrogations. *British Journal of Clinical Psychology* 32(3), 295–301.

Craft, M. (1984) Low intelligence, mental handicap and community. In *Mentally Abnormal Offenders* (Craft, M. & Craft, A., eds). Baillière Tindall, London.

Cullen, C. (1993) The treatment of people with learning disability who offend. In *Clinical Approaches to the Mentally Disordered Offender* (Howells, K. & Hollin, C., eds). Wiley, Chichester.

Cumella, S. & Sansom, D. (1994) A regional mental impaired service. *Mental Handicap Research* 7(3), 257–72.

Day, K, (1988) A hospital based treatment programme for male mentally handicapped offenders. *British Journal of Psychiatry* 153, 635–44.

Day, K. (1993) Crime and mental retardation, a review. In *Clinical Approaches to the Mentally Disordered Offender* (Howells, K. & Hollin, C., eds). Wiley, Chichester.

Deakin, M. (1995) Using relaxation techniques to manage disruptive behaviour. *Nursing Times* 91(17), 40–41.

Department of Health (1989) *Needs and Responses – Services for Adults who are Mentally Ill, who Have Behaviour Problems or who Offend*. HMSO, London.

Department of Health (1990) *Caring for People: the Care Program Approach*. HMSO, London.

Department of Health/Home Office (1992) *Review of Health and Social Services for Mentally Disordered Offenders and Others Requiring Similar Services* (The Reed Report). HMSO, London.

Department of Health and Social Security (1971) *Better Services for the Mentally Handicapped*. HMSO, London.

Donnellan, A. M., La Vigna, G. W., Negri-Shoultz, N., Lassbender, L. L. (1988) *Progress without Punishment*. Teachers College Press, New York.

Emerson, E. (1995) *Challenging Behaviour – Analysis and Intervention in People with Learning Difficulties*. Cambridge University Press, Cambridge.

Fisher, H. (1977) *Report on the Confait Case*. HMSO, London.

Fowles, A. J. (1993) The mentally disordered offender in the era of community care. In *New Direction in Provisions*. Cambridge University Press, Cambridge.

Freeman, C. & Brown, A. (1996) Inquiry into the Care and Treatment of Shaun Anthony Armstrong. Tees Health Authority.

Gardener, M., Kelly, K. & Wilkinson, D. (1996) *Group for Male Sex Offenders with Learning Disability*. NAPSAC Bulletin.

Glancy, J. (1974) *Revised Report on the Working Party on Security in NHS Psychiatric Hospitals*. DHSS, London.

Gross, G. (1984) *Activities of the Developmental Disabilities Adult Offender Project*. Washington State Developmental Disabilities Planning Council, Olympia, WA.

Higgins, J. K. (1981) Four years' experience of an Interim Secure Unit. *British Medical Journal* **282**, 889–93.

Home Office (1990) *Provision for Mentally Disordered Offenders*. Circular 66/90. HMSO, London.

Hopton, J. (1995) Control and restraint in contemporary psychiatric nursing. *Journal of Advanced Nursing* **22**, 110–15.

Kennedy, J., Harrison, J., Hills, T. & Bluglass, R. (1995) Analysis of violent incidents in a regional secure unit. *Medical Science Law* **35**(3), 255–60.

Klimecki, M. & Jenkinson, J. (1994) A study of recidivism amongst offenders with an intellectual disability. *Australia and New Zealand Journal of Development Disabilities* **19**.

Laws, D. R. (1990) *Relapse Prevention with Sex Offenders*. Guildford Press, London.

Lazarus, A. (1976) *Multi Model Behaviour Therapy*. Springer, New York.

Lindsay, W. R. & Smith, A. H. (1998) Responses to treatment for sex offenders with intellectual disability: a comparison of men with 1- and 2-year probation sentences. *Journal of Intellectual Disability Research* **42**(5), 346–53.

Lyall, I., Holland, A. J. & Collins, S. (1995) Offending by adults with learning disability and the attitudes of staff to offending behaviour: implications for service development. *Journal of Intellectual Disability Research* **42**(5), 346–53.

MacEachron, A. E. (1979) Mentally retarded offenders, prevalence and character-istics. *American Journal of Mental Deficiency* **84**(2), 165–76.

McDougall, T. (1995) An emancipatory approach to the therapeutic management of violence and aggression. *Psychiatric Care* **2**(5), 158–60.

McLaren, S., Brown, F. W. A. & Taylor, P. J. (1990) A study of psychotropic medication given 'as required' in a regional secure unit. *British Journal of Psychiatry* **156**, 732–5.

Mansell, J. (1993) *Services for People with Learning Disabilities and Challenging Behaviour or Mental Health Needs.* HMSO, London.

Mayor, S., Bhate, M., Firth, H., Graham, A., Unot, P. & Tyrer, S. (1990) Facilities for mentally impaired patients: three years' experience of a semi secure unit. *Psychiatric Bulletin* **14**, 333–5.

Morrison, P. & Lehane, M. (1995) Staffing levels and seclusion use. *Journal of Advanced Nursing* **22**, 1193–202.

Murphy, G. M., Harnett, H. & Holland, A. J. (1995) A survey of intellectual disabilities amongst men on remand in prison. *Mental Handicap Research* **8**, 81–97.

Nelson, H. E. (1991) *National Adult Reading Test (NART).* NFER, Nelson.

Perkins, D. (1993) Psychological perspectives in working with sex offenders. In *Psychological Perspectives in Sexual Problems: New Directions in Theory and Practice* (Usher, J. M. & Baker, C. D., eds). Routledge, London.

Psychological Corporation (1986) WAIS-R. Psychological Corporation Ltd, 24–28 Oval Road, London NW1 7DX.

Raven, J. C. (1986) *Raven Matrices.* H. K. Lewis, London.

Royal College of Psychiatrists (1980) *Secure Facilities for Psychiatric Patients: Comprehensive Policy.* RCP, London.

Sheppard, D. (1995) *Learning the Lessons.* Zito Trust.

Stilling, L. (1992) The pros and cons of physical restraint and behaviour control. *Journal for the Psychosocial Nurse* **30**(3), 18–20.

Swanson, C. (1986) Modification of destructiveness in the long term in-patient treatment of severe personality disorder. *International Journal of Therapeutic Communities* **7**(3), 155–63.

Swanson, C. & Garwich, G. B. (1990) Treatment for low functioning sex offenders: group therapy and interagency co-operation. *Mental Retardation* **28**, 155–61.

Tarbuck, P. (1992) The use and abuse of control and restraint. *Nursing Standard* **69**(52), 30–20.

Targan, G., Wright, S., Eyman, R. & Keeran, C. (1979) Mentally retarded offenders: prevalence and characteristics. *American Journal of Mental Deficiency* **84**(2), 165–76.

Taylor, J. (1996) The sex offender with a learning disability. *Journal of the Association of Practitioners in Learning Disability* **12**(4), 11–21.

UKCC (1998) *Guidelines for Mental Health and Learning Disabilities Nursing.* UKCC, London

World Health Organisation (1992) *The ICD-10 Classification of Mental and Behavioural Disorder: Clinical Descriptions on Diagnostic Guidelines.* World Health Organisation, Geneva.

Chapter 6

Working with the Personality Disordered Offender

Alison Tennant, Carol Davies and Ian Tennant

INTRODUCTION

Forensic mental health nurses are faced with the contradictory reality of caring for the personality disordered patient. On the one hand nurses are members of a society which appears to regard personality disordered offenders as 'beasts' and 'monsters' and on the other they are expected to see the positive aspects of the individual and support them through the difficult experience of self-awareness and personal change.

This dilemma exists within a profession in which practitioners are not prepared during their nurse training for work with such patients (Moran & Mason, 1996). It is the personal attributes of the individual practitioner together with the practical experience gained within a therapeutic environment that allow the nurse to develop into a confident and credible professional. The development of a therapeutic alliance between nurse and patient will only reach its full potential where the practitioner has the confidence and self-awareness to be able to expose their own vulnerability. It is this 'lack of perfection', together with a consistent unambiguous approach, that provides the opportunity for patient change.

From a clinical nursing standpoint, the debates that continue to rage within the mental health professions have limited practical applicability. These arguments include issues of treatability, diagnostic criteria and the provision of appropriate care environments.

DEFINITIONAL ISSUES

The term 'psychopathic disorder' has had a long and confusing history. It derives from early attempts to delineate pathological personality, such as Prichard's 1837 notion of moral insanity (Paris, 1996). It is used uniquely in the English mental health system as a legal classification and is defined by the Mental Health Act 1983 as:

'a persistent disorder or disability of mind (whether or not including significant impairment of intelligence), which results in abnormally aggressive or seriously irresponsible conduct'.

This legal category of psychopathic disorder is not a clinical diagnosis. While the term is not synonymous with personality disorder, most patients classified as having a psychopathic disorder are diagnosed as suffering from one or more personality disorders. People with personality disorders of this type often pose significant challenges to society and make heavy demands in a wide variety of settings. The challenges they pose are compounded by the differences in terminology and conceptualisation. It is therefore difficult to provide a precise definition of psychopathy. This is reflected in the varying assumptions about psychopathy and the numerous scales that have been developed to measure the disorder (e.g. McCord & McCord, 1964; Hare, 1970; Blackburn, 1975; Cleckley, 1976; Pichot, 1978; Smith, 1978; Doren, 1987).

Psychopathy has been more precisely defined recently by introducing measurements of both personality factors and past behavioural and life-style factors. The most widely accepted method of assessment is the Hare Psychopathy Checklist (Hare, 1991).

Psychopaths are variously described as self-centred, callous people who commit antisocial acts, usually of a recurrent or episodic type. Their lack of empathy and shame is profound and they are unable to sustain relationships with significant others, thus not establishing emotional bonds. From a psychoanalytic perspective, this may well describe someone who lacks conscience or superego, and is sometimes referred to as the primary concept of psychopathy.

Socially, they can be very skilled, with an ability to deceive others. They lack insight and are unable to formulate realistic long-term goals. Their focus is on short-term gains, based on immediate gratification. Behaviourally, they are often described as irresponsible and impulsive, and as having a disregard for moral values. Gunn & Robertson (1976, cited in Dolan & Coid, 1993) point out that there are only five agreed facts about the term 'psychopathic disorder':

- the diagnosis is unreliable
- authors disagree about its definition
- it is used in the vernacular as a term of derogation
- it has legal use in England and Wales
- doctors use it to indicate that a patient is incurable or untreatable

Despite these observations the terms 'psychopath' and 'psychopathic disorder' remain in common use in clinical settings. There has been considerable sentiment in favour of changing the designation from psychopathic to personality disorder, as recommended in a recent working group report on psychopathic disorder (Reed, 1994).

MEDIA REPRESENTATION

There is little doubt that the media influence public opinion. Whilst it would appear that some newspaper editors take this responsibility seriously, others sacrifice balanced reporting to circulation figures. This takes the form of sensationalised reporting and stereotyping of people with mental health problems. On 12 March 1995, the *Sunday Mirror* printed a photograph of a group of men with mental health problems on a rehabilitation day trip to a theme park, Alton Towers. The headline read 'Psycho Towers'.

The central issue in many of the tabloid newspapers is the sensationalisation of the potential for violence. This intrinsically plays upon people's real fears about their personal safety in their own society. It would appear that it is partly the media that are responsible for the creation of a punitive ground swell of opinion amongst the majority of the public.

It is the need for demonstrable reaction on the part of the authorities to such sensationalised incidents that at times seems to generate capricious responses. This may take the form of superficially salient processes of management and treatment of offenders that fail to address the therapeutic agenda. An example of this may be demonstrated in Blom-Cooper's (1996) statements about the Jason Mitchell inquiry, regarding the failure by all clinicians to explore the contributing underlying factors.

There has always been a demand for punishment and retribution policies, with tougher sentencing remaining a popular solution. The media give the public the message that a disposal within the forensic psychiatric system is the 'soft option', allowing the offender to deny the responsibility for his/her actions. In fact, the primary task of working with such offenders is to help them to locate responsibility and to make behavioural changes.

It is within this arena of negative stereotyped images of personality disordered patients that the nurse has to function, both as a member of society, but, more pertinently to this chapter, as a therapeutically optimistic member of a care team. Professional and interpersonal training and support systems are what enable the individual practitioner to maintain a balanced approach to the provision of care within a complex and frequently contradictory mental health-care system.

TREATABILITY ISSUES

The issue of whether or not individuals diagnosed as suffering from a personality disorder are susceptible to treatment interventions continues to be a live debate within mental health care. The efficacy of the differing treatment regimes provides contradictory evidence, further compounding this problem (Dolan & Coid, 1993). The disparity of the clinical presentations of this patient group adds to the complexity of these considerations. There is no one definitive method of treatment interventions supported by all writers/practitioners working in this area.

Recent reviews and meta-analysis by Andrews *et al.* (1990), Hollin (1993), and Antonowicz & Ross (1994) have reached a high level of consensus that effective treatment includes a set of specific factors. These include having a sound theoretical base; multi-faceted programming, based on an individualised assessment of need; targeting of criminogenic needs; the use of active and structured behavioural or social-learning techniques; modelling of pro-social attitudes; and a cognitive behavioural emphasis, including social cognitive skills training. Porporino & Motiuk (1995) argued for the need to address developmental deficits in cognitive and social competence in offenders, particularly with reference to self-control, cognitive style, interpersonal problem-solving, social perspective-taking, values and critical reasoning. Notwithstanding the fascinating nature of this debate, it does little to inform nursing practice on a daily basis. It would be over-simplistic to assume that all nurses without preparatory training and ongoing support would have the skills to work effectively with this patient group.

NURSING PRACTICE

A core principle for nursing is the need to establish trust. This is both a prerequisite for therapy and a target of change for individuals. It requires the nurse to show acceptance of the patient, though not his/her offending behaviour, while at the same time setting limits and external controls, for example the inclusion of a set of ward rules which everyone within the unit must adhere to for health and safety reasons, but especially to create a 'safe' environment to allow therapy/treatment to occur.

It could be argued that many of the skills required to be effective with this group are actually inherent personality traits within individual nurses, rather than acquired skills. This inevitably points towards some nurses coping well with this patient group, whilst others feel vulnerable and afraid and consequently fail to effectively engage in a therapeutic sense (Norton & Hinshelwood, 1996).

A control issue for nursing is to establish a strong, positive, interpersonal relationship with the patient right from the beginning. This may be viewed as having four sequential stages, each with distinct aspects of development. Throughout this process, support systems should be available to both

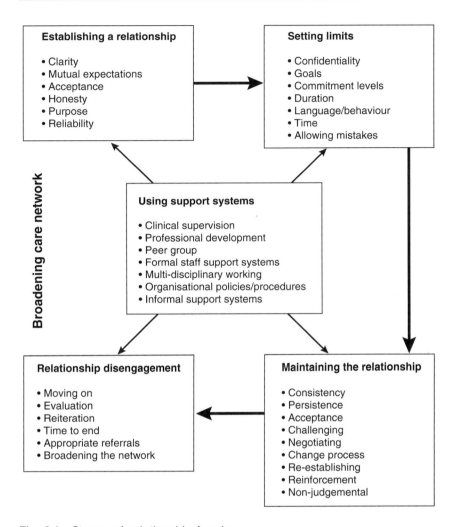

Fig. 6.1 Stages of relationship forming.

parties (Fig. 6.1). The basic principles shown in the diagram may be expanded upon by looking at the four stages individually with their salient components.

ESTABLISHING A RELATIONSHIP

The nature and quality of the therapeutic relationship between the nurse and patient are generally regarded as fundamental components of the helping relationship. Establishing a relationship frequently proves to be the most difficult aspect, with a high risk of the patient rejecting the nurse or at least seeking to contain the engagement at a superficial level. This may reflect the concept of resistance described within psychodynamic therapies. At this stage the nurse's professional skills, together with what Barker (1992) describes as therapeutic use of self, are essential in creating the opportunity for engagement. Nurses are uniquely placed to provide the major therapeutic interventions that lead the way in treating this group effectively within a forensic mental health setting. Goleman's (1985) review of the research concluded that the best predictor of success in the helping relationship was the quality of the relationship between the nurse and the patient. Indeed some authors (Driscoll, 1984; Gelso & Carter, 1985) describe the relationship as a means in itself to a successful outcome, citing collaboration, respect, empathic understanding, genuineness, trust, and challenge with support on the part of the nurse, as a way of promoting these qualities in the patient. This helps the patient use their own resources towards leading a more fulfilled life.

The key factor in forming a relationship is the establishment of *clarity*, the mutual recognition of the purpose and direction of the relationship. A generally held principle in counselling practice is that the patient should set the agenda and the goals of therapy and that the nurse/therapist should neither condone nor condemn behaviour by making judgements. Rogers (1961) advocated that 'The therapist communicated to his client a deep and genuine caring for him as a person with potentialities and caring uncontaminated by evaluations of his thoughts, feelings or behaviour'. Indeed the pre-registration nursing curriculum (mental health) would probably reflect this view. However, many of these key principles have been called into question when related to therapy with sex offenders and in our experience of working with offenders. Crawford concluded: 'Sex offenders are generally regarded as a population unlikely to be responsive to psychotherapy for reasons such as, their denial of guilt, lack of motivation to change and failure to co-operate with voluntary treatment' (Crawford, 1981). Salter (1988) argues that, far from working on the patient's agenda, it is the nurse/ therapist who should set the treatment goals, since the patient will have goals that the nurse does not share, for example to convince the nurse that he/she has changed and will not reoffend and should live in the community. The problem then for nurses, who are solely working towards the patient goals, is that this may involve the patient being discharged from the unit to return to his/her offending behaviour.

It is crucial for the nurse and patient to maintain a clear sight of the objectives/goals of treatment being set. This point may need to be constantly reinforced by the nurse, who will require an inner strength to stay committed to the person, to keep focused on their work and not to punish the patient concerned. To have any success the relationship has to be free of blame, anger, thoughts of revenge and punishment, and must have no hidden agendas. Once a strong, positive relationship has been developed, the most effective reinforcer available to the nurse is the expression and continuation of the positive relationship. The risk of not establishing the clarity of purpose early in the relationship is that the patient may seek the nurse's validation of his experiences as a rationale for avoiding the often unpleasant realities that accompany the heightened self-awareness within the process of change.

The nurse's honesty is a crucial component within the relationship, though at times this can be a difficult process, particularly within early tentative stages. Many patients with personality disorder will report incidents where they perceive themselves as abused, let down or negatively evaluated by those people they trusted. Often nurses who feel ill-prepared for this role, or who lack personal and/or professional confidence, will opt to avoid facing discomfiting and challenging scenarios at the early stages of a therapeutic relationship. It may be that they feel that once a relationship is established is the time to be honest about difficult issues. In reality the patient may view this as simply another form of being 'let down', in short, an abuse of their trust, which may in turn result in their withdrawal from active participation within the relationship.

Moran & Mason (1996) state that the short-term comfort gained by evasion does not support the growth of mutual respect within the relationship. In contrast, honesty, handled as sensitively as possible, results in the patient interpreting the nurse's statements at face value rather than searching for hidden agendas, as may be the case with nurses who try to avoid uncomfortable truths. Reliability and acceptance are the nurse's affirmation of their views of the patient as another human being deserving respect. Acceptance need not be in the form of unqualified validation of all the patient's actions, but rather an acceptance that the patient has a right, reason and rationale for holding beliefs and that the behaviour resulting from these beliefs may need modifying to realise a level of social acceptance for the patient. Reliability should take the form of the nurse consistently maintaining the same stance towards the patient, rather than reacting to the 'mood of the moment'. It may be that this therapeutic alliance forms the supportive bedrock upon which the patient can begin to experiment with change. Without this relationship, the patient may see any change as personal risk-taking and put up physical and emotional barriers to protect his own fragile self-image.

Setting limits

This is the second stage of establishing the therapeutic relationship, perhaps representing the formal aspects of the relationship and the clarification of boundaries and limitations. This approach is simple in theory and difficult in practice. The responsibility for observing limits belongs to the nurse, not to the patient. The nurse must be aware of which patient behaviours they are willing to tolerate and which are unacceptable. This information should be given to the patient at the appropriate time. The major goal of limit setting is to reinforce the patient's sense of identity through enhancing his/her personal boundaries. For the nurse concerned, it is about taking care of oneself, trying to avoid burnout and maintaining honesty as an effective strategy.

Another radical shift in philosophy for the nurse working with offenders is concerned with the nature and degree of confidentiality offered to patients. The issue of confidentiality is considered central to the practice of counselling, since by its very nature counselling encourages patients to disclose the most personal of experiences, thoughts and feelings. These disclosures are made on the understanding that they will not be repeated outside the counselling relationship. Einzig (cited in Bond, 1992) expressed the view of many counsellors when she stated 'all counselling is totally confidential'. However, in working with sex offenders and in our experience of offenders with personality disorders, we concur with the view of many experts (Finkelhor *et al.*, 1986; Salter, 1988; Bolton & Bolton, 1990) that the nurse/therapist must work as part of a team and as a result must ask the patient to agree to give up his right to confidentiality. This can often be a very difficult task for an inexperienced nurse, who may skirt round the subject or say nothing, assuming that the patient knows and accepts this.

In more traditional forms of therapy, the patient is the best source of information and is relied upon to accurately describe his/her experience. The nurse trusts and accepts the patient and their view of the world. However, when working with patients who have a history of offending behaviour, particularly behaviour which is sexually motivated, this is potentially the most damaging and dangerous quality the nurse can bring to the relationship. Dreiblatt (1984, p. 70) describes a personal outlook on this aspect of therapy: 'I tell my clients that I do not operate on a trust basis. Trust is what is abusable, I communicate to them that I have no intention of feeling confident in them. Feeling confident about them can be dangerous'.

Given these conflicting views, is it more helpful to the therapeutic process to suspend one's own way of construing events (Fransella & Dalton, 1990, p. 18) and hence one's values, or to remain anchored in the consensual reality of society's values as a means of challenging and changing the distorted perceptions of the client? This tension raises questions as to whether it is possible or desirable for the nurse working with sex offenders to feel or communicate respect for the patient. Is it possible to view the patient as a person in the 'process of becoming' (Rogers, 1961), to respect them as a human being, to empathise with their pain and to believe in their capacity to change? Salter observed: 'Offenders detect very quickly a sense of respect coming from someone very difficult to manipulate and they respond as though there were something in them worth respecting' (Salter, 1988, p. 93). This view seems to emphasise the importance of the nurse remaining strong and in some way detached. However, in many ways it highlights the fact that the nurse's 'way of being' in the relationship is important, and perhaps reinforces the view of counselling as a social influence process where the characteristics of the therapist have a major impact on therapy outcomes.

The importance of showing commitment to the treatment process is vital, for example by finding issues that will help the patient see the benefits of engaging in therapy and so embarking on the change process. As a minimum the patient must agree to work towards eliminating, for example, aggressive behaviour and building a more worthwhile life. The commitment sought is for the patient to collaborate in the specific treatment interventions selected. One of the reasons for many patients disengaging from treatment is inadequate commitment by either the patient, the nurse or the clinical team. Commitment can, therefore, be viewed as a behaviour itself, something which is elicited, learned and reinforced. It is therefore important that the nursing team look at ways to help this process along.

As part of working together in one-to-one meetings, parameters must be established. In many situations the named nurse assumes two distinct roles in relating to a patient, the first as therapist, the second as generic ward nurse dealing with day-to-day practical aspects of caring for patients. It is important that the patient recognises these differences and respects the limitations this places on the nurse's ability to give time to one individual. For example, his care plan may indicate that he has two 1-hour individual sessions per week to look at a specific issue identified in assessment. The nurse must ensure that whilst the patient gets these sessions he does not waylay the nurse on these issues outside of these agreed times, except in a crisis situation. It is of little benefit to produce a contract specifically relating to the time, place and duration of the individual sessions, but it is important that the patient recognises the two distinct roles. Equally there should be an agreement as to the types of language and behaviours acceptable within the sessions, particularly if they are group settings. A basic rule of thumb could be no verbally threatening or hostile language and definitely no physical violence. However, if such an incident takes place, given the ethos of allowing mistakes, it is important that the incident is openly discussed with the patient rather than simply cancelling sessions.

Maintaining the relationship

Once the relationship has been established and goals have been set and ground rules clarified, then the real purpose of the relationship – helping resolve problems – begins. It is the nurse's role to help the patient gain a realisation of how his thoughts and feelings largely determine his actions. This calls for the nurse to be persistent, accepting and consistent towards often very bizarre and pathological cognitions. However, part of this acceptance must include challenge and the negotiation of alternative strategies, if the nurse is not to be seen to collude with the patient's frequently distorted images of reality. It is important that the nurse recognises all the aspects of the change process for the patient, including the likelihood that the patient's behaviour may deteriorate before it improves. This should not be viewed as failure: the patient requires consistency of approach throughout this stage, together with support in re-establishing his own values and beliefs. Once the goals of the intervention have been achieved, the patient needs support and reinforcement of the benefits of such a change.

Relationship disengagement

There is effectively a 'shelf life' for most therapeutic relationships, after which time the efficacy of the intervention decreases, though aspects of social support may remain high. However, given that the main aim in most cases is for the personality disordered patient to move on towards eventual return to independence in the community, it is important that both nurse and patient acknowledge the need to progress onwards. This should take the form of a planned withdrawal rather than a sudden halt to the session. Essential elements in this process include the following:

(1) The nurse emphasises and praises the progress of the patient, and summarises and evaluates the work so far, what has been achieved, and what further progress can be made.
(2) If the patient is to be referred on to another professional, it is important that they understand the rationale for this referral, otherwise it may be viewed as rejection.
(3) Adequate time should be given to disengagement. This is particularly important since the nurse will inevitably remain on the unit in their more generic role, making it more difficult to terminate than with a professional external to the ward, such as a psychologist. The nurse will continue to play a role in the patient's care, which emphasises that caring for the patient does not stop just because individual work has discontinued.

In summary, the nursing practice role in the care of patients with psychopathic disorders is possibly the most complex of all the care professions. It changes from the provision of basic nursing care through to the complexity of the provision of individual therapy. Included in the custody versus therapy dichotomy, in many instances, it is only with experience that the nurse learns to combine the beneficial aspects of these elements. The combination of challenging, nurturing, controlling and supporting growth in patients should be echoed in the professional development process of nurses.

The case study offered below demonstrates how the theoretical aspects of practice shown in Fig. 6.1 are operationalised in terms of prescribed nursing care. Assessing suitability requires knowledge of both the patient and the particular care provision or environment. Frequently, personality disordered patients are referred to particular care environments and are not willing participants in their treatment. Nurses are aware that active engagement and treatment cannot be taken for granted and that particular skills need to be utilised to foster this, for example:

- an understanding of the patient's difficulties in relating to others
- the knowledge that these difficulties are based upon low self-esteem, ambivalence, fear of intimacy and basic mistrust
- acceptance that these aspects may be understandable and of survival value to the patient given past experiences, but currently are largely maladaptive (Norton & Dolan, 1995).

CASE STUDY

Tom is in his early twenties and has been in hospital for 2 years. His criminal history began in his teenage years and progressed from motoring offences to increasingly serious sexual offences against women and fire-setting episodes.

His personal history described a close family network, whose members maintain good contact. There is no known family history of mental disorder. He reported the following traumatic experiences. From the age of 10 he was sexually abused for a number of years by an older man. He had difficulty with academic work and was suspended from school at the age of 12 and would sniff glue and regularly smoke cannabis. As an adolescent, he became increasingly interested in women, stealing their underwear from washing lines and following women home. This behaviour then progressed to indecent assault and later to sexual offending.

Assessment by the multi-disciplinary team

As part of the multi-modal assessment process, nurses should be responsible for certain aspects of the multi-disciplinary input (Fig. 6.2). Some of the following procedures would be undertaken with supervision from the consultant psychologist involved in Tom's care. The following assessments could be included:

(1)   Interview and structured file review to gather information as part of a functional analysis of problem- and offence-related behaviour.

Fig. 6.2 Multi-disciplinary treatment plan – hypothetical.

Issue	Treatment goal	Intervention	Action by:
Temper control and anger management	To develop and maintain an understanding of triggers for anxiety and increase range of coping skills	Individual sessions to review work	Psychologist Named nurse Patient
		Anger management group	Patient Group facilitator
		Develop effective relaxation techniques	Named nurse Patient
		Distress tolerance group	Group facilitator Patient
		Emotion regulation group	Nursing staff Patient
Social relationship skills, e.g. relationships with women	Increase level of competence in social situations	Interpersonal effectiveness group	Group facilitator Patient
	Reduce socially inappropriate behaviours, e.g. touching, comments	Giving constructive feedback to patient	All staff
Family links	Visit and maintain family links if appropriate	To assess Tom's expectations with regard to his family network	Multi-disciplinary team
Care Programme Approach	Maintain contact with the local authority	Maintain relevant medico/legal documentation as required by organisation	Multi-disciplinary team
	Maintain contact with the health authority	To enable patient to be involved in the care planning process	

(2)   A structured interview and file review to complete the Hare Psycho-pathy Checklist (revised). Specialised training is required to undertake this assessment.

(3)   Standardised psychometric assessments, e.g. impulsivity, empathy, sexual interest and aggression, attribution of blame.

(4)   Structured interview to assess specific problem areas such as: education, work, family, parenting, social relationships, finances, leisure, alcohol and drugs. The interview should consider the potential impact of cultural and ethnic factors on assessment and treatment.

(5)   Pre- and post-intervention psychometric measures are completed by the patient concerned to measure specific factors relating to the type of therapeutic group, e.g. sex offending, arson, anger management.

(6)   As part of the assessment process, the nursing team can monitor and record behaviours in the care setting that the patient may display. This information can be collated for feedback to the patient and to the multi-disciplinary clinical team.

It can be identified that there is an increasing seriousness of behavioural disorder over time. This can be observed from this man's criminal history. Tom, over time, had become very preoccupied with sexual thoughts throughout his adolescence and has been involved in sexual deviant activities, e.g. indecent exposure. It is apparent that elements of planning are evident, which relate to Tom's offences.

Diagnostic formulation

Element 1 – Personality disorder

(1)   He has DSM-IV-R diagnosis of borderline personality disorder.

(2)   He has a score of 28 on the 20-item PCL-R scale, indicating a high level of psychopathy.

Element 2 – Clinical picture

(1)   He has experienced a disturbing traumatic event and highlights evidence of suicidal ideation and high levels of psychological distress. He has a tendency to ruminate about upsetting events and is unable to cope with stress in a rational manner.

(2)   Tendency to adopt careless and impulsive strategies when problem-solving.

(3)   Views dangerous risk-taking as exciting.

(4)   Avoids expressing emotion (see nursing care plan).

(5)   Unassertive and has low self-esteem.

Responsibility

(1) Accepts some responsibility – although externalises blame.
(2) Lacks insight into factors which led to his offending behaviour.

Element 3 – Factors affecting progress in therapy

(1) Tom is easily angered and has difficulty controlling his anger; he has a tendency to react aggressively when challenged.
(2) Tom has been involved in many sexually deviant activities.
(3) He views dangerous risk-taking experiences as stimulating and positive, e.g. joyriding, displays sexually promiscuous behaviour and enjoys gambling.

Treatment goals

Target the following:

(1) Cognitive affective process and interpersonal skills, such as distortions in thinking and deficits in problem-solving processes.
(2) Criminal behaviour through a behavioural analysis, which consists of an examination of the development of the offending behaviour.
(3) Amenability to treatment, e.g. a reliable measure which takes account of:
    (a) the appropriate fit between treatment goals and patient deficits
    (b) history of the patient's response to treatment
    (c) motivation in the treatment process
(4) Personal change rather than 'cure', getting the patient to accept responsibility for his situation.

Treatment outcomes

(1) Evidence that Tom is no longer preoccupied with a particular type of violent or sexual activity.
(2) Evidence of reduced levels of dangerousness, e.g. demonstrates socially appropriate attitude and behaviour towards females.
(3) Socially acceptable responses to others.
(4) Greater tolerance of frustration and stress with a much reduced level of explosive or impulsive behaviour.
(5) Evidence that Tom has improved understanding of what motivates his behaviour, can learn from experience, can take into account the consequences of his actions, and is more mature, reliable and predictable.
(6) Demonstrates concern for others and an ability to see things from the point of view of others.
(7) Able to live in the environment/ward sufficiently well.

USING SUPPORT SYSTEMS

It is only in recent years that the process of clinical supervision has emerged within the repertoire of tools serving to develop quality nursing care within psychiatry (Department of Health, 1994). It has long been a mandatory process in the disciplines of psychology, psychotherapy and social work, both to ensure safe practice and to enable practitioner development. However, it has received a somewhat ambivalent welcome within nursing. Emerging into mainstream nursing, its primary purpose was to ensure safe practice and to a lesser extent the provision of an arena in which practitioners could reflect upon aspects of their practice and attitudes that impact upon their roles (Critchley, 1987).

One of the reasons why the initial evaluation of the introduction of clinical supervision is demonstrating contrasting responses is the lack of a nursing paradigm to support it. This creates a scenario where, even within the same hospital, different priorities and models emerge, resulting in a lack of clarity and consistency. The models of clinical supervision used within nursing exist somewhere along a continuum ranging from personal psycho-therapeutic processes, through to a purely managerial style where success is measured against set objectives by an appraisal system (Faugier, 1996). Working with personality disordered offender patients calls for a balance between the two extremes, creating a fusion between personal support and growth, together with professional development.

Working effectively with personality disordered patients places great emphasis on the psychodynamics of the nurse–patient relationship. Clinical supervision is an essential component in supporting the development and maintenance of this process at a therapeutic rather than custodial level. A high level of anxiety is provoked for an inexperienced nurse working with this patient group (Strong, 1998), almost certainly because:

(1)   There are no definitive frames of reference to guide nursing interventions.
(2)   There is a lack of training at pre-registration level, specific to this patient group.
(3)   The 'giving up of power' that accompanies the empowerment of patients within the therapeutic relationship often creates anxieties for the nurse.
(4)   Nurses are frequently the target of physical and emotional violence, directed at them by patients who fear becoming close to them as a result of their mistrust of anyone who seeks to help. This hostility and rejection from the patient may be the first realisation for an inexperienced nurse that not everyone shares society's views of nurses as caring individuals. This can prove to be a profound challenge to the nurse's self-identity and sense of purpose.

All these issues can be dealt with appropriately, within clinical supervision with a skilled experienced practitioner, as part of a robust training programme designed to enhance the nursing role in the care and management of personality disordered patients. Formal educational strategies contribute towards the development of expertise in caring for this client group, but provide no substitute for the experiential learning gained from clinical practice. The process of clinical supervision serves to enable the nurse to learn from these experiences by analysis and reflection within the safety of the supervision session, as well as providing an arena for dealing with the heavy emotional pressures that arise from working with this patient group.

The planning and development of a specialist service for personality disordered patients must include adequate funding and the availability of time for practitioners to utilise clinical supervision. It cannot be viewed as an *ad hoc* optional process if the 'therapy–security' dilemma (Burrow, 1993) faced by individual nurses is not to interfere with the consistent provision of good quality care.

One of the main concerns faced by nurses beginning clinical supervision relates to an incomplete knowledge of what issues to take to the session and what to expect from the supervisor. Inskipp & Proctor (1994) define three elements of supervision which are commonly accepted as core definitions of supervision in all care professions who undertake this process. These are:

(1) **normative** – the managerial component concerned with efficient and effective care
(2) **formative** – linked to the educational development of the practitioner (skills and knowledge)
(3) **restorative** – addresses the nurse's need for support through stress management

There is a common misconception among nurses about clinical supervision that it represents a purely management tool to direct and control a nurse's work. This leads to a lack of commitment to the process (Platt-Koch, 1986). In fact, clinical supervision should be viewed as both the right and responsibility of every qualified nurse, providing, as it does, the means to develop and refine professional skills whilst at the same time offering the opportunity of personal support within a stressful occupation. In many psychiatric settings, clinical supervision has declined because of the difficulties encountered by focusing on individualised care when the patient turnover is very rapid (Faugier, 1996).

This is not the case within forensic care facilities, where the patient population is more static. However, it may also be argued that, by concentrating solely upon individual care needs, many aspects of the nursing role, particularly with personality disordered patients, are missed, for example group process and dynamics, and inter-professional support strategies. The changing nature of nursing, in particular the extension of responsibilities in clinical practice, needs to be reflected in the scope of issues that can be taken to clinical supervision sessions. In many ways the supervisory relationship's core tenets reflect the nurse–patient relationship. The skilled supervisor (or nurse) will help to guide the supervisee through the process of developing skills, attitudes and the ability to reflect upon their own actions that enables them to reach their best potential. To be effective as a supervisor, the nurse must have a broad repertoire of skills. This range of skills can be demonstrated by Frankam's (1987) model which serves to categorise the roles of a clinical supervisor within a model of 12 roles.

Faugier (1996) catalogues the components of the supervisory relationship. All of these are central to the supervisory process, but some perhaps have additional pertinence for nurses working with personality disordered patients. The hostility and ridicule aimed at individual nurses by such patients often challenge beliefs about nursing as a worthwhile caring profession and may also strike at the very core of the nurse's sense of self. To support nurses through this often very personalised challenge to enable them to emerge as confident and competent practitioners requires very skilled supervision.

Most supervision in nursing takes place in the form of individualised sessions, with the supervisor being a more experienced practitioner than the supervisee. However, there are considerable financial and time implications for this type of approach, so it may be that alternative strategies need to be considered. Group supervision, characterised by a formal meeting with established ground rules, may be a suitable alternative. This should not be mistaken for *ad hoc* mutual peer support sessions that may occur at the end of a shift or following a stressful incident, though this process also has a valuable role in supporting nursing.

The clinical and cost effectiveness of clinical supervision has not, as yet, been empirically proven within a forensic environment (Rogers & Topping-Morris, 1997), though there is much anecdotal evidence to support its benefit in enhancing clinical practice.

A variety of support systems must be utilised. Options may include clinical teams contracting out of the organisation for formal supervision with an experienced facilitator, who may have a greater degree of objectivity towards the task. The multi-disciplinary team may have a role to play in helping the staff member to think clearly about how to conceptualise the patient, the relationship and the application of treatment aims.

STAFF TRAINING AND EDUCATION

Many mental health professionals, some without any formal training and some without even supervision, involve themselves in psychotherapy with offender patients. The negative consequences of this involvement often reflect their level of training and self-awareness. Sallah (1994) surveyed a group of nurses working in high security hospitals and medium secure units with respect to their views on the care and treatment of psychopathic disordered patients. The results of the survey show that nurses as a whole hold the view that this patient group should benefit from care, provided that nurses are appropriately trained – particularly in dealing with difficulties during care management. Nurse training does not on the whole prepare the student for the fact that they may have to face people's emotional distress, painful experiences and despair. The patient can generate very powerful interpersonal pressures which can result in immense emotional stresses and be cognitively incapacitating for the inexperienced clinician. A fundamental problem for student nurses trained in the higher education system may be that learning does not recognise authority based on experience. Instead, it assesses the level of learning based upon academic theories. This can foster a tendency to learn from the literature rather than personally from skilled practitioners (Mollon, 1989). The theory-to-practice gap remains more than a theoretical consideration: it represents the difference between the provision of quality care and merely hypothesising about its provision.

It is generally agreed that effective treatment is linked to well founded theoretical ideas and to individualised treatment targets for each patient (McGuire, 1995). It is important that the contribution which nurses make to the treatment, care and management of these patients is reflected in terms of effective assessment, formulation of accurate care plans and evaluation of the treatment plans. For successful treatment programmes to evolve, there is the requirement for consistency of treatment delivery from all members of staff who contribute to the overall care.

Hughes & Tennant (1996) developed a psychological treatment unit at Rampton Hospital with a treatment regime based on behavioural and cognitive-behavioural principles. An effective strategy for the training of nurses and other ward-based staff was seen as essential in realising this. The training strategy was intended to facilitate the ability of qualified and unqualified nurses to deliver planned care that would enable them to set and target achievable goals. The training needs of this nursing group were based on the following principles.

Assessment

- Assessment of psychosocial history
- Functional analysis of offending behaviour
- Measurement of current patient behaviours displayed on a 24-hour basis

Treatment interventions

- Developing and delivering nursing plans based on behavioural principles

- Understanding and application of psychological strategies, e.g. use of counselling skills and techniques in motivational interviewing
- Skills in monitoring and recording and in giving the patient accurate feedback
- Involving the patient and multi-disciplinary team in the process of treatment planning
- Appropriate knowledge and skills in the principles of cognitive-behavioural therapy techniques
- Understanding of the classification systems for personality disorder and psychopathy
- Understanding basic principles of assertiveness and applying appropriately
- Having a knowledge and understanding of the assessment of risk and dangerousness
- Understanding psychological approaches to anger management strategies

Group treatment

- Understanding the principles of group processes and being competent to lead psycho-educational therapeutic groups
- Understanding functional analysis of both past and presenting behaviour problems
- Having a working knowledge of clinical supervision and reflecting on their own practice during supervision

The training strategy outlined above was based on a model proposed by Gardner (1981) and recommended by Hollin *et al.* (1995). It was proposed that staff be trained through three different levels. The first level of development would be represented by nursing assistants working under close supervision. They should have an understanding of the assessment process and basic behavioural principles and be able to record and monitor patient behaviours on a daily basis. Accurate observation and communication skills are a fundamental part of this role in passing on information to other staff about a particular patient.

'Technicians' are then trained to function at the second level. This training would take approximately one year through work experience and educational input. Nurses working at this level should be involved in the assessment process and in developing and delivering treatment intervention based on behavioural principles. Having an understanding of group work and being able to co-facilitate a group in a structured format under supervision would play a major part in their training programme.

The final stage of the training would involve nurses facilitating cognitive-behavioural skills group programmes. These 'specialists' should be able to link assessment to treatment and risk analysis. A major part of this role would be to liaise and consult with the multi-disciplinary team in terms of the development in the treatment planning process. This training could take up to 2 years.

The need for undergraduate programmes for accredited health-care workers was identified as an essential development for those working in the forensic setting (Reed, 1994). There presently exist several routes of study up to and including diploma level in the care and management of the mentally disordered offender, and the BA(Hons) Health Care Practice (Forensic) has been developed for nurses working in this specialist area.

THE LEARNING ENVIRONMENT AND TREATMENT ETHOS

The aim of any unit is to develop an environment which is therapeutic in all aspects. Having a clear working philosophy that the ward team is part of is crucial to the success of skills-based training. Unit management must develop treatment methods that rely upon the creation of a culture of enquiry or reflective practice for their therapeutic efficiency. Staff should be encouraged to question and to seek help and advice from peers and other professions. To allow this to happen, staff need the time and space to read and reflect on their practice. This learning milieu is essential to avoid extreme and polarised views about particular patients' maladaptive behaviour, to minimise the impact of patient-generated splits in the staff team. The emphasis for staff working in these environments is to avoid punishing, shaming or blaming patients, and to develop a more thoughtful stance. To facilitate this process, effective communication systems need to be established throughout the day and night. Attention should be paid to staff's mutual support and self-examination through staff meetings, clinical supervision, support groups and multi-disciplinary meetings.

FUTURE DIRECTIONS

Linehan (1993) describes a treatment model for borderline personality disorder which encompasses training in emotional awareness, distress reduction and emotion regulation skills. Recently developed therapeutic models for borderline personality disorder, in particular Linehan's (1993) dialectical behaviour therapy, may be pertinent to work with the severely personality disordered person. The major focus of this work is on establishing interventions which target life-threatening behaviours that interfere with the process of therapy, quality-of-life issues and, lastly, resolving post-traumatic stress, self-validation and self-respect.

The role of dysfunctional concepts of masculinity have been suggested as a useful target for treatment with offenders (Chapman & Maitland, 1995).

Many of those dysfunctional ideas about what it takes 'to be a man' inter-fere with problem resolution within therapy. Nurses who work with male offenders may therefore require training in relation to gender awareness and in anti-discriminatory work (Lloyd, 1996). Similar consideration would need to be included where working with women, ethnicity and disability. Men's traditional place in the world is being affected by major changes in the workplace and social and economic structures, and is having a sig-nificant impact on their lives and the way they perceive themselves. These changes challenge men to think about their roles and to examine their assumptions about themselves and others, which affect their attitudes and behaviours. If we are asking our patients to examine and change their atti-tudes and behaviours, then it seems logical that nurses should do the same. It is important that they reconsider some of their attitudes and behaviours, placing themselves in a better position to enable the patient to consider a wider range of choices that impact on relationships with others and their behaviour as men.

Some of the issues that may arise out of working with men and that need to be considered in relation to the therapeutic context are that men may have typical styles and psychological issues that they bring to treatment. Traditional methods of one-to-one psychotherapy were developed mostly to treat female patients. Within counselling relationships we see that very few of the traditional concepts of masculinity are conducive to requesting treatment or indeed asking for help. Whilst receiving therapy, patients are expected to discuss their problems, which involves personal self-disclosure and an exploration of how they feel. Men generally have little experience of this. On the whole, strategies that men employ to solve problems include an emphasis on thought over feelings, to distract themselves or learn how to avoid the issue. Nurses working with men need to be sensitive to these issues, as asking men to do these things can be a very uncomfortable process and may well be a factor as to why men drop out of treatment at an early stage. This environment can be aversive for many men; several theorists have suggested that structured and psycho-educational approaches be considered as an alternative to one-to-one psychotherapy. Chapman & Maitland (1995) have developed a structured group programme, which allows men to do what they rarely do otherwise, share feelings, talk about their inner life and express the parts of self that are repressed by traditional concepts of masculinity.

CONCLUSION

The strategies described in this chapter are vehicles to keep the treatment frame in existence while the patient learns how to be different. The diverse skills and aptitudes of practitioners indicate that they will be more effective with differing types of individual patient and the problems that they present. Some readers will appropriately say, 'This field of nursing is not for me'. Others do not share this perspective and find that helping the patient to change his/her attitudes and behaviours is a rewarding challenge.

It is our belief that the goals of therapy should not be for a complete cure in the sense that the character of the person will be changed dramatically and that the patient will lose their desire to offend. A more realistic expectation would be some degree of emotional cognitive and behavioural change that will enable the person to have a quality of life that is more socially integrated and fulfilling.

The emphasis of this chapter is on a learning process for both staff and patients. For patients it is important that they learn to recognise their maladaptive thinking and behaviour patterns and to recognise situations that may put them at risk of acting out. Through the learning process they begin to see people as humans who have feelings and whom they may hurt, rather than as objects that they can use.

Working with this patient group is a constant learning process. We must strive to minimise our prejudices and stereotypes and develop a clear professional vision if we are to be effective in understanding and managing this group of people. Success in the treatment arena may allow for improvement of management skills. Personality disordered patients remain the most exacting of all client groups.

In conclusion this chapter serves to provide the reader with a brief overview of the issues relating to the nursing care and management of the personality disordered patient. It is hoped that it may guide the reader into studying in greater depth this field of nursing with an enhanced awareness of the difficulties that they may face in practice, and point to potential solutions to these dilemmas.

REFERENCES

Andrews, D. A., Zinger, I., Hodge, R. D. *et al.* (1990) Does correctional treatment work? A clinically relevant and psychologically informed meta-analysis. *Criminology* **28**, 369–404.

Antonowicz, D. H. & Ross, R. R. (1994) Essential components of successful rehabilitation programmes for offenders. *International Journal of Offender Therapy and Comparative Criminology* **38**, 97–104.

Barker, P. (1992) Psychiatric nursing. In *Clinical Supervision and Mentorship in Nursing* (Butterworth, T. & Faugier, J., eds). Chapman & Hall, London.

Blackburn, R. (1975) An empirical classification of psychopathic personality. *British Journal of Psychiatry* **127**, 456–60.

Blom-Cooper, L. (1996) Case of Jason Mitchell. *Report of the independent panel of enquiry.* Duckworth, London.

Bolton, S. R. & Bolton, F. G. Jr (1990) Meeting the challenge: legal dilemmas and considerations in working with the perpetrator. In *The Incest Perpetrator: A Family Member No One Wants To Treat* (Horton, A. L., Johnson, B. L., Roundy, L. M. & Williams, D., eds). Sage, Newbury Park, CA.

Bond, T. (1992) Confidentiality, counselling, ethics and the law. *Employee Counselling Today* 4(4), 4–9.

Burrow, S. (1993) The role conflict of the forensic nurse. *Senior Nurse* 13(5), 20–25.

Chapman, T. & Maitland, A. (1995) *Stop, Think and Change: An Integrated and Progressive Programme of Change for High Risk Offenders*. Probation Board for Northern Ireland, Belfast.

Cleckley, H. (1976) *The Mask of Sanity*, 5th edn. Mosby, St Louis, MO.

Crawford, D. A. (1981) Treatment approaches with paedophiles. In *Adult Sexual Interest in Children* (Cook, M. & Howells, K., eds). Academic Press, New York.

Critchley, D. (1987) Clinical supervision as a learning tool for the therapist in milieu settings. *Journal of Psychosocial Nursing* 25(8), 18–22.

Department of Health (1994) *Working in Partnership: A Review of Mental Health Nursing*. HMSO, London.

Dolan, B. & Coid, J. (1993) *Psychopathic and Anti-social Personality Disorder. Treatment and Research Issues*. Gaskell, London.

Doren, D. (1987) *Understanding and Treating the Psychopath*. Wiley, New York.

Dreiblatt, L. (1984) Cited in: Knopp, F. H. (1984) *Retaining Adult Sex Offenders: Methods and Models*. Safer Society, Orviell.

Driscoll, R. (1984) *Pragmatic Psychotherapy*. Van Nostrand Reinhold, New York.

Faugier, J. (1996) Clinical supervision and mental health nursing. In *Perspectives in Mental Health Nursing* (Sandford, T. & Gournay, K., eds). Baillière Tindall, London.

Finkelhor, D. and Associates (1986) *A Source Book on Child Sexual Abuse*. Sage, Newbury Park, CA.

Frankam, H. (1987) *Aspects of supervision, counsellor satisfaction, utility and defensiveness and the tasks in supervision*. Unpublished dissertation, University of Surrey, Roehampton.

Fransella, F. & Dalton, P. (1990) *Personal Construct Counselling in Action*. Sage Publications, London.

Gardner, J. M. (1981) *Training Non-Professionals in Behaviour Modification*. Witwatersrand University Press, Johannesburg.

Gelso, C. J. & Carter, J. A. (1985) The relationship in counselling and psychotherapy; components, consequences and theoretical antecedents. *Counselling Psychologist* 13, 155–243.

Goleman, G. (1985) Cited in: Egan, G. (1990) *The Skilled Helper* (4th edn). Brooks/Cole, Monterey, CA.

Gunn, J. & Robertson, G. (1976) Psychopathic personality: a conceptual problem. *Psychological Medicine* 6, 631–4. Cited in: Dolan, B. & Coid, J. *Psychopathic and Antisocial Personality Disorders*. Gaskell, London.

Hare, R. D. (1970) *Psychopathy: Theory and Research*. Wiley, New York.

Hare, R. D. (1991) *The Hare Psychotherapy Checklist*. Multi-Health System, Toronto.

Hollin, C. (1993) Advances in the psychological treatment of delinquent behaviour. *Criminal Behaviour and Mental Health* 3. 142–57.

Hollin, C., Kendrick, D. & Epps, K. (1995) *Managing Behavioural Treatment. Policy and Practice with Delinquent Adolescents.* Routledge, London.

Hughes, G. & Tennant, A. (1996) A training and development strategy for clinically based staff working with people diagnosed as having psychopathic disorders. *Psychiatric Care* 3(5), 194–9.

Inskipp, F. & Proctor, B. (1994) *The Art, Craft and Tasks of Counselling Supervision.* Cascade, London.

Linehan, M. (1993) *Cognitive Behavioural Treatment of Borderline Personality Disorder.* Guildford Press, New York.

Lloyd, T. (1996) The role of training in the development of work with men. In *Working With Men* (Newburn, T. & Mair, G., eds). Russell House Publishing, Dorset.

McCord, W. & McCord, J. (1964) *The Psychopath: An Essay on the Criminal Mind.* Van Nostrand, New Jersey.

McGuire, J. (1995) *What Works: Reducing Re-offending Guidelines from Research and Practice.* Wiley, Chichester.

Mollon, P. (1989) Narcissus, Oedipus and the psychologist's fraudulent identity. *Clinical Psychology Forum* 23, 7–11.

Moran, T. & Mason, T. (1996) Revisiting the nursing management of the psychopath. *Journal of Psychiatric and Mental Health Nursing* 3, 189–94.

Norton, K. & Dolan, B. (1995) Acting out and the institutional response. *Journal of Forensic Psychiatry* 6, 317–32.

Norton, K. & Hinshelwood, R. D. (1996) Severe personality disorder treatment issues and selection for in-patient psychotherapy. *British Journal of Psychiatry* 16, 723–31.

Paris, J. (1996) *Social factors in personality disorders: a biopsychosocial approach to etiology and treatment.* Cambridge University Press, Cambridge.

Pichot, P. (1978) Psychopathic behaviour: a historical overview. In *Approaches to Research Psychopathic Behaviour* (Hare, R. D. & Schalling, D., eds). Wiley, Chichester.

Platt-Koch, L. (1986) Clinical supervision for psychiatric nurses. *Nursing Management* 4(5), 13–15.

Porporino, F. J. & Motiuk, L. L. (1995) The prison careers of mentally disordered offenders. Special Issue. International Perspectives on Mental Health Issues in the Criminal Justice System. *International Journal of Law and Psychiatry* 18(1), 29–44.

Reed, J. (1994) *Report of the Department of Health and Home Office Working Group on Psychopathic Disorder.* Department of Health, London.

Rogers, C. (1961) *On Becoming a Person.* Houghton Mifflin, Boston.

Rogers, P. & Topping-Morris, B. (1997) Clinical supervision for forensic mental health nurses. *Nursing Management* 4(5), 13–15.

Sallah, D. (1994) Views on the future: care of psychopathically disordered patients. *Psychiatric Care* 1(4), 129–32.

Salter, A. C. (1988) *Treating Child Sex Offenders and their Victims. A Practical Guide.* Sage, Newbury Park, CA.

Smith, S. (1978) *The Psychopath in Society.* Academic Press, New York.

Strong, S. (1998) Sentenced to care. *Nursing Times* 94(2), 26–32.

Chapter 7
The Experience of Black Mentally Disordered Offenders

Anne Aiyegbusi

INTRODUCTION

A chapter about the experience of black people in a text aiming to examine forensic mental health nursing practice must get to the heart of the matter if it is to be relevant in the real world of clinical work with patients. Indeed, if black patients are to benefit, reality must be faced in a way which does not alienate them or their caregivers. Such is the emotional sensitivity of this subject area that a delicate pathway has necessarily been taken through territory which has tended to baffle professionals while arguably maintaining a suboptimal service to black mentally disordered offenders and their families.

In an attempt to move forward within the limited space of this small contribution, historical perspective is integrated with psychological theory. This leads to a logical and theoretically valid clinical formulation, recognising the longstanding consequences of disconnection, the inflicted humiliation of racism, and emotional invalidation about the fear, anger and pain this causes. Conceptualised as a particular form of psychological trauma, the toxic dynamics of chronic racism are also likely to pervade forensic services when a black perspective is lacking.

Awareness and commitment to tuning into the pain black patients feel may represent one vital step along the way to healing inter-racial wounds which threaten collaborative working and the strong therapeutic relationships forensic nurses must develop with all patients.

In light of research that has established a consistent picture of over-representation by African Caribbean males as patients in forensic mental health services, this population form the primary focus for the chapter. The experiences of other minority ethnic groups cannot be entirely generalised from its content but the principles of appreciating and working with diversity and difference will be of value when approaching the needs of any patients whose backgrounds are in the minority.

This chapter aims to provide a framework for assisting the development of forensic mental health nursing as a discipline which manages to validate patients equally and with the flexibility and insight to manage racial boundaries with empathy and understanding.

BLACK PEOPLE AND MENTAL HEALTH – AN OVERVIEW OF THE RESEARCH

Despite a degree of statistical variation, psychiatric studies consistently find elevated rates of psychosis among black people when compared with white people in the United Kingdom (Carpenter & Brockington, 1980; Bebbington *et al.*, 1981; Cochrane & Bal, 1987; McGovern & Cope, 1987a, b; Thomas *et al.*, 1993; McGovern *et al.*, 1994; Takei *et al.*, 1998). Relatively low levels of less severe mental health problems are diagnosed for black people when compared with white people according to the research. No satisfactory explanation has been found to account for this or the fact that personality disorder diagnoses are rarely formulated for members of the black community.

King *et al.* (1994) compared annual incidences of psychosis amongst people of different ethnic groups in the catchment area of a London psychiatric hospital. Schizophrenia and other major psychoses were more prevalent among all minority ethnic groups. This pattern was attributed to personal and social stressors associated with belonging to any minority ethnic group living in the United Kingdom. In contrast, low levels of minor disorder such as anxiety states and alcohol dependence were diagnosed when compared with whites. Other research has consistently found that the African Caribbean community experiences the highest rates of schizophrenia and other major psychoses, also receiving low rates of minor mental disorder according to patterns of psychiatric diagnoses.

Over recent decades a variety of explanations have been proffered to explain why the black community suffers such relatively poor mental health. They have included both the stress of migration and the possibility that those who migrate are amongst the most psychologically vulnerable individuals in a society and subsequently experience profound mental health problems upon settlement. Such theories, linking migration with mental health breakdown, have been discussed in detail by Littlewood & Lipsedge (1997, pp. 83–103).

Culturally specific manifestations of distress, misdiagnosed as psychotic illnesses in the setting of Eurocentric diagnostic criteria and the possibility of racial stereotyping whereby the more exuberant behavioural characteristics of blacks are misinterpreted and labelled as 'illness' have been hypothesised and are also discussed in detail by Littlewood & Lipsedge (1997, pp. 104–23). While these reasons may appear superficially plausible,

Littlewood & Lipsedge's (1997) conclusions correspond with research by McGovern *et al.* (1994) in suggesting that they cannot be regarded as strong enough to cause the previously described profile of mental health problems.

In accordance with the observations of King *et al.* (1994), the ongoing stress of racial discrimination has frequently been discussed and cited as a main variable in severe mental breakdown. Because little elaboration has tended to take place in clearly defining what the stress of racial discrimination actually entails in human terms and how it contributes to severe psychosis, its status as a causative factor remains vague.

BLACK PEOPLE AND FORENSIC MENTAL HEALTH SERVICES – AN OVERVIEW OF THE RESEARCH

In order to acquire some insight into the reasons why black people are so consistently over-represented in forensic mental health services, a multitude of interrelated factors need to be unravelled. In so doing, inferences can be made about what actually happens within the system to inadvertently but continually maintain such a pattern. As we have seen, there is a clear picture of black people experiencing significantly higher rates of severe psychological breakdown than whites in the United Kingdom. There then appears to be a pathway from this position to one where black people, especially males, are over-represented in populations characterised by both severe mental health problems and dangerousness. The relationship between those two variables is fairly clear within the forensic literature whereby untreated, acute psychotic symptoms consistently mediate violent and illegal acts (Link & Stueve, 1994). The question remains as to what possible mediating factors could result in such high levels of untreated, acute psychotic illness among black people.

In a very thorough paper, Boast & Chesterman (1995) explore many individual areas of thought and discussion to arrive at a putative model for explaining in a comprehensive way why there is an over-representation of black people detained in forensic mental health services. By employing research evidence from the fields of psychiatry and criminology, these authors critically analyse various factors previously associated with the forensic picture. They conclude that no deliberate, systematic bias operates against black people in the criminal justice and mental health systems. However, black people experience substantial disadvantage across a range of other spectrums. When these areas of disadvantage accumulate and interact, they clearly contribute to the tragedy which is now such a familiar fixture in forensic mental health work. In summary, Boast & Chesterman (1995) describe black people suffering socio-economic disadvantage in the form of material wealth, housing, education, employment opportunities and various support and care services. This picture is used to explain their relatively poor mental health and also their high arrest rates as both factors are increased in deprived populations.

Boast & Chesterman (1995) recognise relationships between untreated, acute psychotic symptoms, violence and crime. In relation to untreated acute symptoms, they suggest that 'mutual disenchantment' between psychiatric employees and black patients is a possible reason why patterns of early discharge and poor after-care feature so often. This trend is linked to high numbers of black mentally ill people eventually offending and receiving periods of compulsory detention. That is, psychotic illness remains untreated, so symptoms then escalate, increasing the risk of violence and offending.

Sellwood & Tarrier (1994) studied demographic factors associated with extreme non-compliance with depot medication in a population with schizophrenia. They found that gender and ethnicity were significant and that African Caribbean males were the group most likely to completely refuse prophylactic medication and they were almost twice as likely to do so than other groups. Sellwood & Tarrier (1994) link their finding about non-compliance with conditions found to characterise contacts black people have with mental health services in other research. Their experiences include frequent relapses and contact with services at a late stage in their illness when symptoms are most severe. Those particular factors have in turn been related to compulsory detention, increased likelihood of police intervention, high doses of neuroleptic medication being prescribed and the use of seclusion and restraint.

Perkins & Moodley (1993) noted that compliance with medication and treatment was associated with how people construe their difficulties. In a study of how recently admitted psychiatric patients understood their problems, these authors found that African Caribbeans tended to deny having any problems at all. Related to this, ethnicity determined how problems were construed and also legal status on admission whereby African Caribbeans were more likely to be compulsorily detained.

McGovern *et al.* (1994) followed up a sample of African Caribbeans and white people who had received a diagnosis of schizophrenia on their first admission. Black people had a worse clinical outcome with 25% detained in secure facilities at the time of follow-up compared with no white patients. More black people had been admitted from prison on forensic sections of the Mental Health Act 1983 when compared with white people during the period between first diagnosis and follow-up. Four variables were associated with the poor clinical outcome. They were living alone, unemployment, prior criminal conviction and a period of imprisonment, all occurring prior to first admission. The authors found that the African Caribbean patients were also significantly more likely than their white counterparts to have been separated from their parents for more than one year during childhood and also to have left home by the time of the follow-up study.

Much of the research so far described corresponds with what Littlewood & Lipsedge (1997) describe as those epidemiological studies which 'are largely concerned with "serious mental illness" which necessitates hospital admission (and thus easy collection of figures)'. Such research is favoured when grants are awarded, and as a result there is a failure to motivate academics towards exploring what causes the patterns so consistently uncovered by epidemiological research from more detailed or informed social and psychological perspectives. Disappointingly, little effort has been invested in the direction of identifying alternative treatment programmes to those which the black community clearly find so unattractive.

Numerous different descriptions of how black people fail to comply with the services offered to them can be found in the research. In formal academic terms, detail referring to what actually happens within the services appears to be decidedly light. The risk is that psychopathology will be regarded as the mediating factor. The forensic mental health system will be further examined within this chapter. Before that, the scene will be set by a review of relations between blacks and whites from a historical perspective in an attempt to analyse the background to what is now manifest in the state of black people's psychological health and the ill-fitting nature of services primarily designated to provide care and treatment in response.

BLACK PEOPLE AND MENTAL HEALTH – INTEGRATING THE HISTORICAL CONTEXT

Slavery

The forces which motivated European interest in Africa and its people can be safely described as economic. Columbus had discovered the Caribbean, and a means of capitalising on the natural resources of the islands was all that stood between Europeans and untold wealth. As history reveals, a source of labour was found in the people of Africa who were enslaved and trafficked by Europeans to be worked, often to death, in the sugar, tobacco and cotton plantations of southern American states and the Caribbean. It was here that African slaves, assuming they survived the treacherous sea crossings, were set to endure mercilessly brutal, physical, psychological and social conditions. Being torn from home and family and deliberately placed with others who did not share language or tribal customs was routine. This resulted in a disconnected race of people, dispossessed of their cultures, languages and other traditions as well as their families and social relationships. The ties that naturally bound people together were entirely shredded. The daily choice became that of 'submit or die' as the systematic process of dehumanisation began by destroying any evidence of individuality in mind, body or spirit (Grier & Cobbs, 1992).

The experience of slavery was worse for women by virtue of their gender. Rape and having children taken away to be sold elsewhere into a life many believed to be far worse than death were among many of the particular threats which conspired to keep slave women in a perpetual state of terror.

EARLY PSYCHIATRY

Given the above situation, it may seem unsurprising that running parallel with the exploitation of Africans by Europeans for material gain, the powerful institutions of religion, medicine and law uniformly declared the inferiority of black people when compared with whites. A position supposedly determined by God and nature was subsequently legitimised by man. Due to obvious gains in maintaining the status quo, pseudo-ideology underpinned this position and was largely unchallenged. Psychiatry, biased as it was by socio-economic rich pickings, endorsed a view of biologically determined inferiority, espousing research findings to justify a social order reliant on a belief in the subhuman mental functioning of black people.

Littlewood & Lipsedge (1997) describe how, in the early days of slavery, black people were considered incapable of suffering mental illness and this was attributed to the fact they were somehow naturally insane. This theory was reinforced by beliefs that blacks could retain their equilibrium only as long as they existed in primitive simplicity. Supposedly, freedom from slavery could only result in a decline in the slaves' mental health status. Later, they were found to be vulnerable to experiencing specific mental illnesses including drapetomania which was 'diagnosed' by the presence of an irresistible urge to run away from the plantations.

Dysaethesia Aethiopis was another illness which slaves were particularly vulnerable to. This condition was said to include the 'symptoms' of wastefulness, destructiveness and disregard for the rights of property. This condition was considered to be brought about by freedom (Fernando, 1991). These 'diagnoses' from the nineteenth century serve as early examples of how the struggles of black people, in the face of appalling circumstances, were classified and pathologised while ignoring the social and interpersonal context in which they occurred.

Despite the atrocities perpetrated upon black people during slavery, European academics and social reporters freely espoused not only the biological and spiritual inferiority of blacks but also their supposed moral ineptitude. Howitt & Owusu-Bempah (1994) in their lively text about the racism of psychology quote a narrative by the Scottish philosopher David Hume (1711–1776). Hume, when commenting upon the intrinsic inferiority of black people, observed:

'They are characterised by idleness, treachery, nastiness and intemperance. They, that is the Negroes, are strangers to every sentiment of compassion, and are an awful example of the corruption of man left to himself.'

It is worth bearing in mind factual details about the context of these remarks. That is, black people, after being forced into bondage, were routinely beaten, raped and murdered by white people who were ruthlessly and savagely wringing from them virtually any essence that could indicate life. Regardless of given rationalisations, this was actually for no other reason than material gain. By the time of Hume's remarks, slavery had been a deeply embedded fact of life. Dynamically, Hume's narrative is undoubtedly a sample of the kind of collective projective process so typical of racism. Unconsciously, unacceptable and intolerable aspects of a group or society are psychologically split off and attributed to another collective who are in turn regarded as suitable receptacles for these projections and who then act as host. Victims of racism can be expected to unconsciously project their power, independence, competence and dominance into the racial oppressors. Such processes deplete all concerned.

POST-COLONIALISM

Following the abolition of slavery, black people were subjected to almost a century and a half of colonialism. Ironically, approximately 400 years after slavery began, it was again labour that motivated the British government to invite young adults from the Caribbean to emigrate to the 'Mother Country'. With a shortage of labour and a booming economy following the Second World War, African Caribbeans were felt to be a useful source of labour for supporting further post-war developments (Bryan *et al.*, 1985). Once again this population were considered 'units of easily accessible labour' (Williams, 1996). In their turn, African Caribbeans were said to have regarded Britain as variously, 'The land of milk and honey', with 'streets paved with gold'. This may be all the more understandable given their observations of everything of material value being exported from their own lands to Europe where anybody of power was known to have originated (Bryan *et al.*, 1985).

IMMIGRATION TO POST-WAR BRITAIN

Dreams were not fulfilled. Far from finding a welcoming 'Mother Country', these black people found hostile rejection. Rather than streets paved with gold, the grey and dismal landscapes of inner city Britain were largely the only places they could afford to live and it is indeed in these communities that the majority settled. Housing, health, child care and educational requirements were afforded little consideration by a government whose priority was simply to find labour for low status work which the indigenous population were reluctant to do (Bryan *et al.*, 1985; Williams, 1996).

So, metaphorically speaking, the rich, plump and bejewelled 'Mother Country' oozed no milk and no honey. Instead, a cold and mocking nightmare unfolded for too many people who, once in its grip, rejecting as it was, would wait a long time before they were to feel at home again. This particular 'mother' was no more prepared to give or to share what was good than she had ever been.

Because early immigrants from the Caribbean were generally young adults, many had left children behind as part of their plans of short-term work, sacrifice and separation for longer term gain and advancement. As history shows, Britain's economic boom was short lived. When in a financial position to do so, parents were able to send for their children. In many cases this was accelerated by the pending Immigration Act of 1969 (Bryan *et al.*, 1985).

It must be noted that British society had recently been devastated by two world wars in relatively quick succession. De Zulueta (1993) describes how in 'what appears to be a socially induced form of psychological defence, patriotic stoicism was encouraged, with the result that pre-war funeral and mourning customs were abandoned' after the First World War and into the aftermath of the second. In such a social context, the sense of grief and loss, often unresolved but nevertheless felt by the indigenous population should not be undermined in relation to their ability to welcome an influx of black immigrants from the Caribbean. No account of these predictable difficulties appears to have been taken by the government of the day.

THE EXPERIENCE OF CHILDREN

The bitter journey of African Caribbean children was typically and understandably traumatic. Young children were separated from their parent or parents at the time of initial emigration from the Caribbean. They were likely to be separated again from surrogate caregivers and attachment figures to join parents they could sometimes barely remember after years apart from them. Sometimes, adjustments had to be made for whole new families of brothers and sisters. The bewilderment, trauma and profound sense of loss experienced by this generation of black children were compounded by requirements that they adapt to the cold, run-down and depressing inner city environments which were in stark contrast to the warm sunshine of home (Bryan *et al.*, 1985). Williams (1996) notes how these circumstances diametrically oppose the ideological perspectives of the time,

based on important observations by the eminent English child psycho-
analysts, John Bowlby and D. W. Winnicott. Their work clearly describes
the extreme and largely long-term emotional difficulties experienced by
young children who are separated from their mothers or other primary
attachment figures for significant periods. In his groundbreaking attachment
theory, Bowlby (1988) refers to 'the secure base'. Its loss is recognised as a
major psychological trauma, with the potential to profoundly damage
mental health and abilities to develop and maintain relationships with
others (van der Kolk, 1987).

These children often experienced a loss of caregiving relationships on
two occasions during their earliest and most delicate developmental phases.
The second of these phases took them to a grossly unsupportive social
environment. A secure social environment is key to positive adaptation
following such enormous loss (Bowlby, 1988). While these circumstances
could and clearly have been survived by many, others with the risk of
damaged attachment systems already high, may have simply found the
adjustment required of them too much to psychologically manage.

Schooling, usually in the worst conditions the UK could possibly offer,
was unlikely to have included meaningful sensitivity to their plight. Predictably disoriented, they were plunged into an environment of prolonged,
routine hostility, consisting of verbal, physical and psychological assaults
on their sense of identity (Bryan *et al.*, 1985). Children, with their immature
psychological defence systems, were certainly unlikely to have an emotional
vocabulary through which they could make sense of or communicate their
confusion and feelings of vulnerability. Logically and clinically, childhood
depression was almost certainly commonplace in the midst of an invalidating social environment which failed to properly acknowledge or contextualise their distress. Albeit retrospective, this hypothesis is theoretically
viable and clinical experience suggests it reflects the cases of many black
people who have subsequently found themselves using forensic mental
health services. Their stories are so painfully similar. At the time, such
thoughts were obviously a long way from the minds of those agencies
tasked with the children's welfare, particularly in schools where teachers,
firmly in possession of their own racial stereotypes, were unlikely to have
had much scope in the way of alternative reference points. However, this
stage in history seems to have been neither satisfactorily explored nor
explained (Williams, 1996).

CONTINUING THE 'MENTAL INFERIORITY OF BLACKS' DEBATE

Early attempts to describe the inferiority of black people were undoubtedly
cruel and damaging. With the passage of time, though, they were also easily

identified as communicating much about racist priorities of the era. By the 1950s and 1960s scientific rigour had emerged as a tool to convey legitimised and more subtle messages about the mental unsophistication of black people and how this was the cause of their downtrodden position in a natural social order. Influential psychologists such as Arthur Jensen in America and Hans Eysenck in England forcefully promoted their findings that intelligence was attributed by race. The implication was that, due to the limited capacity of black people's minds resulting from inferior genetic endowment, efforts to improve their lot were a waste of time and energy as they did not have the fundamental neurophysiological equipment to do anything constructive with such opportunities (Fernando, 1991; Howitt & Owusu-Bempah, 1994; Richards, 1997). These particular theories have since been discredited. Nevertheless, in their time they were powerful forces which were sufficiently credible that when explanations for the poor academic performance of black children were sought, it was thought necessary to look no further than their race (Howitt & Owusu-Bempah, 1994).

The academic underachievement of black schoolchildren was considered by Bernard Coard (1971) to be a byproduct of an interaction between culturally alienated, frightened children and the British education system. Coard observed the education system to be completely insensitive to their needs. It was felt to do little more than further distress the children. Coard (1971) delivers a stinging response to the trend of placing black children into schools for the educationally subnormal on the basis of IQ test results and the recommendations of educational psychologists. He locates the source of poor results in the manner of assessment and cultural differences between typical classroom behaviour in Britain compared with the Caribbean. This meant that the quieter, more compliant African Caribbean child was perceived as subnormal or simmeringly hostile when the more competitive, garrulous behaviour which typified British children was taken as the normative standard.

Despite comments by people like Coard, the trend of black failure had begun. It is unfortunate that again the focus of clinical attention about psychological observations had shifted from actual social experience to biological conjecture. It is notable that consideration about the effects of early loss and separation on this generation of children seems to be strangely absent from the literature. None the less, these experiences must have been felt at an emotional level as abandonment and depersonalisation. When psychological trauma is complicated by adverse environmental factors, severe emotional distress, manifest in behavioural disturbance and cognitive impairment, is a fairly predictable outcome (de Zulueta, 1993). However, psychological trauma and its effects have only been formally acknowledged by the international mental health community in relatively recent years, and the significance of chronic trauma, especially during childhood, remains an area of continuing debate (Herman, 1992; Pynoos et al., 1996).

It seems clear that, in the context of widespread distress, failure and even behavioural disturbance by black children, British establishments were prepared either directly or indirectly to attribute this to inherent racial inferiority (Williams, 1996). With hindsight, psychological trauma provides an appropriate and meaningful model, but surprisingly in academic circles little effort has been made to apply it in a formal and valid way despite the fact that vague descriptions of social stress are commonly used as an explanation for the high rates of severe mental health problems experienced by black people in adult life.

THE SECOND GENERATION

By the mid 1970s a new generation of British born and raised black children were approaching adolescence and in the context of social change on both sides of the Atlantic were able to experience a more positive self-image. Fuelled by media-generated opportunities to defend against the often dour realities of poor, working-class British culture, escapism and a more satisfying sense of identity were possible through the comparatively uplifting influences of the time, including concepts such as 'Black Power'. Unfortunately, as Bryan *et al.* (1985) point out, this increased self-esteem was met with societal suspicion and obsession with the idea of black criminality such as 'mugging' and other acts of violence against white people and white society. Excessive cannabis usage could be added to these stereotypical suspicions. So, far from achieving an increased sense of belonging or assimilation, as is often assumed, those who are referred to as 'second generation' merely faced a different set of barriers, both socially and psychologically, than their parents did. In many ways this was heaped on top of long-term invalidation and rejection by a wider society with whom they would never fully belong but dare not be separate from either. Predictably, this would result in severe stress arising from maintaining a less threatening but false self, to avoid envious attacks. It amounts to a form of subjugation. As McGovern & Cope (1987b) noted, the second generation experienced even worse mental health than the first generation of African Caribbeans in the United Kingdom.

BLACK PEOPLE EXPERIENCING CONTEMPORARY MENTAL HEALTH SYSTEMS – IN SHARPER FOCUS

Research is at best unfocused and vague about the experiences black people have within mental health systems. Importantly, methodological shortfalls mean that interpersonal phenomena are not captured.

Public inquiry reports provide an additional source of information and their nature is such that a different, perhaps sharper lens can be applied to inspect the routine care and treatment experiences that black people have. A series of well publicised inquiry reports are referred to here and it is strongly suggested that the conditions found are representative of a wider system, contrary to the conclusions of researchers such as Boast & Chesterman (1995).

Ashworth Inquiry 1992

The Report of the Committee of Inquiry into allegations of brutality to patients at Ashworth high security psychiatric hospital revealed the presence of an overtly racist culture in parts of the hospital where some nurses were members of extreme right-wing racist organisations. Their doctrines were evident and a small minority of staff members allegedly intimidated patients and colleagues alike. Evidence suggested that black male patients were sometimes regarded in a stereotypical way, as though they were all the same, by clinical teams who confused one case with another (Blom-Cooper *et al.*, 1992).

Ashworth Hospital HAS Report, 1995

Further public scrutiny into Ashworth Hospital occurred in 1994 in the form of a review by the Health Advisory Service. In the report (HAS, 1995), the team comment upon the hospital's response to 'cultural and ethnicity issues'. The fact that the hospital is essentially 'a white establishment' was recognised and while attempts to address the needs of patients from diverse ethnic and cultural backgrounds was welcomed, the review team note:

'Discussions with a wide range of groups and individual staff members on cultural and ethnic issues, revealed to the review team, a marked tendency to collapse the issues into considerations of language, diet or religion.'

Inquiry considering the deaths of three African Caribbean male patients at Broadmoor Hospital, 1993

The sub-title 'Big, Black and Dangerous' reflects the way this term was frequently used to describe black, mostly African Caribbean, male patients according to the inquiry report (SHSA, 1993). Culturally, Broadmoor high security psychiatric hospital was reportedly a white, mostly middle class establishment which was unable to make contact with black inner city experience, despite the backgrounds of its African Caribbean patients.

While not in touch with, or able to understand their experiences, the hospital was also unable to understand how subtle racism operated. This position was problematic to some patients who reported that their complaints were met with dismissal and suggestions that they were based on delusional thought. Furthermore, in relation to the previous deaths, black patients revealed to the inquiry team that they were often frightened that they were being 'killed off'.

The report makes a number of observations about the care and treatment of black patients which experience suggests cannot be confined to Broadmoor Hospital. They include an all-round lack of emphasis on getting to know black patients as individuals, reliance on tranquillising medication to control behavioural disturbance; and failure to consider psychotherapy or counselling interventions. Diet, therapies and other activities reflected lack of thought about the emotional impact detention in the alien environment of a high security psychiatric hospital had on black patients who were admitted there for long periods of time.

Diagnostic problems in regard to the black mentally disordered population were recognised and an affective dimension to psychotic illness was discussed. The confidence psychiatrists typically placed on black patients' alleged cannabis abuse being significant to their mental health was noted, as was the lack of attention to what were seen as more obvious variables such as the experience of growing up in inner city environments.

In relation to Orville Blackwood, whose death in a seclusion room provided the main focus for investigation, the circumstances described above apply, as does the fact that he was regarded as having some degree of learning disability or low intelligence despite the fact that psychological testing carried out in the hospital's own psychology department had revealed a higher than average IQ score. His intellect was verified by a number of witnesses, including family members who knew him whereas it was undermined by some professionals. Reportedly, his talents and interests were not encouraged while his expressions of anger and frustration were seemingly met with oppression and control.

Inquiry into the case of Christopher Clunis, 1994

The Report of the Inquiry into the Care and Treatment of Christopher Clunis (Ritchie *et al.*, 1994) identified a cumulation of problems. Christopher Clunis had received many short admissions, without after-care, seemingly for what were regarded as acute episodes of psychosis but which were clearly all part of a longstanding severe illness. In the five and a half years between Christopher Clunis's first contact with psychiatry services and the manslaughter of his victim, Jonathan Zito, no real attempt was made by mental health services to understand who he was. His sister reported to the inquiry that, despite continual family involvement, no service had ever contacted family members to clarify his history, despite the fact that he often gave blatantly false information.

A psychological characteristic of Christopher Clunis which neither mental health services nor, in any meaningful way, the inquiry team picked up has been illustrated (Harris, 1994). That is, the way loss or separation from important attachments had an observedly 'profound effect' upon his mental health. In the case of Christopher Clunis, the inquiry team note the willingness with which mental health services were prepared to attribute his disturbed presentation to misuse of drugs despite there never being any evidence to support this. In fact the reverse was so in repeated negative results of drug screens. Harris (1994) is critical about both these observations which typify the experience of black people using psychiatry services where their experience of depression is overlooked while drug-induced explanations are accepted with too much readiness. It seems quite clear that, from the patients' perspective, clinical approaches of this nature would predictably drift in a direction of control, domination and invalidation. Suspicion leading to further intrusion, and humiliating disempowerment rather than discontinuing the approaches when they prove to be fruitless, typically seal this curious cycle.

LOCATING A VOID BETWEEN RESEARCH AND REALITY

Some consistent themes can be observed throughout the literature. Put simply, an obvious social and psychological void has been maintained over time in regard to actual black experience and the official picture painted by clinical and academic disciplines. Sadly, this picture, shallow and distorted as it undoubtedly is, informs the way services are delivered. Their long-standing failure to achieve basic aims, such as developing interventions to effectively treat and at least alleviate the psychological distress experienced by large numbers of black people in a way which enables them to engage in a meaningful lifestyle, can be understood in terms of that void. The suggestion is that rather than reducing dangerousness, an absence of engagement and trust through positive therapeutic relationships runs the risk of prolonging or even increasing it.

INTRODUCING A BLACK PERSPECTIVE

Harris (1994) describes 'the Black perspective' in the following terms:

'The Black perspective is both analytical and perceptual. The very act of living and attempting to survive in a racist society has provided Black people with a unique and valuable body of empirical knowledge. The Black perspective derives both its insight and inspiration from this source.'

Realistically, the void between the reality of black people's experience and the picture indicated by both research and clinical practice surrounding their distress can be understood as stemming from an absence of 'the black perspective' in terms of shaping academic debate and influencing clinical practice. Essentially, to effectively provide a service to black people, a basic requirement is an ability to see and experience the world in the way in which black people do. To date this seems not to have happened to any extent that significantly impacts on policy, service design or delivery. The roots of the prevailing void can be located in the domain of inter-racial relationships.

ASSESSMENT AND MANAGEMENT

Relationships

In order to assess black mentally disordered patients, it is critical to understand black history and to validate it as a real human experience. To do otherwise leads to constricted, biased interpretation, inevitably to the detriment of black patients. When this happens, it is accompanied by a high risk of denial or minimisation about the way specific, adverse psychosocial factors have influenced psychological development and eventually impacted upon clinical presentation. This perpetuates a traditional pattern of attributing psychopathology entirely to individual vulnerability. Alternatively, or in fact additionally, there is a risk of considering the stress of racism as only relevant to the patient's experience with other people or agencies when it is also likely to be relevant in the 'here and now'. This possibility is difficult to think about, as professionals tend to vigorously defend against entertaining ideas of themselves as racist. Meanwhile, the consequences of defensively invalidating and denying what the patient may be feeling is clearly unhelpful and undoubtedly anti-therapeutic with all the hallmarks of racial oppression.

A useful paradigm is proposed by Dalal (1993) who suggests race may be more usefully viewed as a dynamic process rather than as a static entity. When this model is adopted, it becomes impossible to separate the experience of black people from their relationship with white people and vice versa. This position appears to have no less relevance today than at any other point in history. In clinical situations, psychodynamic processes of transference and counter-transference provide a more therapeutic way of understanding what is going on within inter-racial relationships and indeed intra-racial ones, especially in terms of understanding what the patient is feeling. Equally, a psychodynamic formulation would aim to increase professionals' awareness of their own feelings and behaviour.

In need of a working formulation

Any attempt to assess or manage the needs of black mentally disordered offenders must take into account 'the Black perspective'. To do so involves validating the prolonged victimisation which is an inherent part of black experience in the United Kingdom. How it influences crime and mental health requires further research but the existing literature provides sufficient clues to inform at least a loose hypothesis. In turn, acceptance of such a hypothesis seems justifiable as by far surpassing that which is currently available and which fails badly.

As Grier & Cobbs (1992) point out, black people have 'no special psychology or exceptional genetic determinants'. The psychological defence mechanisms of black people are the same as those employed by anyone else. However, history and the context in which they occur are different from those of white people or indeed other minority ethnic groups, and this shapes the current clinical picture during episodes of mental ill health. Necessarily, the interplay between ethnic groups is important, and in this context the relationship between black and white people is critical to understanding the way black people experience forensic mental health services. Racially specific power and privilege differentials dictate that black people are far more likely to be patients while professional groups are predominantly white. The experience of black professionals who work in or have contact with forensic services represents a separate though related issue which is beyond the scope of this chapter with its focus on patients. Nevertheless, it is worth mentioning that the toxicity of directly received, personal racist encounters and those which are vicariously experienced through bearing witness to, and necessarily identifying with, patients' dilemmas, hardly encourages black professionals to work within forensic mental health services. It is suggested that this is a serious problem in many services but one that remains largely unexplored.

To regard the level of psychopathology experienced by black people as unrelated to social position and their experience of a lifetime of inflicted humiliation is too simple. While formal diagnostic issues will remain complicated as long as the present practice of psychiatry prevails, this preoccupation is probably less relevant to the theory and practice of forensic mental health nursing with its key role of developing and maintaining interpersonal relationships with patients. As such, it is likely to be more critical for nurses to gain insight into patients' internal worlds. This invariably involves appreciating the role of loss at an individual and also a generational level, in addition to what a lifetime of repeated racial abuse and discrimination entails from a developmental perspective and how this influences the patient's relationships with those of the same race as their tormentors. The African American feminist writer and therapist, Bell Hooks (1995) formulates this as often amounting to 'profound debilitating life-threatening psychological pain'. Hooks is referring to the consequence of prolonged racism, personally and vicariously, to the extent that chronically low self-esteem, humiliation and the expectations that go with these devastating feelings are internalised into the developing personality structure and form part of the self. Ultimately, negative projections are internalised by the recipient who acts them out in identification.

While forensic patients primarily present as offenders or perpetrators, the link with past victimisation is also a part of clinical work. The discipline of forensic psychotherapy, while making no reference to the existence of black people in its publications so far, nevertheless emphasises the victim in the offender. Indeed, in order to understand the offender, it is often necessary to clarify the significance of that person's experience of being a victim given that it is likely to be played out or re-enacted within their relationships, in the offence situation and repeatedly thereafter within therapeutic relationships. This pattern is summed up in the term 'cycles of abuse and deprivation' whereby individuals repeatedly re-create the conditions of their own deprivation and abuse as either victim or perpetrator, in literal or disguised form (Herman, 1992; de Zulueta, 1993). Mediated by the attachment system, these cycles are typically perpetuated throughout generations of families unless they can be discontinued.

Welldon (1993) describes the aim of forensic psychotherapy as:

'...the psychodynamic understanding of the offender and their consequent treatment regardless of the seriousness of the offence. It involves understanding the unconscious motivation in the criminal mind which underlies the offences.'

Psychopathological features associated with early abuse and deprivation are set out by Welldon (1993) in terms of:

- a need to be in control which is evident from the moment they are seen
- vulnerability to anything reminiscent of the original conditions of abuse and deprivation
- a desire for revenge expressed in sado-masochism as an unconscious need to inflict harm
- eroticisation or sexualisation of the act
- manic defence against depression

These psychopathological features provide an insight into how early experiences of abuse and deprivation are manifest in specific personality characteristics, shared by individuals who later offend and who may also experience significant mental health problems. In order to apply a 'black perspective' to this, it is obviously important to understand not only the experience of individual patients but also those experiences which are specific to the black population. These are likely to include a generational trauma, prolonged victimisation in the form of racist abuse and discrimination and an expectation, borne out through lengthy past experience, of invalidation by whites. This invalidation is likely to be particularly apparent as far as denial of blacks' anger and rage about racism is concerned, while their pain is defensively 'tuned out' by whites (Hooks, 1995) who simply cannot tolerate it. Complications such as abandonment with subsequent fostering or adoption by white families are far from uncommon and equally relevant in understanding the psychopathology of individual patients. The same applies to patients of mixed race parentage who present a different constellation of factors which in turn influence their self-image as well as their particular view of racial boundaries.

It is the contention of this chapter that damaging scenarios are repeatedly played out in the psychological dynamics between black and white people in forensic mental health services. Literal re-enactments of common racial dramas are not discounted but they are more likely to be evident, dynamically, in disguised form, especially through the transferences and counter-transferences operating within the social environments of secure units and hospitals, in turn reflecting the wider society.

Examples include such projective processes as splitting whereby excessive concerns about antisocial impulses, organised criminal activity and sexual danger are mainly, if not exclusively, focused towards black patients. We can also cite many examples of envious spoiling when black people are seen to be enjoying themselves, especially with each other. This scenario is all the more poignant because, through the centuries of unbearable suffering, black people necessarily found release internally, relying on an enhanced relationship with their more spiritual or esoteric human capacities in order to survive psychically. This quality has remained evident over the generations and is manifest culturally in an inherent liveliness and exuberance arising from an everyday focus on inner experience as well as external events, on accommodating for possibilities beyond the logical, mechanical and functional as a way of adapting to the struggle to find meaning and enjoyment in life. All too often this is regarded as threatening and so it is stifled in forensic services. The consequences of denying black people the opportunity to express themselves is a further example of subjugation and arises unconsciously out of envy and the need to defend against primitive anxiety aroused by difference.

In terms of understanding the emotional deadlock dictating the slow pace of change, Campling (1989), when discussing the absence of black people either as clients or therapists in a Leicester psychotherapy department, seems to grasp the point. She states:

'We cannot open the doors to black patients and hope to exclude the pain and hurt of racism from our therapeutic encounters. It is this we resist and I believe worries about "cultural sensitivity" are in part a rationalisation.'

This emotional deadlock can also be understood by employing a trauma paradigm. As Herman (1992) explains: 'The conflict between the will to deny horrible events and the will to proclaim them aloud is the central dialectic of psychological trauma'.

Herman (1992) also points out that victims of trauma, by the way they attempt to tell their stories sometimes through symptoms or in a disjointed verbal narrative, are prone to being disbelieved by those who are required to bear witness. According to Herman: 'Denial, repression and dissociation operate on a social as well as an individual level'.

These dynamics are key to understanding the difficulties which underlie attempts to effectively assess and manage the racially specific clinical needs of black forensic patients. They are central to many therapeutic relationships. The way that re-enactments occur has been emphasised by Davies (1996) who writes about the internal world of the offender and how this gets acted out unconsciously by multi-disciplinary teams. Davies (1996) describes how professionals '. . . who deal with offenders are not free agents but actors who have been assigned roles in the individual offender's own re-enactment of their internal world drama'. And, according to Davies (1996), 'The professionals have the choice not to perform but they can only make this choice when they know what the role is they are trying to avoid'.

It seems quite logical, therefore, that if the role of racial abuser is to be avoided, patients' past experience and the high risk of this being re-enacted in the 'here and now' must be understood and acknowledged before effective care and treatment can occur. Because it is sensitive and requires open-mindedness and self-awareness to a degree that may involve painful self-reflection, support for professionals is much needed too. It could be reasonably argued that this is in the nature of forensic mental health nursing. If so, an important drawback in regard to managing the emotional challenge where race is concerned lies with the absence of a theoretical framework which enables the relevant issues to be worked through in a supportive way.

A WAY FORWARD?

Herman (1992) has described how understanding psychological trauma begins by rediscovering history. This seems like a good point to close this chapter. It is hoped that the work presented here does in fact go some way towards 'rediscovering history' as far as the African Caribbean community are concerned, and that it leads to a greater understanding at an individual and a collective level of black people who are also forensic patients. In so doing, perhaps thought and action may be stimulated towards enabling further clarity, especially in a quantifiable way, focusing upon racially specific psychological trauma and its generational roots. In the meantime, this paradigm should provide something of a platform from which forensic mental health nurses can begin to appreciate and validate how black patients feel about being in their care, and in so doing recognise what occurs within the important space of therapeutic relationships.

REFERENCES

Bebbington, P. E., Hurry, J. & Tennant, C. (1981) Psychiatric disorders in selected immigrant groups in Camberwell. *Social Psychiatry* **16**, 43–51.

Blom-Cooper, L., Brown, M., Dolan, R. & Murphy, E. (1992) *Report of the Committee of Inquiry into Complaints about Ashworth Hospital.* HMSO, London.

Boast, N. & Chesterman, P. (1995) Black people and secure psychiatric facilities: patterns of processing and the role of stereotypes. *British Journal of Criminology* **35**(2), 218–35.

Bowlby, J. (1988) *A Secure Base: Clinical Applications of Attachment Theory.* Routledge, London.

Bryan, B., Dadzie, S. & Scafe, S. (1985) *The Heart of the Race: Black Women's Lives in Britain.* Virago, London.

Campling, P. (1989) Race, culture and psychotherapy. *Psychiatric Bulletin* **13**, 550–51.

Carpenter, L. & Brockington, I. F. (1980) A study of mental illness in Asians, West Indians and Africans in Manchester. *British Journal of Psychiatry* **137**, 201–205.

Coard, B (1971) *How the West Indian Child is Made Educationally Subnormal in the British School System.* New Beacon, London.

Cochrane, R. and Bal, S. S. (1987) Migration and schizophrenia: an examination of five hypotheses. *Social Psychiatry* **22**, 181–91.

Dalal, F. N. (1993) Race and racism: an attempt to organise difference. *Group Analysis* **26**, 277–93.

Davies, R. (1996) The interdisciplinary network and the internal world of the offender. In *Forensic Psychotherapy: Crime, Psychodynamics and the Offender*, Part 2, pp. 133–44 (Cordess, C. & Cox, M., eds). Jessica Kingsley, London.

de Zulueta, F. (1993) *From Pain to Violence: The Traumatic Roots of Destructiveness.* Whurr, London.

Fernando, S. (1991) *Mental Health, Race and Culture.* Macmillan, London.

Grier, W. H. & Cobbs, P. M. (1992) *Black Rage*, 3rd edn. Basic Books, USA.

Harris, V. (1994) *Review of the Report of the Inquiry into the Care and Treatment of Christopher Clunis: A Black Perspective.* Race Equality Unit, London.

Health Advisory Service (1995) *With Care in Mind Secure.* HMSO, London.

Herman, J. L. (1992) *Trauma and Recovery: From Domestic Abuse to Political Terror.* Basic Books, London.

Hooks, B. (1995) *Killing Rage: Ending Racism*. Penguin, London.

Howitt, D. & Owusu-Bempah, J. (1994) *The Racism of Psychology: Time for a Change*. Harvester-Wheatsheaf, Hemel Hempstead.

King, M., Coker, E., Leavey, G., Hoare, A. & Johnson-Sabine, E. (1994) Incidence of psychotic illness in London: comparison of ethnic groups. *British Medical Journal* 309, 1115–19.

Link, B. J. & Stueve, A. (1994) Psychotic symptoms and the violent/illegal behaviour of mental patients compared to community controls. In: *Violence and Mental Disorder: Developments in Risk Assessment* (Monahan, J. & Steadman, H. J. P, eds), pp. 137–59. University of Chicago Press, Chicago.

Littlewood, R. & Lipsedge, M. (1997) *Aliens and Alienists: Ethnic Minorities and Psychiatry*, 3rd edn. Routledge, London.

McGovern, D. & Cope, R. V. (1987a) The compulsory detention of males of different ethnic groups, with special reference to offender patients. *British Journal of Psychiatry* 150, 505–12.

McGovern, D. & Cope, R. V. (1987b) First psychiatric admission rates of first and second generation Afro Caribbeans. *Social Psychiatry* 22, 139–49.

McGovern, D., Hemmings, P., Cope, R. & Lowerson, A. (1994) Long term follow-up of young Afro-Caribbean Britons and white Britons with a first admission diagnosis of schizophrenia. *Social Psychiatry and Psychiatric Epidemiology* 29, 8–19.

Perkins, R. E. & Moodley, P. (1993) Perceptions of problems in psychiatric patients: denial, race and service usage. *Social Psychiatry and Psychiatric Epidemiology* 28, 189–93.

Pynoos, R. S., Steinberg, A. M. & Goenjian, A. (1996) Traumatic stress in childhood and adolescence: recent developments and current controversies. In *Traumatic Stress: The Effects of Overwhelming Experience on Mind, Body, and Society*, pp. 331–58 (van der Kolk, B. A., McFarlane, A. C. & Weisaeth, L., eds). Guildford Press, New York.

Richards, G. (1997) *'Race', Racism and Psychology: Towards a Reflexive History*. Routledge, London.

Ritchie, J. H., Dick, D. & Lingham, R. (1994) *Report of the Inquiry into the Care and Treatment of Christopher Clunis*. HMSO, London.

Sellwood, W. & Tarrier, N. (1994) Demographic factors associated with extreme non-compliance in schizophrenia. *Social Psychiatry and Psychiatric Epidemiology* 29, 172–7.

Special Hospitals Service Authority (1993) *Report of the Committee of Inquiry into the Death in Broadmoor Hospital of Orville Blackwood and a Review of the Deaths of Two Other Afro-Caribbean Patients: 'Big, Black and Dangerous?'*. SHSA, London.

Takei, N., Persaud, R., Woodruff, P., Brockington, I. & Murray, R. M. (1998) First episodes of psychosis in Afro-Caribbean and white people. An 18-year follow-up population-based study. *British Journal of Psychiatry* 172, 147–53.

Thomas, C. S., Stone, K., Osborn, M., Thomas, P. F. & Fisher, M. (1993) Psychiatric morbidity and compulsory admission among UK-born Europeans, Afro-Caribbeans and Asians in Central Manchester. *British Journal of Psychiatry* 163, 91–9.

van der Kolk, B. A., ed. (1987) The separation cry and the trauma response: developmental issues in the psychobiology of attachment and separation. In *Psychological Trauma*, pp. 31–62. American Psychiatric Press, Washington.

Welldon, E. V. (1993) Forensic psychotherapy and group analysis. *Group Analysis* **26**(4), 487–502.

Williams, F. (1996) 'Race', welfare and community care: A historical perspective. In *'Race' and Community Care* (Ahmad, W. I. U. & Atkin, K., eds), pp. 15–28. Open University Press, Buckingham.

Chapter 8
Risk Assessment and Management

Mike Doyle

INTRODUCTION

In recent years there has been growing interest in the risks associated with people with mental disorder. Assessing and managing risk to others is fundamental to the practice of mental health professionals in forensic services. Evidence has been growing that mentally disordered people are a risk to others as a result of their mental disorder (Swanson *et al.*, 1990; Monahan, 1992; Coid, 1996). Forensic mental health nurses (FMHNs) play a key role in risk assessment and risk management, which are seen as advanced forms of nursing intervention (Royal College of Nursing (RCN), 1997a). How these advanced interventions are implemented is not entirely clear. This chapter provides an overview of risk assessment and risk management in relation to forensic mental health services. First the characteristics of risk will be briefly considered to try to elucidate the components of risk and how they relate to forensic mental health services.

Despite the importance of the subject area there still appears to be a scarcity of valid and reliable frameworks for assessing and managing risk. The risk management cycle is presented as a simple problem-solving framework to assist FMHNs to identify, assess and manage risk. Combining this cycle with a systematic approach to the delivery of care via the Care Programme Approach will be discussed.

The risk to others posed by people with mental disorder is of great concern to the public and mental health professionals alike. The raison d'être of forensic services is to assess those individuals perceived as dangerous or a risk to others as a result of their disorder and provide care, treatment and management. Evidence for the link between mental disorder and harm to others is reviewed and factors associated with an increased risk to others are considered with recommendations on which information FMHNs need to assimilate in order to reliably inform their clinical judgement.

Although risk to others is the principal reason for the development and expansion of forensic mental health services, those who come into contact with these services usually have a multiplicity of problems which may place them at risk to themselves. The risk of self-harm and suicide will be considered in relation to individuals who are in contact with forensic services.

Risks to self and others, perhaps understandably, tend to be viewed as the main risks that mental health services are expected to focus upon. However, users of mental health services are subjected to many risks which are not necessarily viewed as priorities for action by services. These risks tend to have a significant impact on the individual's well-being, quality of life and ability to function as a 'normal' citizen. The relevance of these risks is highlighted in the hope that they will receive due consideration in the future.

ROLE OF THE FORENSIC MENTAL HEALTH NURSE IN CLINICAL RISK MANAGEMENT

Risk assessment is an inexact science. Ultimately the decision on level of risk is based on clinical judgement. From the legal perspective the judgement of the responsible medical officer is paramount, although ideally in practice decisions on risk should be made by a multi-disciplinary team involving all the clinicians involved in the care of the individual being assessed. Either directly or indirectly FMHNs play a pivotal role in the assessment and management of risk.

In in-patient settings FMHNs are a major source of clinical information which should be considered by the nurse and the team as a whole when assessing risks. Mental health nurses in in-patient settings have access to 24-hour observation of behaviour and have greater opportunities than other professionals to develop relationships with service users and their family/carers (Allen, 1997). FMHNs are constantly making decisions based on the level of risk to and/or from service users in these environments. For example, they are involved in managing crises as they arise, controlling freedom of movement within and outside the secure facility, and maintaining safe levels of supervision and observation. This unique position makes the role of the FMHN crucial to the process of assessing and managing risk.

In the community, FMHNs tend to have a more autonomous role in assessing and managing risk to and/or from service users. This is especially true if the FMHN is identified as the keyworker in accordance with the requirements of the Care Programme Approach (Department of Health, 1990). Mental health nurses are most often identified as keyworkers (Boyd *et al.*, 1996). FMHNs in the community are often at the forefront of mentally disordered offender schemes where their expertise as practitioners gives them a key position in the process of screening (RCN, 1997a), especially when working in court diversion schemes. These relatively new roles have significant implications for FMHNs as they identify, assess and manage risk, not just because their individual legal responsibility may increase (Gupta, 1995) but also because their professional judgement will inevitably be subjected to closer scrutiny.

FMHNs often have advanced competencies in interventions employing behavioural and cognitive therapies, counselling, psychodynamic therapies and family therapy (RCN, 1997a). They may also have long experience working with particular client groups including sex offenders, people with personality disorders, people who self-injure and persistent offenders. Clearly the knowledge, skills and experience that FMHNs possess are crucial to clinical interventions involved in the process of assessing and managing risk.

The role of the FMHN is pivotal in the assessment and management of risk, whether as part of a multi-disciplinary team or as an autonomous practitioner, in in-patient settings or in the community. Advanced practices and professional development should equip FMHNs to fully participate in all the stages of assessing and managing risk.

CHARACTERISTICS OF RISK, RISK ASSESSMENT AND RISK MANAGEMENT

Risk means different things to different people. A typical dictionary definition may explain risk as the possibility of meeting danger or harm (*Oxford Popular Dictionary*). Definitions of risk nearly always include reference to the likelihood ('possibility') of a harmful outcome ('danger or harm'). Risk defined in this way is sometimes referred to as 'pure' risk. However, some definitions make reference to the likelihood of outcomes that may be beneficial. For example, risk is 'the possibility of beneficial and harmful outcomes and the likelihood of their occurrence in a stated timescale' (University of Manchester, 1996). This is sometimes referred to as speculative risk. This definition is particularly pertinent for clinicians making decisions that involve taking risks. Risk-taking is commonplace in clinical mental health services. Reaching a decision about what interventions are required to reduce or eliminate risk involves carefully weighing up the harms and benefits associated with those interventions. Most approaches to risk management initially concentrate on identifying and assessing 'pure' risks in order to reduce or eliminate the likelihood of harmful outcomes. Risk-taking arises in clinical practice when decisions need to be made about what measures should be implemented to reduce risks, especially when attempting to promote the independence of service users (Ryan, 1993).

THE PROCESS OF CLINICAL RISK ASSESSMENT AND MANAGEMENT

Approaches to risk management usually progress through the stages of identification, assessment, control/management, monitoring and review (Box 8.1). The stages of clinical risk assessment and management may be conceptualised as an ongoing process. This process has been described as a risk management cycle (Doyle, 1998) and is usually implicit to the provision of good quality health care and linked to systematic approaches to mental health care such as the care programme approach (Fig. 8.1).

Box 8.1 Stages of the risk management cycle

(a) *Identification*
Clinicians need to identify the potential for harm or identify a situation, task or condition that has the potential for harm before assessing the risk.

(b) *Risk assessment*
The risk assessment is concerned with establishing the level of risk. Consideration of the following questions will assist this process:

- What is the likelihood of the harm occurring?
- How immediate is the risk?
- How often is the harm likely to occur?
- Over what timescale is the risk being assessed?
- What are the possible outcomes if the harm occurs?
- Under what circumstances is the risk likely to increase/decrease?
- Who is at risk?

It is unlikely that there will be definite answers to these somewhat 'unfathomable' questions. However, considering these questions should help to inform clinical judgement. At this stage actuarial (statistical) and clinical factors that may be associated with an increase or a decrease in the risk of harming others should be considered.

(c) *Rating risk*
It is unlikely that the level of risk will be measured exactly. The risk rating will prioritise the risk and should determine the risk management measures and interventions required.

(d) *Implement risk management measures*
Risk management measures are the means by which the risk of harm is minimised. These measures should be part of an overall plan of care which

---

Contd.

is produced in collaboration with the service user where possible. A review date should be agreed to review the measures implemented usually as part of the care planning review process.

(e)   *Monitoring of risk management measures*
Risk management measures need to be monitored to ensure that they are being implemented as planned and in order to keep updated on progress between reviews.

(f)   *Risk assessment review*
The review should be concerned with evaluating whether the measures implemented have eliminated or reduced the risks.

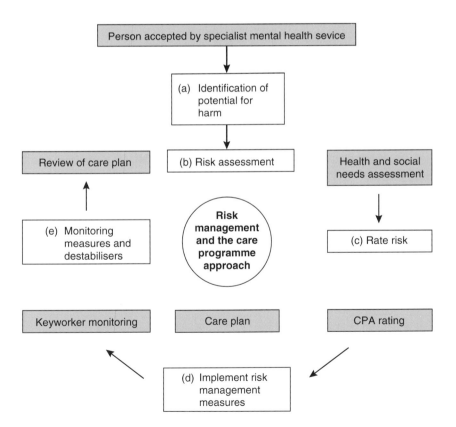

Fig. 8.1   Relationship between the stages of the risk management cycle and the stages of the care programme approach.

Accumulating information is the basis of any assessment. Mental health nurses use a number of methods to elicit useful information. Doyle (1996) explored what methods community mental health nurses (CMHNs) used to assess risk of violence. These included:

- interviews
- observation
- record reviews
- liaison with others – clinicians, other agencies, family, significant others
- via the therapeutic relationship
- intuition

Psychometric tests and rating scales are now increasingly used to assess risk. These can prove very useful and efficient although they should be used with caution. Ultimately tests and scales of this type can help to inform clinical judgement, not replace it. The methods used by the FMHNs to elicit information and assess risk will ultimately depend upon the circumstances in which the assessment is conducted. It is important wherever possible to have a multi-disciplinary framework for assessing and managing clinical risk which identifies how the risk assessment will be undertaken and sets out interventions and outcomes that need to occur in a sequential and timely fashion. Any framework needs to make the process of assessment and management explicit.

Effective frameworks must be:

- developed so that the process of clinical risk assessment and management is explicit in service users' records
- evidence/experience based
- organised around relevant ideas and research literature commonly understood by all disciplines and agencies
- linked to established practice and in accordance with systematic approaches to care provision (e.g. the CPA)
- designed with time constraints in mind
- sensitive to the dynamic nature of risk
- monitored and reviewed regularly

ASSESSING THE RISK TO OTHERS FROM PEOPLE WITH MENTAL DISORDER

Risk factors

In order to reach a decision about the level of risk to others and implement the necessary risk management measures, FMHNs need to assimilate a wide range of information. Focusing on the factors associated with an increase/decrease in risk to others is essential for this process. If a valid array of risk factors for risk of harm to others could be reliably identified and incorporated into routine practice then the accuracy of clinical risk assessment and management should increase (Monahan & Steadman, 1994). There are many factors which clinicians working in forensic services take into account when assessing the risk to others. The RCN (1998) produced guidance for mental health nurses when assessing and managing the risk of harm to others from people with mental health problems. In the USA the MacArthur Foundation has recently completed research into the relationship between violence and mental disorder in its violence risk assessment study (see Monahan & Steadman, 1994). They have focused on risk factors which are thought to have a positive association with an increased risk of violence (Box 8.2). At the time of writing, the full findings from the research have not been published. However, Steadman *et al.* (1998) recently published findings from the study which considered whether people discharged from acute mental health facilities were more or less likely to be violent than others living in the same neighbourhood. The study found that the patients discharged who did not abuse alcohol and illegal drugs had a rate of violence no different from that of their neighbours in the community. They also found that a higher proportion of discharged patients were more likely to abuse substances than others in their neighbourhood.

The information on risk factors provided in Box 8.2 may prove a useful guide to some of the key risk factors that FMHNs need to consider when assessing the risk to others. Some of these key risk factors will now be considered.

Box 8.2   Risk factors in the MacArthur violence risk assessment study

Personal Factors	A. Demographic
	B. Personality
	(1) Impulsiveness
	(2) Anger
	(3) Personality style
	(4) Psychopathy
	C. Cognitive
	(1) Neurological impairment
	(2) IQ
Historical Factors	A. Social history
	(1) Family history
	(2) Work and educational history
	(3) Physical and sexual abuse

Contd.

          B. Mental hospitalisation history
          C. History of crime and violence
              (1) Arrests and incarcerations
              (2) Self-reported violence
              (3) Violence toward self

Contextual Factors   A. Perceived stress
                       B. Social support
                           (1) Living arrangements
                           (2) Perceived support
                           (3) Social networks
                       C. Means of violence (i.e. guns)

Clinical Factors   A. Symptoms
                           (1) Delusions
                           (2) Hallucinations
                           (3) Symptom severity
                           (4) Violent fantasies
                       B. Diagnosis
                       C. Functioning
                           (1) Activities of daily living
                           (2) Global assessment of functioning
                       D. Substance use
                           (1) Alcohol
                           (2) Other drugs
                       E. Treatment
                           (1) Type
                           (2) Coercion
                           (3) Compliance

MENTAL DISORDER AND THE RISK OF HARM TO OTHERS

The notion that people are a risk to others due to their mental disorder is commonly accepted by the general public (Monahan, 1992; Reda, 1996) and traditionally contested by clinicians and service user advocates. In recent times the view taken by mental health professionals that service users are no more likely to cause harm to others than non-mentally disordered people from similar backgrounds has been increasingly questioned by research (Monahan, 1992). The Epidemiological Catchment Area (ECA) survey carried out by Swanson and colleagues (Swanson *et al.*, 1990) involved a sample of over 10 000 people randomly selected from five sites in the USA. Each of the respondents was interviewed using the Diagnostic Interview Schedule (DIS) (Robins *et al.*, 1981) and diagnosed accordingly.

They were then asked five questions to elicit whether they had been violent in their adult lifetime and in the previous 12 months. The results revealed that, controlling for demographic characteristics (age, gender, socio-economic status), people with mental disorder were up to five times more likely to have been violent in the previous year than those with no disorder. The conclusion from this study suggests that mental disorder may be a robust and significant risk factor for violence (Monahan, 1992). A closer look at the data from the ECA survey reveals that the link between mental disorder and violence depends upon the presence of active symptoms of serious mental illness and the prevalence of substance abuse. Hiday (1997) suggests that the association between mental disorder and harm to others is modest. The mentally ill account for only a small proportion of the total violence in society and not all display higher rates of violence, just those with a major mental illness and active symptoms (Link & Stueve, 1995).

Active symptoms and risk of harm to others

The link between mental disorder and harm to others depends greatly upon the presence, type and severity of psychotic symptoms. Existing research suggests that auditory hallucinations (especially command hallucinations) may be related to violence as part of a presentation of acute psychosis, along with impaired reality testing and poor judgement (McNiel, 1994). Junginger (1995) concluded that non-dangerous commands were more likely to be acted on than dangerous ones and that voices patients recognised were more likely to be heeded. Taylor (1985), in a study of 121 prisoners, found that command hallucinations can result in violent behaviour, and Rogers *et al.* (1990) reported that nearly 6% of a forensic hospital sample had committed their offence in response to command hallucinations. An underlying consideration is the fact that the majority of dangerous commands are not followed (Hiday, 1997). Even so, a consideration of the content of auditory hallucinations is clearly warranted in risk assessment (Yarvis & Swanson, 1996). The importance of command hallucinations in risk assessment is dependent on a number of concomitant factors such as associated delusions, recognition of voice, preoccupation with voice, distress caused and level of control over voice. Fear of the consequences of non-compliance and perceived threat from others should be the main considerations.

Link & Stueve (1994) suggest that symptoms which cause feelings of personal threat and involve intrusion of thoughts which override self-control are closely associated with increased risk of violence in mentally disordered people. It is suggested that these threat/control override (TCO) symptoms result in 'rationality-within-irrationality' where the person may take a pre-emptive strike to prevent harm to themselves (Link & Stueve, 1994). Behaviour constraints are likely to be overridden and violence is more likely when a disordered person believes he or she is gravely threatened by others who intend harm and believes that others are dominating his or her mind. Swanson *et al.* (1996) provide evidence supporting this hypothesis. They reviewed the findings of the ECA survey (Swanson *et al.* 1990) and compared the rate of violence by the psychotic symptoms present (see Box 8.3). They found that among a sample of people diagnosed as suffering from schizophrenia those who believed one of the following: (1) your mind is dominated by forces beyond your control; (2) thoughts are put in your head that are not your own; (3) there are people who wish to do you harm; and (4) others are following you, were twice as likely to be violent as those who did not (see Fig. 8.2).

There is now evidence to support the association between the presence of TCO symptoms and the increased risk of violence (Swanson *et al.*, 1997). The presence of TCO symptoms may also explain the prevalence of harm to others in non-schizophrenic populations. For example, Malmquist's (1995) literature review of the link between affective disorders and violence concluded that concomitant psychotic symptoms, such as persecutory and nihilistic delusions, rather than the affective symptoms such as despondency and hopelessness, promoted violence. Dolan & Parry (1996) found, in a special hospital in-patient sample of people with personality disorder who committed homicide, that the most common motives for killing included revenge and retaliation where a persecutory or hostile view of society or the world was prominent.

Clearly fear of the harmful intent of others, whether real or perceived, is an important risk factor associated with an increased risk to others. It may also be an important factor in non-psychotic and personality disordered samples.

Box 8.3   Prevalence of violence in past year by presence of schizophrenia and psychotic symptoms (Swanson *et al.*, 1996)

Sample with:	*% violent*
No symptoms	3%
Hallucinations only	7%
Delusions only	12%
Hallucinations and delusions	18%

TCO symptoms twice as likely to engage in violence than those with other psychotic symptoms (see Fig. 8.2) (Swanson *et al.*, 1996)

Past history of harming others

The old adage that nothing predicts future behaviour better than past behaviour (Kvarceus, 1954; Gunn, 1993) holds true. Monahan (1981)

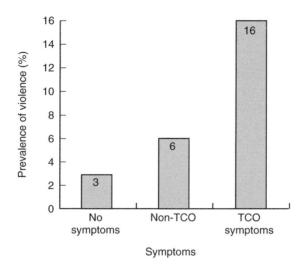

Fig. 8.2 Comparison between threat/control override symptoms and other psychotic symptoms and prevalence of violence (Swanson *et al.*, 1996). TCO = Threat control override.

reminds us that the probability of future crime increases with each prior criminal act. Risk assessments undertaken by FMHNs must also take account of past history, even if this risks reducing the objectivity of the assessment interview. Reviewing past history may be the best way of anticipating future conduct, especially if efforts are made to ascertain the pattern of events that led to each incident (Vaughan & Badger, 1995). Recent inquiries into tragedies involving people with serious mental illness have referred to the need for improved history-taking (Ritchie *et al.*, 1994; Blom-Cooper *et al.*, 1995, 1996). It is important to consider the number of incidents of behaviour which have resulted in harm to others, together with immediacy, frequency, severity and pattern of events (University of Manchester, 1996).

The importance of history-taking is clear. Clark *et al.* (1993) describe a methodology for the actuarial assessment of risk based on the analysis of past history to predict how prisoners will behave in a secure environment. At the very least, historical analysis should provide clinicians with an insight into what to expect.

Despite the importance of past history it is worthwhile considering the concerns of Gunn (1996) who suggested that it is myth that previous violence predicts future violence. The problem is that while retrospective statistical data reinforce the link between past history of violence and prospective group activity it tells us nothing about which members of which group will do what (Gunn, 1996).

Anger and hostility

The occurrence of harm to others usually corresponds to an increase in anger and hostility. Although anger is often a concomitant of violent behaviour, it is not essential for violence to occur. Therefore the degree to which anger constitutes a risk factor hinges on its operation as a mediator of the relationship between aversive events (occurrences the person would choose to avoid) and the harming behaviour (Novaco, 1994). Assessing the level of anger needs to take account of the cognitive, physical and behavioural aspects of anger. Novaco (1994) describes the development of the Novaco Anger Scale which measures the determinants and consequences of anger.

Closely linked to anger is the concept of hostility. Robinson *et al.* (1996) report attempts to develop and validate nursing assessments of potential dangerousness. Included in this research is the Buss–Durkee Hostility Inventory (BDHI) (Buss & Durkee, 1957), a self-report questionnaire on aggression. Initial results show that the BDHI reflected high levels of overt and covert aggression (Robinson *et al.*, 1996). This scale should make a valuable contribution to the risk assessment process and prove useful for informing clinical judgement.

Impulsivity

Impulsivity relates to the ability to control thoughts and behaviour. Problems of impulse control are implicated in a number of mental disorders. The role of impulsivity in risk to others is apparent. Segal *et al.* (1988) found a strong correspondence between perceptions of impulse control and perceptions of dangerousness. This association suggested that psychiatric patients in their study were not thought to be dangerous unless they had deficiencies in impulse control. As with anger and hostility the challenge for clinicians is how to assess the extent of an individual's impulsivity. Generally speaking, people who are highly impulsive tend to feel an increasing sense of tension or arousal before committing an act. This can be followed by great feelings of relief and gratification. Webster & Jackson (1997, p. 18) outline five categories which describe impulsive people. These are interpersonal dysfunction and lack of plans; further, esteem of self is distorted and there is rage, anger and hostility and taxing irresponsibility. Webster & Jackson (1997, p. 31) have also developed a 20-item Impulsivity Checklist to evaluate impulsivity in individuals using a simple 0, 1, 2 scoring system.

The Barratt Impulsiveness Scale (Barratt, 1994) has three sub-factors of impulsiveness. These are:

(1)   motor – acting without thinking
(2)   cognitive – making quick decisions
(3)   non-planning – lack of concern for the future

These frameworks should prove useful for FMHNs in clinical assessment of risk to others and self. As a minimum these scales provide a guide to the areas which need to be considered.

Antisocial personality traits

Very often FMHNs will be involved in the care and treatment of service users who do not have a 'formal' mental illness, but where problems and needs arise due to disorders in personality. Antisocial hostile traits are evident in the majority of personality disorders. There is evidence to suggest that individuals with mental illness who commit acts likely to cause harm to others are different from non-offending mentally ill individuals in that they have a history of antisocial traits preceding the onset of their illness (Hafner & Boker, 1982).

Antisocial personality disorder (ASP) is a recognised diagnosis in DSM-IV (American Psychiatric Association, 1994). Also referred to as psychopathy and sociopathic and dyssocial personality disorder, it is a disorder with a distinctive pattern of interpersonal, affective and behavioural symptoms (Hart & Hare, 1996). There have been criticisms of the classifications for being no more than the medicalisation of bad behaviour (Hart *et al.*, 1994) and debate continues regarding the pejorative nature of the term. Despite this it seems likely that FMHNs will continue to see people with ASP. Much progress has been made in developing a reliable scale to measure psychopathy. The Hare Psychopathy Checklist – revised (Hare, 1991) and more recently the Psychopathy Checklist: Screening Version (PCL: SV) (Hart *et al.*, 1995) have been used in contemporary research to predict violent behaviour (Monahan & Steadman, 1994).

Findings suggest that psychopathy can be a reliable predictor of harm to others from people with mental disorder, including schizophrenia (Harris *et al.*, 1993). It is not exactly clear why psychopathy is such a significant risk factor. Hart & Hare (1996) suggest that it may be that psychopathic individuals have cognitive schemata that predispose them to perceive hostile intent in the actions of others; they are prone to violence due to a general pattern of impulsivity; or psychopaths have a generalised emotional deficit that prevents them from experiencing empathy, fear and guilt which normally inhibit the expression of violent impulses. The MacArthur Violence Risk Assessment Study (Monahan & Steadman, 1994) used the PCL: SV in their research. Early indications are that high scores on this scale are consistently associated with high risk of subsequent violent behaviour (Swanson, 1994). With the necessary training and supervision the PCL: SV may prove a useful risk assessment tool for FMHNs.

Substance abuse

Substance abuse is linked to an increased risk to others whether a person is mentally disordered or not. Substance abuse is a much greater risk factor for violence than any mental illness (Swanson *et al.*, 1990). There is increasing interest in people with serious mental illness who abuse substances. The term 'dual diagnosis' has been applied to this group of people who meet the diagnostic criteria for both a substance misuse disorder and severe mental illness. There is evidence that people with a psychotic illness who abuse substances are more likely to be hostile and/or violent than those who are psychotic only (Bartels *et al.*, 1991; Cuffel *et al.*, 1994; Scott *et al.*, 1998; Steadman *et al.*, 1998; Swanson *et al.*, 1990, 1996). Alcohol and stimulants have been found to be the substances most closely associated with an increased risk.

There are a number of reasons why substance abuse is associated with an increased risk to others. Substances such as alcohol may impair perception, interfere with judgement, act as disinhibitors of aggressive impulses, contribute to the development of concurrent antisocial personality disorder and exacerbate psychotic symptoms (University of Manchester, 1996). The use of substances, especially illicit substances, may also draw persons into threatening and hostile environments and render individuals less responsive to and compliant with services (Swanson *et al.*, 1996). This may be significant when considering the prevalence of substance abuse in society and impact on the risks posed by people with mental illness (Scott *et al.*, 1998). Recent findings from the MacArthur Violence Risk Assessment Study (Monahan & Steadman, 1994) conclude that people discharged from an acute mental health facility are no more likely to be violent than others in their neighbourhood, unless they abuse substances (Steadman *et al.*, 1998).

Other risk factors

It is impossible to cover all the factors that indicate an increase in risk to others from people with mental disorder. The risk factors referred to reflect the most common areas for consideration when assessing risk to others. However, there are many other factors that could be considered. These include situational/contextual factors, availability of weapons, noncompliance, homelessness and personal characteristics such as motivation, acceptance of responsibility for behaviour and remorse.

FRAMEWORKS FOR ASSESSING RISK TO OTHERS

Literature and research on clinical risk assessment and management in mental health services is available yet despite this there are few if any systematic efforts to incorporate this information into useful frameworks for clinical risk management (Borum, 1996). However, there are some frameworks available which have been developed to assist mental health professionals carrying out risk assessments. A list of some useful frameworks is provided in Box 8.4.

Box 8.4   Some useful frameworks for assessing risk to others

- Assessment and clinical management of risk of harm to other people. (Royal College of Psychiatrists, 1996)
- Behavioural Status Index and BDHI-D (Robinson *et al.*, 1996, Collins & Robinson, 1997)
- HCR-20 (version 2) – Assessing Risk for Violence (Webster *et al.*, 1997)
- Management of Imminent Violence (RCP, 1998)
- Overt Aggression Scale (Yudofsky *et al.*, 1986)
- Psychopathy Checklist: Screening Version (Hart *et al.*, 1995)
- RAMAS – Risk Assessment and Management Audit System (O'Rourke *et al.*, 1997)
- Risk Assessment: Guidance for Mental Health Nurses: Assessing and Managing the Risk of Harm to Others from People with Mental Health Problems (RCN, 1998)
- SHAPS: Special Hospitals Assessment of Personality and Socialisation (Blackburn, 1982)
- Violence Prediction Scheme (Webster *et al.*, 1994)
- Weighted Risk Indicator (Worthing Priority Care NHS Trust, 1995)

ASSESSING THE RISK OF SELF-HARM AND SUICIDE

Problems with definition

The term 'self-harm' is subject to debate. Behaviour intended to take one's own life and non-lethal self-harming behaviour are not necessarily considered as the same phenomena. Evidence suggests that they are largely different populations but there are also data to suggest considerable overlap (MacLeod *et al.*, 1992). While accepting that it can be very difficult to distinguish between self-harming behaviour on the basis of ultimate intention, the focus here is on assessing and managing the risk of self-harm which is likely to result in life-threatening injury or death. Self-mutilation and self-injurious behaviour are very common problems in forensic services. A significant proportion of people who self-injure are at a greatly increased risk of committing suicide at some later date.

Suicide

Suicide is legally defined as '...the intentional act of self destruction committed by someone knowing what he/she is doing and knowing the probable consequences of his/her action' (Bluglass & Bowden, 1990). Suicide is a major cause of death in Britain accounting for 1% of all deaths annually. It is likely that the rate of suicide is even higher (Health Advisory Service (HAS), 1994, p. 9).

All categories of mental disorder carry an increased risk of self-harm and suicide. In 1992 the Health of the Nation White Paper selected mental illness as a key area for action with the objective of reducing ill-health and death caused by mental illness. The aim was to reduce the overall suicide rate by 15% and by 33% in the severely mentally ill by the year 2000 (Department of Health, 1993). Effective risk assessment and management may help achieve these targets.

The rate of suicide amongst the prison population is three to four times higher than in the general population and suicide amongst prisoners has increased considerably over the past 15 years (Liebling, 1993). Specific factors associated with prison-type secure environments are thought to contribute to suicidal behaviour. These include prospect of long-term detention, inability to cope, lack of communication with the outside world and failure of appeals against detention (Dooley, 1990). Clearly forensic mental health environments place similar pressures upon a population already classed as high risk due to mental disorder. Effective approaches to identifying, assessing and managing the risk of self-harm in forensic services are of paramount importance.

Risk factors

As with all risk assessments there is a need to identify factors which are associated with an increased risk. Extensive data exist on demographic and biological correlates of risk of self-harm and suicide (HAS, 1994, p.10; University of Manchester, 1996, p. 53). These correlates are impressive in describing risk trends but have limited utility in clinical settings. In a clinical setting FMHNs will be concerned with assessing the risk in the short to medium term. If an initial screening indicates that there is a risk of self-harm, further risk factors must be considered. According to Morgan (1994) three main diagnostic groups pose the highest suicide risk. These are people with:

- depression – especially with sleep difficulties, self-neglect, impaired memory or agitation
- schizophrenia – particularly younger people who are unemployed and have serious recurrent illness

- problems with alcohol abuse – especially men with high level of dependency and a long drinking history

Current presentation

In order to assess the risk of self-harm it is advisable that the following areas are covered through careful questioning:

- Hopes that things will turn out well
- Feels hopeful from day to day
- Sees a point to it all
- Feels that it is impossible to face the next day
- Wishes it would all end
- Has thoughts of ending life; if so how persistently?
- Feels able to resist any suicidal thoughts or intentions; and has any thoughts about what would make them disappear
- Gets pleasure out of life
- Feels able to face each day
- Ever despairs about things
- Feels life to be a burden
- Knows why he or she feels this way (e.g. wants to be with a dead person)
- Has ever acted on any suicidal thoughts or intentions

More specific factors which need to be considered include (Doyle, 1998):

- Current suicidal intent
- Current suicidal ideation
- Hopelessness
- Recent loss or anniversary of loss
- Substance abuse
- Past history of self-harm/suicide attempts
- Low mood
- Non-compliance with treatment
- Recent failure or rejection

Some of these factors will now be considered in more detail.

Current suicidal intent

Suicidal intent is the most powerful predictor of whether an individual will attempt suicide. Questions that need to be considered include:

(1) Is there a suicide plan?
(2) Are the means for suicide/self-harm available?
(3) Is there a 'contract' not to self-harm?

Clinicians need to be vigilant when assessing suicidal intent as it is common for those intent on committing suicide to deny and/or minimise their ultimate intentions.

Hopelessness

There is evidence that future directed thinking is in some way different in those who contemplate suicide. Studies have shown that hopelessness about the future plays a significant role in mediating between people who are depressed and have suicidal intent (Salter & Platt, 1990). The lack of rewarding short-term routines as well as long-term plans and goals may be an important component (MacLeod *et al.*, 1992).

Previous suicide/self-harm attempts

A history of previous attempts at self-harm/suicide is obviously significant when assessing the level of risk. When analysing past history it is important to consider the following:

- Immediacy (the more recent the higher the risk)
- Severity (the more severe the higher the risk)
- Antecedents/precipitants
- Consequences
- Frequency (the more frequent the higher the risk)
- Pattern
- Details of attempt – especially any efforts made to avoid/ensure discovery

It is hoped that the above sections on risk of self-harm will serve as a useful basis for developing frameworks for assessment.

Assessing imminent risk

The factors that need to be taken into account when assessing the risks that service users pose to themselves or others are similar whether assessing risk in the short or longer term. However, there may be differences in emphasis between in-patient and community settings. The risks assessed in in-patient settings are usually short term in nature to reflect the day-to-day functioning of the service user in the ward environment. In the community imminent risk is equally important although the risk assessment may be undertaken to reflect the prospect of a medium-/-long-term community placement and longer periods between contacts. Risk factors relating to past history, present mental state and social functioning will remain vital to any risk assessment. The imminent risk of harm to the individual and others may be more of a concern in in-patient settings where the patient's condition may be in an acute state.

Research has identified behaviour which precedes violent aggressive acts by service users (Powell *et al.*, 1994). Clinical practice guidelines have been produced by the Royal College of Psychiatrists (1998) on the management of imminent violence. Risk factors associated with imminent violence include demographic factors, past history, age, sex, clinical variables, substance abuse, active symptoms, antisocial explosive personality traits and situational factors, extent of social support and the availability of weapons. Whittington & Patterson (1996) aimed to enhance the assessment of imminent violence by identifying typical verbal and non-verbal behaviour that preceded aggressive acts. They found that much of the behaviour that preceded aggressive acts also occurred in the absence of aggression. Despite this, approaches aimed at identifying overt signs of imminent aggression may prove useful in preventing and/or reducing the risk of harm to others. The types of behaviour which indicate an increasing risk to others include:

- Anger
- Hostility
- Verbal abuse
- Verbal threats
- Aggression to objects
- Threatening gestures
- Alcohol and/or substance abuse
- Glaring eye contact
- Confusion/disorientation
- High overall activity
- Standing uncomfortably close

Where a significant risk of self-harm is recognised, further assessment should consider behaviour indicating an increase in risk. The assessment of the imminent risk of self-harm should include monitoring for symptoms such as (Clark, 1990):

- Anhedonia (lack of pleasure)
- Increasing anxiety
- Alcohol/substance abuse
- Diminished concentration
- Insomnia
- Panic attacks

MANAGING THE RISK TO SELF AND OTHERS

Risk management involves introducing measures which have a reasonable likelihood of minimising the risk. Risk management measures should contribute to an individual's overall plan of care. In order to reduce the risk and manage risk effectively, the response to the risk needs to reflect the circumstances of the risk, taking into account different levels of intervention. Roughly speaking there are four levels of intervention:

- primary – proactive and aim to prevent harm occurring
- secondary – taken during and immediately after an adverse incident

- tertiary – to reduce the risks which arise as a consequence of any adverse incident
- externally imposed – legislation and guidelines may be imposed

The harms and benefits of implementing risk management measures need to be weighed against the harms and benefits of inaction (Carson, 1990). This is very important for the service user. Careful consideration and documentation of the harms and benefits of a decision will also improve the defensibility of the clinician if something goes wrong. Risk decisions need to be made in a manner which can readily be justified (Carson, 1996). The need for careful consideration of the measures implemented is highlighted by Pilgrim & Rogers (1996, p. 183) who outline the risks posed by psychiatric services, i.e. loss of freedom and access to material and social resources and iatrogenic risks.

Risk to others

The management of risk to others encompasses clinical, health and safety, and public protection (political) issues. Effective risk assessment should be part of risk management and vice versa. Behaviour likely to cause harm to others may be symptomatic of many disorders and therefore unlikely to be susceptible to any single intervention. Harris & Rice (1997) distinguish between several types of risk management intervention:

- static – involves preventing harm via such things as video monitoring, seclusion and locked doors
- dynamic – aims to reduce harm, e.g. control and restraint techniques
- situational – attempts to restrict access to the means of violence or potential victims, e.g. paedophile having restricted contact with children
- pharmacological – involves using sedatives or other drugs
- interpersonal – mainly by talking using de-escalation techniques
- self-control – psychotherapeutic or pharmacological means to control behaviour

Closely examining the factors which have contributed to harm to others will also prove fruitful in identifying targets for treatment which may reduce risk, for example: poor anger control – anger management; substance abuse – drug/alcohol therapy; persecutory delusions – cognitive and pharmacological interventions.

Risk to self

Before considering measures to reduce risk of self-harm it is worth considering the problems of suicide prevention. James (1996) highlighted the dilemma of having to implement effective measures to prevent suicide while also preserving the individual's quality of life. Measures aimed at physically reducing the suicide risk may make the individual worse. Morgan (1994) argues that life-enhancing measures should be adopted instead of physically preventative measures, even if this results in a marginally increased risk. This balancing act is not an easy one for FMHNs and it is strongly recommended that decisions about implementing risk management measures are made in collaboration with other clinicians, in particular the responsible medical officer.

In the ward environment where high-risk individuals are likely to reside, it is sensible to carry out regular inspections to ensure hazards such as the means for self-harm (e.g. razors, glass, chemicals, ropes, hooks) are not available and the hazards of the physical layout are identified. Efforts should be made to improve observation and reduce access to areas where high-risk individuals can avoid detection

From an interpersonal perspective it has been found that people who attempt suicide have certain deficits in their psychological functioning. Studies examining psychological processes involved in suicidal behaviour have revealed deficits in problem-solving, appraisals about the future (hopelessness) and reduced ability to regulate emotions (MacLeod *et al.*, 1992). These deficits should provide FMHNs with targets for treatment which will minimise the risk of self-harm and suicide. At the very least, emotional and practical support needs to be available for those who are identified as high risk.

Self-neglect

Due to the nature of some mental health problems some service users may be at risk of neglecting themselves. In fact risk of severe self-neglect has been cited as the criterion for inclusion on the Supervision Register (NHSME, 1994). In forensic services the risk of self-neglect is high whether due to lack of skills or motivation or the negative symptoms of psychotic illness. It is important to respect the self-determination and freedom of choice of individuals although it is advisable to cover a number of areas through the assessment process.

Areas to be considered when assessing risk of self-neglect may include:

- Inadequate diet
- Poor hygiene
- Infestation

- Unsafe residence
- Lack of necessary warmth
- Non-compliance with prescribed physical care/treatment

High risk of self-neglect may also be synonymous with high risk of self-harm.

Assessing other clinical risks

Ryan (1998) carried out research to explore the perceptions of risks associated with mental illness. He discovered six factors of perceived risk,
namely being in an underclass, medical disempowerment, threat, vulnerability, self-harm and dependency. He concluded that stakeholders (mental
health professionals, service users, carers, general public) have a wider perception of risk than defined through current policy. The research broadens
the concept of risk from that focused on in media and government circles.
Other common risks associated with forensic mental health services include
risk of:

- abuse to service user
- alienation
- exploitation
- falling
- HIV infection

- homelessness
- relapse
- side-effects of medication
- unemployment

The stages of clinical risk assessment and risk management remain the
same although there will be specific factors that need to be taken into
account when assessing these risks.

CONCLUSION

Risk assessment and risk management pervade much of the activity of
FMHNs. Although clinical risk management is usually implicit to recognised good practice, it is becoming increasingly important for FMHNs
to clarify and demonstrate approaches to clinical risk decision-making.
The level of risk is dependent on the context. In clinical practice there
needs to be an emphasis on systematic structured approaches to identification, assessment, rating, management, monitoring and review of risk
rather than prediction. Such an approach should enable the identification of
risks specific to the service user rather than focusing solely on risk to self
and others.

There are many risks which arise which may be more worthy of
intervention and viewed as more relevant by service users. Integrating a
systematic approach to assessing and managing risk with care planning
processes such as the CPA should enhance decision-making. Evidence-based
frameworks for risk management need to be developed to reflect service
needs, although existing tools and scales are available which may prove
useful. It is important for FMHNs to ensure that any framework adopted
has been tested for practical utility.

The challenge for FMHNs is how to apply their knowledge, skills and
experience in ensuring that risks are assessed and managed to enhance the

well-being of the service user while protecting the wider public interests. Useful areas for future inquiry include:

- exploring how FMHNs make judgements about risk
- the role of the FMHN in interdisciplinary risk decision-making
- the education and training needs of FMHNs in order to equip them to assess and manage risk effectively
- risk communication between forensic and non-forensic CMHNs
- integration of useful frameworks into routine clinical practice

CASE STUDY: RISK TO OTHERS

The person referred to in the following case study is fictitious.

Jake is a 50-year-old man with a 25-year history of paranoid schizophrenia. When he was 22 he killed his older brother in response to command hallucinations. He has spent 20 years in a special hospital and later a medium secure unit. He has been in the community in a residential care home for 2 years subject to conditional discharge under Section 41 of the Mental Health Act 1983. He is due his multi-disciplinary case review and the FCMHN has been asked to assess the risk to others from Jake. The framework outlined in Box 8.5 was used to guide the assessment. The following is the summary report.

Box 8.5   Framework for risk assessment

(1)   Source of information
Interview
Observation
Record reviews
Rating scales/psychometric tests
Liaison with others
Other – please specify

(2)   Past history of harm to self/others
Is there evidence of a history of behaviour resulting in harm to self/others?
Details?
Immediacy
No. of occurrences
Frequency
Most severe outcome
Is there a pattern to past harmful behaviour?
If yes/maybe, please list any possible precipitants or triggers
Indicate if they are present now

Contd.

(3) Mental health
Diagnostic category
Symptomatology

(4) Current presentation

(5) Observations of behaviour

(6) Alcohol and substance use

(7) Social circumstances
Type of present accommodation
Does the person have any family and/or friends who offer support?
Does the person value the support offered by family and friends?
Are there any professionals involved in support and supervision?

(8) Other relevant information
Rating scales/tests
Information from third party

(9) Summary
Risk factors
Current protective factors (restraining factors associated with decrease in risk)

(10) Risk rating
Based on the best available information
Likelihood?
Likely severity of harm should it occur?
Overall risk rating – low, medium, high, very high
Specific person or group of persons at risk
Detail circumstances under which the risk is likely to:
(a) Increase
(b) Decrease

(11) Risk management plan
Recommended measures to minimise risk:
Method(s) of monitoring
Date of review and venue
Include name of assessor(s), designation, signature, date completed

Source of information

Weekly interviews with Jake
Review of medical records since index offence
HCR-20 scheme (version 2)

Liaison with social worker and responsible medical officer
Interviews with proprietor of care home

Historical analysis

No. of incidents known:	1 (one incident of harm to others)
Frequency:	1 (very infrequent)
Severity:	4 (death)
Recency:	1 (more than 4 years ago)
Presence of known triggers for violence	3 (at least one known trigger present)
Score	10/20 (low to moderate risk to others)

HCR-20 version 2 (Webster *et al.*, 1997)

Historical score	10/20
Clinical score	5/10
Risk management score	6/10
Total	21/40 (low to moderate risk for violence)

Risk factors present

Escalating conflict with fellow resident
Active symptoms – command hallucinations, persecutory delusions
Overall hostility
Increasing stress

Protective/restraining factors

Intensive professional support
Age
24 years since previous harm to others
Ability to disobey command hallucinations
Remorse for index offence
Psychomotor retardation
Intent to stay out of trouble
Insight into personal consequences of harming others

Risk rating

Medium – several risk factors present with several restraining factors in place. Need to involve all disciplines in deciding the number of risk categories, defining them and criteria used. This may involve non-mental health agencies, e.g. judges, probation workers, other carers and managers (Monahan & Steadman, 1994).

Factors which may increase risk

Escalation in conflict with fellow resident
Substance abuse
Increasing anxiety due to mental state
Deteriorating mental state

Factors which may decrease risk

Resolution of problems with fellow resident
Increased control over positive symptoms
Controlled drinking

Risk management measures

Continue monitoring relationship with fellow resident
Address relationship problems in sessions
Plan early alert system with proprietor and confirm crisis intervention plan
Close liaison with other professionals
Monitor alcohol abuse
Continue work on reducing distress and increasing control of psychotic symptoms
Review in multi-disciplinary major review, 12/12/00

Name: A. N. Other   Date: 11/11/00

REFERENCES

Allen, J. (1997) Assessing and managing risk of violence in the mentally disordered. *Journal of Psychiatric and Mental Health Nursing* 4, 369–78.

American Psychiatric Association (1994) *DSM-IV: Diagnostic and Statistical Manual of Mental Disorders*, 4th edn. APA, Washington.

Barratt, E. (1994) Impulsiveness and aggression. In *Violence and Mental Disorder: Developments in Risk Assessment* (Monahan, J. & Steadman, H., eds), pp. 61–80. University of Chicago Press, Chicago.

Bartels, S., Drake, R., Wallach, M. & Freeman, D. H. (1991) Characteristic hostility in schizophrenic outpatients. *Schizophrenia Bulletin* 17, 163–71.

Blackburn, R. (1982) The special hospitals assessment of personality and socialisation (SHAPS) and the personality deviation questionnaire. Park Lane Hospital, Maghull. Unpublished.

Blom-Cooper, L., Grounds, A., Guinan, P., Parker, A. & Taylor, M. (1996) *The Case of Jason Mitchell: Independent panel of inquiry.* Duckworth, London.

Blom-Cooper, L., Hally, H. & Murphy, E. (1995) *The Falling Shadow: One Patient's Mental Health Care 1978–1993.* Duckworth, London.

Bluglass, R. & Bowden, P. (1990) *Principles and Practice of Forensic Psychiatry.* Churchill Livingstone, Edinburgh.

Borum, R. (1996) Improving the clinical practice of violence risk assessment. *American Psychologist* 51(9), 945–56.

Boyd, W., Simms, A., Brooker, A., *et al.* (1996) *Boyd Report: Report of the Confidential Inquiry into Homicides and Suicides by Mentally Ill People.* Royal College of Psychiatrists, London.

Buss, A. & Durkee, A. (1957) An inventory for assessing different kinds of hostility. *Journal of Consulting Psychology* 21, 165–74.

Carson, D. (ed.) (1990) *Risk Taking in Mental Disorder: Analyses, Policies and Practical Strategies.* SLE Publications, Chister.

Carson, D. (1996) Risking legal repercussions. In *Good Practice in Risk Assessment and Risk Management* (Kemshall, H. & Pritchard, J., eds), pp. 3–12. Jessica Kingsley Publishers, London.

Clark, D. (1990) Suicide risk assessment and prediction in the 1990s. *Crisis* 11(2), 104–12.

Clark, D., Fisher, M. & McDougall, C. (1993) A new methodology for assessing the level of risk in incarcerated offenders. *British Journal of Criminology* 33(3), 436–47.

Coid, J. (1996) Dangerous patients with mental illness: increased risks warrant new policies, adequate resources, and appropriate legislation. *British Medical Journal* 312, 965–9.

Collins, M. & Robinson, D. (1997) Measuring aggression in forensic care. *Psychiatric Care* 4, 67–70.

Cuffel, B., Schumway, M., Chouljiam, T. & MacDonald, T. (1994) A longitudinal study of substance use and community violence in schizophrenia. *Journal of Nervous and Mental Disease* 182, 704–708.

Department of Health (1990) *The Care Programme Approach for people with a mental illness referred to the specialist psychiatric services.* HC(90) 23/LASSL (90) 11, DH.

Department of Health (1993) *Health of the Nation Key Area Handbook: Mental Illness.* HMSO, London.

Dolan, M. & Parry, J. (1996) A survey of male homicide cases resident in an English special hospital. *Medicine, Science and Law* 36(3), 249–58.

Dooley, E. (1990) Prison suicides in England and Wales 1972–1987. *British Journal of Psychiatry* 156, 40–45.

Doyle, M. (1996) Assessing risk of violence from clients. *Mental Health Nursing* 16(3), 20–23.

Doyle, M. (1998) Clinical risk assessment for mental health nurses. *Nursing Times* 94(17), 47–9.

Gunn, J. (1996) Let's get serious about dangerousness. *Criminal Behaviour in Mental Health Supplement* 51–64.

Gunn, J. (ed.) (1993) Dangerousness. In *Forensic Psychiatry: Clinical, Legal and Ethical Issues* (Gunn, J. & Taylor, P., eds), pp. 624–45. Butterworth Heinemann, London.

Gupta, N. (1995) Keyworkers and the Care Programme Approach. The role and responsibilities of community workers. *Psychiatric Care* 1, 239–42.

Hafner, H. & Boker, W. (1982) *Crimes of Violence by Mentally Abnormal Offenders*. Cambridge University Press, New York.

Hare, R. (1991) *Manual for the Hare Psychopathy Checklist – Revised*. Multi-Health Systems, Toronto.

Harris, G. & Rice, M. (1997) Risk appraisal and management of violent behaviour. *Psychiatric Services* 48(9), 1168–76.

Harris, G., Rice, M. & Quinsey, V. (1993) Violence recidivism of mentally disordered offenders: the development of a statistical prediction instrument. *Criminal Justice and Behaviour* 20, 315–35.

Hart, S. & Hare, R. (1996) Psychopathy and risk assessment. *Current Opinion in Psychiatry* 9, 380–83.

Hart, S., Cox, D. & Hare, R. (1995) *The Hare PCL: SV: Psychopathy Checklist: Screening Version*. Multi-Health Systems, New York.

Hart, S., Hare, R. & Forth, A. (1994) Psychopathy as a risk marker for violence: Development and validation of a screening version of the revised psychopathy checklist. In *Violence and Mental Disorder: Developments in Risk Assessment* (Monahan, J. & Steadman, J., eds), pp. 81–98. University of Chicago Press, Chicago.

Health Advisory Service (1994) *Suicide Prevention: Mental Health Services – the Challenge Confronted*. HMSO, London.

Hiday, V. (1997) Understanding the connection between mental illness and violence. *International Journal of Law and Psychiatry* 20(4), 399–417.

James, A. (1996) Suicide reduction in medium security. *Journal of Forensic Psychiatry* 7(2), 406–12.

Junginger, J. (1995) Command hallucinations and the prediction of dangerousness. *Psychiatric Services* 46, 911–14.

Kvarceus, W. (1954) *The Community and the Delinquent*. New York, World Books.

Liebling, A. (1993) Suicides in young prisoners: A summary. *Death Studies* 17(5), 381–409.

Link, B. & Stueve, A. (1994) Psychotic symptoms and the violent/illegal behaviour of mental patients compared to community controls. In *Violence and Mental Disorder: Developments in Risk Assessment* (Monahan, J. & Steadman, H., eds), pp. 137–60. University of Chicago Press, Chicago.

Link, B. & Stueve, A. (1995) Evidence bearing on mental illness as a possible cause of violent behaviour. *Epidemiologic Reviews* 17, 1–9.

MacLeod, A., Williams, J. & Linehan, M. (1992) New developments in the understanding and treatment of suicidal behaviour. *Behavioural Psychotherapy* 20, 193–218.

McNiel, D. (1994) Hallucinations and violence. In *Violence and Mental Disorder: Developments in Risk Assessment* (Monahan, J. & Steadman, H., eds), pp. 183–202. University of Chicago Press, Chicago.

Malmquist, C. (1995) Depression and homicidal violence. *International Journal of Law and Psychiatry* 18, 145–62.

Monahan, J. (1981) *Predicting Violent Behaviour*. Sage Library of Social Research, Vol. 114, Sage Publications, Beverley Hills.

Monahan, J. (1992) Mental disorder and violent behaviour: perceptions and evidence. *American Psychologist* **47**(4), 511–21.

Monahan, J. & Steadman, H. (eds) (1994) *Violence and Mental Disorder: Developments in Risk Assessment*. University of Chicago Press, Chicago.

Morgan, H. (1994) How feasible is suicide prevention? *Current Opinion in Psychiatry* **7**, 111–18.

National Health Service Management Executive (1994) *Introduction of supervision registers for mentally ill people from 1st April 1994*. NHSME HSG(94)5.

Novaco, R. (1994) Anger as a risk factor for violence among the mentally disordered. In *Violence and Mental Disorder: Developments in Risk Assessment* (Monahan, J. & Steadman, H., eds), pp. 21–60. University of Chicago Press, Chicago.

O'Rourke, M., Hammond, S. & Davies, E. (1997) Risk assessment and risk management: the way forward. *Psychiatric Care* **4**(3), 104–106.

Pilgrim, D. & Rogers, A. (1996) Two notions of risk in mental health debates. In *Mental Health Matters* (Heller, T., Reynolds, J., Gomm, R., Muston, R. & Pattison, S.), pp. 181–5. Macmillan, London.

Powell, G., Caan, W. & Crowe, M. (1994) What events precede violent incidents in psychiatric hospitals? *British Journal of Psychiatry* **165**, 107–12.

Reda, S. (1996) Public perceptions of former psychiatric patients in England. *Psychiatric Services* **47**(11), 1253–5.

Ritchie, J., Dick, D. & Lingham, R. (1994) *The Report of the Inquiry into the Care and Treatment of Christopher Clunis*. HMSO, London.

Robins, L., Helzer, J., Croughan, J. & Ratcliffe, K. (1981) National Institute of Mental Health diagnostic interview schedule: its history, characteristics and validity. *Archives of General Psychiatry* **38**, 381–9.

Robinson, D., Reed, V. & Lange, A. (1996) Developing risk assessment scales in forensic psychiatric care. *Psychiatric Care* **3**(4), 141–7.

Rogers, R., Gillis, J., Turner, R. & Frise-Smith, T. (1990) The clinical presentation of command hallucinations in a forensic population. *American Journal of Psychiatry* **147**, 1304–1307.

Royal College of Nursing (1997a) *Buying Forensic Mental Health Nursing: an RCN Guide for Purchasers*. RCN, London.

Royal College of Nursing (1997b) *The Management of Aggression and Violence in Places of Care: An RCN Position Statement*. RCN, London.

Royal College of Nursing (1998) Risk assessment: Guidance for mental health nurses: Assessing and managing the risk of harm to others from people with mental health problems. Draft paper. RCN, London.

Royal College of Psychiatrists (1996) *Assessment and Clinical Management of Risk of Harm to Other People*. RCP, London.

Royal College of Psychiatrists (1998) Management of imminent violence: Clinical practice guidelines to support mental health services. Occasional paper OP41.

Ryan, T. (1993) Therapeutic risks in mental health nursing. *Nursing Standard* **3**(24), 29–31.

Ryan, T. (1998) Perceived risk associated with mental illness: beyond homicide and suicide. *Social Science and Medicine* **46**(2), 287–97.

Salter, D. & Platt, S. (1990) Suicidal intent, hopelessness and depression in a parasuicide population: the influence of social desirability and elapsed time. *British Journal of Clinical Psychology* **29**, 361–71.

Scott, H., Johnson, S., Menezes, P., Thornicroft, G., Marshall, J., Bindman, J., Bebbington, P. & Kuipers, E. (1998) Substance misuse and risk of aggression and offending among the severely mentally ill. *British Journal of Psychiatry* **172**, 345–50.

Segal, S., Watson, M., Goldfinger, S. & Averbuck, D. (1988) Civil commitment in the psychiatric emergency room: eleven mental disorder indicators and three dangerousness criteria. *Archives of General Psychiatry* **45**, 753–8.

Steadman, H., Mulvey, E., Monahan, J., Clarke Robins, P., Appelbaum, P., Grisso, T., Roth, L. & Silva, E. (1998) Violence by people discharged from acute psychiatric inpatient facilities and by others in the same neighbourhoods. *Archives of General Psychiatry* **55**, 393–401.

Swanson, J. (1994) Mental disorder, substance abuse and community violence: an epidemiological approach. In *Violence and Mental Disorder: Developments in Risk Assessment* (Monahan, J. & Steadman, H., eds). University of Chicago Press, Chicago, IL.

Swanson, J., Borum, R., Swartz, M. & Monahan, J. (1996) Psychotic symptoms and disorders and the risk of violent behaviour in the community. *Criminal Behaviour and Mental Health* **6**, 309–29.

Swanson, J., Estroff, S., Swartz, M., Borum, R., Lachicotte, W., Zimmer, C. & Wagner, R. (1997) Violence and severe mental disorder in clinical and community populations: the effects of psychotic symptoms, comorbidity and lack of treatment. *Psychiatry* **60**, 1–22.

Swanson, J., Holzer, C., Ganju, V. & Jono, R. (1990) Violence and psychiatric disorder in the community: Evidence from the epidemiological catchment area surveys. *Hospital and Community Psychiatry* **41**, 762–70.

Taylor, P. (1985) Motives for offending among violent and psychotic men. *British Journal of Psychiatry* **147**, 491–8.

University of Manchester (1996) *Learning Materials on Mental Health Risk Assessment*. School of Psychiatry and Behavioural Sciences.

Vaughan, P. & Badger, D. (1995) *Working with the Mentally Disordered Offender in the Community*. Chapman & Hall, London.

Webster, C. & Jackson, M. (1997) A clinical perspective on impulsivity. In *Impulsivity: Theory, Assessment and Treatment* (Webster, C. & Jackson, M., eds), pp. 13–31. Guildford Press, New York.

Webster, C., Douglas, K., Eaves, D. & Hart, S. (1997) *HCR-20: Assessing Risk for Violence – Version 2*. Simon Fraser University, British Columbia, Canada.

Webster, C., Harris, G., Rice, M., Cormier, C. & Quinsey, V. (1994) *Violence Prediction Scheme: Assessing Dangerousness in High Risk Men*. Centre of Criminology, University of Toronto.

Whittington, R. & Patterson, P. (1996) Verbal and non-verbal behaviour immediately prior to aggression by mentally disordered people: enhancing the assessment of risk. *Journal of Psychiatric and Mental Health Nursing* **3**, 47–54.

Worthing Priority Care NHS Trust (1995) Weighted risk indicator. Internal Document.

Yarvis, R. & Swanson, A. (1996) Psychiatric aspects of homicide. *Current Opinion in Psychiatry* 9, 389–92.

Yudofsky, S., Silver, J., Jackson, W., Endicott, J. & Williams, D. (1986) The overt aggression scale for the objective rating of verbal and physical aggression. *American Journal of Psychiatry* 143(1), 35–9.

Chapter 9
Developing Community Services

Michael Coffey

INTRODUCTION

People with serious mental illness present a challenge to mental health services in that they require a diverse range of services. These patients are often beset with problems of poor accommodation, poor finances, and reduced opportunities for daytime activities and for meaningful relationships. As challenging as this may be for services, the combination of serious mental illness and a 'forensic' history can present a formidable range of needs.

Community psychiatry has in recent years attracted significant controversy in Britain. On both local and national levels public fear often provoked by failures of care and fed by media speculation has prompted many reviews in policy. Mentally disordered offenders living in the community give particular cause for concern. It is often this group of patients who have demonstrated the type of behaviour that has labelled them 'forensic'. This label creates much anxiety even among professionals who understand by it only that it must mean 'dangerous'. The community supervision of this group therefore requires sensitive handling, a sound knowledge of mental health law and a firm understanding of the management of risk. This chapter, while recognising the diverse range of roles of forensic community mental health nurses (FCMHNs) is primarily concerned with the development of evidence-based services for mentally disordered offenders living in the community.

The Reed Report (Department of Health/Home Office, 1992) recommendation of treating patients in the least restrictive environment, which if brought to its logical conclusion includes the community, has effectively become government policy. More recently the UK government has set out plans for a comprehensive review of mental health services (Department of Health (DoH), 1998). With this in mind it is useful to explore strategies for managing these patients in the community in a safe, effective and evidence-based way.

Swanson *et al.* (1996) acknowledge that a tension exists between treatment effectiveness and patients' rights. It is a tension which FCMHNs cope with on a daily basis. Operating on the continuum between overt coercion and humanistic therapeutic intervention, forensic nurses have to a large degree incorporated into practice a conceptual framework which although still in its infancy is nevertheless functional and pragmatic. It is the contention of this chapter that the community treatment and supervision of forensic patients should be based around a comprehensive case management approach which incorporates relevant evidence-based practice and risk management strategies.

ESTABLISHING A ROLE FOR FCMHNs

Defining the role of FCMHNs is in its early stages but efforts to do this may usefully prompt debate about the role and its development. Evans (1996, p. 35) believes: 'A forensic community mental health nurse provides ... care for patients both inside and outside the secure environment, dependent upon the individual's needs' and that this care involves 'collating information as an integral member of the multidisciplinary clinical team to develop a comprehensive risk assessment leading to a risk management strategy'.

Evans suggests that there is some value for the community nurse in seeing the patient throughout their stay in hospital. The patient can be seen when unwell and as they start to improve. This will give the nurse a greater understanding of how the patient presents when unwell and will facilitate identification of early signs of relapse. This process may help later engagement with the patient.

Burrow (1993, p. 904) suggests that forensic mental health nursing involves 'highly informed, ethical skills-based practice until the client's individual risk to the public has been minimised', and that forensic nurses are 'better able to detect signs of dangerousness arising out of their patients' relationships, social circumstances and mental state'. It is questionable if there is any evidence for the latter assertion. 'Better able' than whom? It could be argued that the nurse may have more frequent contact with the patient and will therefore be best placed to make such assessments. Gournay (1995, p. 343) suggests that the seriously mentally ill should be offered services by clinically focused case managers and that 'mental health nurses because of the breadth and depth of their training have an obvious first claim on this role'.

In a critique of a report collating the findings of inquiries for the Zito Trust (Sheppard, 1996) Petch & Bradley (1997) outline a number of areas to which mental health services need to pay close attention. Essentially the lessons are that services improve liaison and communication, improve training for staff, adopt assertive follow-up, do not discharge patients in ignorance of their current circumstances and have contingency plans included in care plans. They also argue that inquiries have not been able to demonstrate that service failures are associated with patient homicide in any systematic way. This of course does not mean that service failures are not implicated, only that it has not been demonstrated. Deficiencies may exist in some services which have experienced no homicides while the same deficiencies may not exist in services who have experienced homicides.

MENTALLY DISORDERED OFFENDERS

The literature available on mentally disordered offenders provides useful information for informing and developing practice. Robertson (1988), for instance, reports his study of remand prisoners which included 91 men with mental illness and 76 men without mental illness. He found that prior to the offence for which they were on remand the vast majority of those men with schizophrenia were living alone. This compared to those men who had affective disorders of whom 20% were living with partners prior to offending and 49% of the non-violent group without mental illness. Forty-three per cent of the mentally ill were homeless prior to their offence. These findings while not generalisable to the whole population of those with mental illness are interesting. The lack of social networks for those with mental health problems has been highlighted by other researchers, and the implication is that it is positively associated with offending behaviour (Estroff *et al.*, 1994).

While it is a commonly held belief that detaining patients on hospital orders leads to reduced dangerousness, this has rarely been demonstrated. The reasons for this are the problems inherent in longitudinal studies, for example tracing patients. While prolonged incarceration may reduce dangerous behaviour due to reduced opportunity, it is when patients have returned to community living that realistic assessments of long-term risk behaviours can be conducted.

Gibbens & Robertson (1983) conducted a 15-year follow-up study of men receiving hospital orders (without restriction) in the years 1963–64 to determine reoffending, convictions, hospital admissions and death. There were 249 patients alive 15 years later and of these 42% had had no court appearances, 28% had one or two court appearances and 30% had had three or more. Of those who reoffended, two patients had committed homicide, one had committed arson, six wounding with intent or grievous bodily harm (GBH), and 24 aggravated bodily harm (ABH). Half of all convictions were within 12 months of leaving hospital. Gibbens & Robertson (1983) conclude that the 'results do not suggest that hospital orders failed to protect the public from dangerous offenders'.

DEVELOPING EVIDENCE-BASED INTERVENTIONS FOR MENTALLY DISORDERED OFFENDERS IN THE COMMUNITY

Mentally disordered offenders face problems of social reintegration. The transfer between secure and open settings in many ways mirrors that of the long-term mentally ill. Shepherd (1993, p. 166) acknowledges the similarity between the long-term mentally ill and mentally disordered offenders in that they have similar needs which 'can only be met by co-operation between a number of different agencies'. Dvoskin & Steadman (1994, p. 680) note that these patients require continuous rather than episodic care and 'regular monitoring to contain the individual situational factors that may result in violence'.

For many clinicians forensic patients living in the community present challenges which seem beyond the scope of current services. This can be particularly the case with patients over whom there is no legal sanction. Developing an intensive and collaborative service delivery system may be appropriate and case management is one such system. The recent government emphasis on using an assertive outreach model is essentially one of aggressive application of the case management model of care (DoH, 1998). Holloway *et al.* (1996) carried out a controlled trial using clinical case management in a deprived inner London area. The experimental group consisted of 35 'hard to treat' patients with functional psychosis. This well resourced team offered direct treatment including family interventions, cognitive-behavioural treatments aimed at decreasing distressing symptoms and crisis intervention. Although no figures are provided, the authors state that the team were able to maintain contact with the 'hard to treat' group, and anecdotal evidence provided suggests that this form of service delivery was acceptable to the patients.

Rose (1998) has suggested that as we near the end of the twentieth century the primary function of mental health services is coercion and control rather than cure. Case management may deliver a suitable alternative. Dvoskin & Steadman (1994, p. 680) suggest that case management can be an appropriate strategy for management of risk 'if individual case managers are responsible for small caseloads and if a comprehensive array of services are available in the community'. They argue that patients in the community are often those who have not had long hospital stays. They will not therefore have learnt compliant behaviours and are likely to be difficult to follow up and treat. Case management may therefore be one way of providing services to these patients. It is noted that although patients may, as Dvoskin & Steadman (1994) suggest, regard services as their enemies, restricted patients do not have the luxury of choosing to stay in contact with services. They report findings from a number of US studies which suggest that intensive case management can reduce risk of harmful behaviour. Dvoskin &

Steadman (1994, p. 682) note that the studies are far from definitive but that they 'provide preliminary empirical support for an association between intensive case management and reduced violent behaviour by high risk clients in the community'. They conclude that case management is the 'key to managing the risk of violence in the community among people with mental illness'. In Britain Cooke *et al.* (1994) reported on a group of eight patients with a history of offending and serious mental illness. Most of the patients lived in residential care, and had little income, no jobs and poor family contacts. Hence Cooke and colleagues argue these patients had little to lose by offending and appearing in court. The case management approach offered to these patients initially concentrated on building supportive relationships with the patient rather than confronting their behaviour. Cooke *et al.* (1994) suggest that their patients would offend to get admission to hospital. Involvement with a case manager while not condoning offending behaviour ensured that when the patients felt they needed admission this was arranged for them. Case managers stayed in contact with the patient even if they were convicted and sent to prison so that follow-up could recommence once they were released. In the 18-month period for which data are provided three patients were reconvicted of offences. One patient was placed on a probation order as a result of the support of the case manager. The study suggests a trend towards less episodes of violent behaviour but given the sample size and lack of control group the authors acknowledge the limitations of interpreting these results. Cooke *et al.* (1994) make clear that case management is unlikely to reduce offending where this behaviour is part of a criminal subculture in which offending actions have meaning. One positive outcome, however, was that all patients stayed in contact with the services over the period of the study.

In their study of intensive case management of 47 patients with serious mental illness Ford *et al.* (1996) demonstrated improvements in social functioning, perceived social support, less risk behaviour and increased involvement with activities. Non-significant improvements in mental state and quality of life are also reported. Case management has also demonstrated an increase in treatment uptake, contact with services, satisfaction with services, decrease in family burden, improvement in symptomatology and decrease in the number of bed days used (Stein & Test, 1980; Muijen *et al.*, 1992; Hoult, 1993). It appears therefore that using a case management approach with forensic community patients may at the very least improve the supervision these patients receive. Keeping forensic patients in contact with services may not on its own reduce the potential for risk behaviour. It is arguable whether this is the province of health professionals. What can be gleaned from the literature, however, is that regular contact will enable early intervention should the mental health of these patients deteriorate. In such cases risk behaviour related to deteriorating mental health may be minimised.

CONCEPTS OF CASE MANAGEMENT

There are mixed results for the efficacy and cost-effectiveness of case management. Studies while employing rigorous methods have been largely conducted on small though clearly defined groups of patients for a limited time only. It is important to note that case management works at least as well as conventional treatments and is largely successful in maintaining contact with patients who otherwise would drop out of treatment. The success of case management in managing the symptoms of serious mental illness may largely depend on the type of components inherent within individual programmes.

Gournay (1995) notes that those working with the seriously mentally ill group must have the necessary skills in observation and the ability to form and sustain a therapeutic relationship. The concept of engagement is perhaps one of the most crucial tasks of working with those with serious mental illness. Essentially it involves establishing contact and meaningfully engaging with the person to facilitate later work. Many people with mental illness can lack insight into their condition and are keen to put the experience behind them and do not want the help that is offered. Many mentally disordered offenders are not offered a choice on these matters and this can compound the difficulties in forming a relationship with the worker. Some workers still attempt to engage with a patient of whom they know little but such an approach does not accord with sound risk management procedures. Onyett (1992) reports that his team collected information on a standardised registration form at the point of referral, with the case manager filling in any important gaps in information before meeting the patient for the first time. In regard to forensic patients it is imperative to establish as much information about the person before meeting them. Onyett (1992) makes the point that the patient needs to place the worker in context and that workers should make themselves real people when approaching the patient. It is therefore important to make contact through an established source. This can smooth the path for FCMHNs to establish a relationship with the patient without the antagonism that often occurs when patients are approached 'cold'. Repper *et al.* (1994) investigated the strategies used by mental health nurses who worked as case managers, in establishing relationships with seriously mentally ill patients. A number of areas were important in the initial stages of the relationship with the patient. Case managers referred to the effectiveness of being able to demonstrate their usefulness to the patient. This was particularly important when patients were wary of the case manager. Repper *et al.* (1994) found that the emphasis in the early stages of the relationship was aimed at achieving practical tasks and this served to both clarify the worker's role and provide the foundations for the relationship. Engagement with the patient requires persistence, skill and imagination (Holloway *et al.*, 1996). Both Onyett

(1992) and Holloway *et al.* (1996) emphasise the importance of a respectful approach to the patient. Repper *et al.* (1994) found that the first principle of working with the seriously mentally ill was to establish realistic expectations from the outset with the patient. This enables the patient and the worker to reduce the feelings of frustration and failure, which can envelop the process. Engagement is not only about the initial linking with the patient but also about keeping the patient in contact with the service. Case management involves assertively following the patient into the community and linking with them in whatever venue is appropriate. The engagement process may not be easily achieved. Dvoskin & Steadman (1994, p. 681) note that 'developing a personal relationship with a client takes a great deal of time'. Repper *et al.* (1994) argue that the case management role allows for this consistent and persistent contact over a long period of time. This is a fundamental factor when working with community-based mentally disordered offenders. Engagement, while primarily involving establishing a relationship with the patient, will also involve the process of assessment. An approach which is sensitive to the patient's needs while addressing pertinent issues of assessment should be adopted during this engagement process.

Shepherd (1993) argues that case management is not a panacea for safe management for mentally disordered offenders living in the community. Without adequate resources and support, case managers are unlikely to be able to deliver the hoped-for treatment gains which may be possible with community forensic patients. Shepherd (1993, p. 173) has highlighted that 'treatment in the community is not a substitute for treatment in hospital, it is complementary to it' and this reality must especially be acknowledged when working with mentally disordered offenders.

In many services intensive clinical case management is not possible due to resource issues or ideological differences. It is probably therefore wiser to adopt the best practice principles of case management to deliver services to mentally disordered offenders living in the community. Forensic community mental health nurses can act as keyworkers (Gupta, 1995) under the Care Program Approach (DoH, 1990). They can then prompt or complete assessments of need, deliver services, initiate reviews of care, link the patient into other services they require and offer assertive outreach as required. These functions along with collaborative inter-agency working and liaison should ensure that the services offered are appropriate and comprehensive. Using the principles of case management may help achieve the goal of sustained community tenure coupled with sound risk management.

If the management of mentally disordered offenders in the community is to be a success, it appears that close attention will also have to be given to caseloads. It must be understood, however, that in advocating smaller caseloads FCMHNs must be prepared to keep their end of the deal. That is, specifically, to produce quality patient outcomes, which involves offering specific treatments and support to patients over and above monitoring of mental state and administration of medication. Harris & Bergman (1988) suggest an optimum caseload of 1:12–1:15 for providing case management services to the seriously mentally ill living in the community. This is based on their experience of providing services to seriously mentally ill patients with a mean contact with services of 16 years, 75% of whom had schizophrenia or paranoid schizophrenia. They suggest that caseload ratios of this range are important if clinical outcomes are envisaged. Caseloads for FCMHNs attached to medium secure units in England and Wales currently range between nil and 80 patients (mean = 13.15) per FCMHN (Coffey, 1998a). The expectation that FCMHNs can deliver improvements in outcomes for these patients while carrying large caseloads is improbable.

IMPROVING ADHERENCE TO TREATMENT

With the current emphasis in mental health nursing now centring on a positivist bio-medical model, FCMHNs will be expected to adopt a range of interventions targeted at the seriously mentally ill. This will include not only improved monitoring of medication side-effects but also strategies to improve adherence to treatment and by implication reduce relapse. While it is common in health service delivery for patients to omit medication (Pullar *et al.*, 1990), within forensic mental health the consequences of such behaviour are potentially disastrous. There is now a growing body of evidence and some debate about exactly why patients do not take medication as prescribed. Mortimer (1994) suggests that as many as 75% of patients on neuroleptics may experience extra-pyramidal side effects. One of the main reasons suggested for non-adherence with prescriptions is side effects (Buchanan, 1992). The assumption within the professional literature appears to be that atypical anti-psychotics will be more acceptable to patients because of the lower risk of extra-pyramidal side effects (Gournay & Gray, 1998). This assertion assumes without clear evidence that extra-pyramidal side effects are of most concern to the patients themselves. In fact clinicians views of patients' experience of side effects remain problematic. Day *et al.* (1995) found that clinicians tended to underestimate the severity of distress associated with side effects of medication. Bennett *et al.* (1995) found that community psychiatric nurses were poor at detecting many of the common side effects of anti-psychotic medication. This combination of poor knowledge and underestimating the severity of distress makes it difficult to imagine how patients will be convinced that newer atypical anti-psychotics will have potential benefits for them. Chaplin & Potter (1996) found that the majority of psychiatrists were concerned that informing patients of potential side effects would lead to adherence problems. It seems that without conclusive evidence to the contrary it is assumed that extra-pyramidal side effects are associated with patients not taking their medication. In terms of side effects, how the patient perceives these may be of prime importance in determining compliance (Hogan *et al.*, 1983). Clinical experience would suggest, however, that side effects such as impotence have an important part to play in poor adherence to treatment. Sensitive handling by clinicians of patients' experiences of side effects which does not dismiss them as irrelevant and which aims to involve the patient in reviewing medication levels may go a long way towards improving medication management in schizophrenia. A collaborative approach which does not ignore patient concerns will improve the credibility of the clinician and boost the patient's confidence in the information provided (Hughes *et al.*, 1997).

PSYCHO-EDUCATION

Educating patients and their carers about medication, its uses and its side effects may contribute towards improved adherence to prescriptions (Hogarty *et al.*, 1991). Patients themselves would like more information. Withington & Renoden (1997) surveyed 50 patients attending a clinic for administration of depot injections about knowledge of their medication. While all the patients knew what medication they were on, just under half knew the side effects associated with their medication. Only 30% of the patients surveyed said that they had been given information on their medication and approximately 40% felt that they would like more information.

Improving adherence to treatment may not be sufficiently addressed by providing more information. Hornung *et al.* (1998) offered psycho-educational training in medication management to out-patients with schizophrenia. This group was compared with a group of patients who had not received the intervention. At one-year follow-up the groups did not differ in terms of medication management. The patients receiving the intervention did, however, have reduced fear of side effects and increased confidence in their medication. In the patients not receiving the intervention, confidence in the medication declined and fear of side effects increased. Education may therefore improve attitudes about medication but not necessarily effect adherence. Giving patients information about their treatment does not equate to them understanding and conceptualising the information in the same way as those providing it (Hughes *et al.*, 1997). If the patient already has erroneous beliefs or information about the illness, then facts about the treatment will be incorporated within those beliefs and be similarly misunderstood. Schizophrenia itself can lead to impaired cognitive abilities and this must be recognised in providing education on any aspect of the illness. Further, a subset of patients with low IQ and high levels of negative symptoms do not benefit from psycho-education (MacPherson *et al.*, 1996). Broader educational programmes aimed at providing easily understood information about the illness and its treatment may be indicated. The challenge for FCMHNs is to incorporate education about illness and its treatment into a framework in which implicit coercion to take treatment is common.

MOTIVATIONAL INTERVIEWING

Adversarial approaches to encouraging patients to take prescribed medication are unlikely to be effective (Rollnick *et al.*, 1992). Hughes *et al.* (1997) also suggest that labelling patients as 'lacking in insight' and viewing this behaviour as being somehow deviant will again do little to encourage the spirit of collaboration which is required for successful management of serious mental illness.

One intervention for improving adherence which has been suggested is termed 'brief motivational interviewing' (Rollnick *et al.*, 1992). This technique helps people work through their ambivalence to change. The premise is that patients do not enter therapeutic sessions in a state of readiness to change. The use of straightforward advice-giving is therefore unlikely to effect changes in behaviour. Advising the patient to take medication may push them into a defensive position. This creates an adversarial dynamic within what should ideally be a collaborative therapeutic alliance. Brief motivational interviewing neatly sidesteps this problem by encouraging the patient to articulate the positive and negative elements of the behaviour change, in this instance taking medication. The intervention encourages empathic understanding from the interviewer and is essentially non-directive. That is, the patient is never told or advised what to do but encouraged to explore the benefits or otherwise of behaviour change (accepting treatment) (Rollnick *et al.*, 1992). Whether the use of brief motivational interviewing in people with schizophrenia would result in improvements in medication adherence remains to be seen. Similarly whether such an approach could be operationalised within the field of forensic mental health remains unknown but is worthy of further exploration. Research which compared the use of brief motivational interviewing with intensive psycho-educational interventions in schizophrenia would be enlightening.

PREVENTING RELAPSE THROUGH EARLY INTERVENTION

The development of crisis or contingency plans for forensic community patients summarising past history including risk behaviours, early signs of relapse, current medication and contact numbers of carers and professionals may assist in preventing relapse. These plans can be developed in conjunction with the patient and the carer and included in the care plan. Primm (1996, p. 225) suggests that teams should anticipate crises with patients and implement crisis prevention strategies. Primm (1996, p. 225) states that 'focusing on prevention of crises lowers the likelihood that a crisis will occur'. The use of early signs monitoring and early interventions for each patient can also contribute towards relapse prevention and early resolution (Birchwood *et al.*, 1989). Information learned from this process can then be incorporated into crisis plans so that nurses can be aware of relapse patterns of the patients they work with. Early intervention may also require the development of out-of-hours crisis services for forensic patients (Coffey, 1998b).

Staff providing crisis services may have to deal with many difficult and complex problems. Access to senior staff for advice and direction is important so that staff feel supported and are able to ratify decisions with someone with more experience.

There are other benefits for forensic patients in having an out-of-hours support service for crises. In some cases it can improve the chances of finding accommodation for these often difficult to place patients (Coffey & Chaloner, 1997).

OUT-OF-HOURS PROVISION

With recent UK government intentions it would seem that community-based forensic patients will require an efficient out-of-hours crisis service (DoH, 1998). Many forensic patients living in the community do not currently have 24-hour support and supervision (Coffey & Chaloner, 1997). The literature suggests a need for out-of-hours crisis services for patients with a history of violence. Dvoskin & Steadman (1994, p. 681) state that services 'must be available 24 hours a day, either individually or via teams'. The reason they give for this is that many violent incidents occur when services are closed. It has been identified that provision of out-of-hours working within forensic community mental health nursing is patchy but increasing (Coffey & Chaloner, 1997). Issues of perceived need should be weighed against resource implications when providing out-of-hours provision. The type of service to be provided will reflect this. The range of options for out-of-hours crisis provision includes on-call telephone support to multi-disciplinary on-call emergency teams providing domiciliary visits.

Emergency psychiatric services generally are of two main types. These are either a centralised specialised psychiatric team specifically for emergency work, or a decentralised locality-based team in which emergency work is an integral part of a comprehensive service. While these models may overlap, the broad categories still apply (Johnson & Thornicroft (1995, p. 17). Difficulties remain in demonstrating the efficacy of emergency mental health services. Johnson & Thornicroft (1995, p. 32) note that 'the empirical case for these forms of care remains largely unproven'. There is little evidence in the literature of evaluative research in this area. In forensic psychiatry evidence is particularly scarce. Attempts to evaluate crisis work have been mostly in model programmes. The aim is often to demonstrate gains for the patient coupled with a decrease in bed usage and therefore cost savings. Stein & Test (1980) believe that a service must be prepared to go to the patient and offer treatment wherever the patient is. Their service provided 24-hour cover, and patient programmes were individually drawn up based on assessment of needs. While improvements in symptomatology and social functioning were demonstrated, little detail was given about the out-of-hours portion of the service (Stein & Test, 1980). Muijen *et al.* (1992) offered alternatives to admission to people with long-term mental illness in south London. The project provided assertive home treatment and follow-up. Muijen *et al.* (1992) demonstrated an 80% reduction in hospital stay in the experimental group. This reduced length of stay did not lead to an increase in readmissions. Improvements in symptoms, social adjustments and patients' and relatives' satisfaction were demonstrated. In some cases services have demonstrated reduction in bed use without resorting to offering out-of-hours crisis work. Merson *et al.* (1992) managed to reduce bed occupancy without providing crisis response or 24-hour cover. This suggests that planning care and early intervention may be as effective as offering 24-hour support and advice. This is, however, unlikely to be adequate in terms of risk management of forensic community patients. There is evidence to support the notion that most users of out-of-hours crisis services are already known to services (Cooper, 1979). The implication is that these crises may have been preventable. Johnson & Thornicroft (1995) suggest that better planning, support, education and relapse prevention with these patients may reduce episodes of crisis.

HEALTH POLICY AND LEGISLATION

The traditional practice of community support and follow-up of discharged psychiatric patients, i.e. an out-patient appointment and referral to a community mental health nurse, is unlikely to be sufficient for forensic patients. As more forensic patients are discharged into the community there has been a corresponding increase in the number of forensic community mental health nurses (Brooker & White, 1997). This suggests that follow-up should be comprehensive, assertive and based on sound principles of risk assessment and management. The Care Programme Approach has provided a basic format for what are essentially case management principles. While these fundamentals will possibly see an improvement in the supervision and treatment of discharged patients, no content of the care to be provided is specified. As a response to concerns such as this the Clinical Standards Advisory Group (CSAG, 1995) detailed standards of care. As the seriously mentally ill are considered largely synonymous with forensic patients, these standards of care are worthy of consideration and incorporation into practice by FCHMNs.

IMPACT OF HEALTH POLICY

There is a lack of evidence for Supervised Discharge Orders (DoH, 1995), Supervision Registers (DoH, 1994) or the Care Programme Approach (DoH, 1990) for reducing reoffending or risk of violence. This may be because the research has yet to catch up with these policy changes. In terms of the supervised discharge legislation, concerns have been raised in regard to its potential to deliver the improvements in risk management of the seriously mentally ill (Fulop, 1995; Wells, 1998). In the United States, however, Keilitz (1990) looked at 24 empirical studies which investigated Involuntary Outpatient Commitment (IOC), a power similar to supervised discharge. Nine of these studies looked at outcomes. The results were mixed, and Keilitz (1990) concluded that the success of particular programmes depended on the features of the individual process, the specific programme, and those participating in it. This suggests that how Section 25 is interpreted will be an important factor. Miller & Fiddleman (1984, p. 150) suggest that the success of IOC was hampered by staff resistance: 'non-medical personnel tend to be less authoritarian than are physicians and therefore less comfortable with coerced treatment'. Hiday & Scheid-Cook (1987, p. 230) found that some community mental health centres had an 'unofficial policy' of not using the powers because they were opposed to using coerced treatment.

This raises the point of the willingness of staff to use these powers. Miller & Fiddleman (1984) concluded in their study of services in North Carolina in the United States that IOC was not successful because community staff were ideologically resistant to the concept. Hiday & Scheid-Cook (1987, p. 231), however, conclude that it is working for a group of patients who would otherwise 'refuse treatment, become dangerous, would be hospitalised and consequently would experience a greater deprivation of liberty'.

In the UK Sensky *et al.* (1991a, p. 792) have argued that the success of community care depends on: 'the willingness of people vulnerable to serious psychiatric breakdown to co-operate with their treatments'. They make the point that patients discharged from hospital 'are sometimes unwilling to continue with their treatment' (Sensky *et al.*, 1991a, p. 792). In their retrospective study of patients being treated on extended leave, Sensky *et al.* (1991a) found that these patients had reduced total length of time spent in hospital and had shorter admissions. However, the number of admissions for this group was not significantly altered. The patients being treated on extended leave showed improved compliance with out-patient appointments and medication. The authors conclude that a community treatment order giving the power of recall to hospital would 'benefit a small group of patients with severe mental illness in improving their compliance as out-patients and reducing the time they spend in hospital' (Sensky *et al.*, 1991b, p. 799). This it is argued would mean patients spending less time in hospital, resulting in less interference in their lives. Patients would not therefore be removed from the community for long periods of time and would maintain contact with friends and relatives preserving these important social support networks. Sensky *et al.*'s (1991a) assertion that the success of community care is dependent on the co-operation of the patient ignores the issue of resourcing of community care which MIND (1995) argues is as important. However, it appears again that UK mental health policy may be moving towards greater coercion of those with mental illness living in the community and this, coupled with the avowed intention to improve services, may yet make the biggest impact on how FCMHNs deliver care in the future (DoH, 1998).

COMMUNITY FOLLOW-UP OF SPECIAL HOSPITAL PATIENTS

Evidence from the follow-up of discharged special hospital patients can shed little light on what approaches may be useful with forensic community patients. Bailey & MacCulloch (1992) followed up 112 discharges from a special hospital and found that 37% had committed a fresh offence, and 17% (of the total) had committed serious offences, i.e. homicide, assault, rape, arson, robbery and indecent assault. Patients given a conditional discharge were less likely to be reconvicted. There were similar differences between mentally ill patients and those with personality disorder. That is, mentally ill patients were less likely to be reconvicted than personality disordered patients. Patients of both groups discharged conditionally were less likely to offend than their counterparts. If a mentally ill patient was not reconvicted within 30 months, then the chances of this happening were reduced to 'virtually nil'. No information on the content of the care offered is provided, however. The relevance of this research to community follow-up of forensic patients is that they mirror very closely those patients seen by FCMHNs in daily practice.

INDIVIDUAL RESPONSIBILITY FOR THE PATIENT'S ACTIONS

The development of health policy initiatives in regard to forensic patients living in the community has prompted concerns that responsibility for patient actions may move to clinicians. Burrow (1996, p. 918) notes 'the focus on the shortcomings of the community care programme represents a move away from holding the non-compliant patient responsible for any disastrous deterioration in his/her health'.

However, Kennedy & Jones (1996, p. 209) acknowledge that in English law there is 'generally no duty of care owed by a person for the conduct of a third party' and that the courts have been reluctant to impose such a duty. In the United States, most states have what has become known as a Tarasoff ruling. This followed a case of a patient who told his psychotherapist of his plan to kill a woman, Tatiana Tarasoff. The psychotherapist did not warn the woman who was subsequently killed by the patient. Her parents sued on the basis that the therapist was negligent in not warning the victim. The court held that a duty of care existed towards any potential victim of one of his patients. Across the United States other rulings followed this line of reasoning. Kennedy & Jones (1996) argue that with problems in the implementation of community care there is an increasing pressure on courts in the UK to introduce a duty of care on professionals. Should this happen the implications for both patients and those looking after them will be far-reaching. Kennedy & Jones (1996, p. 215) note that in the United States 'the fear of being sued has an impact on the process of deciding when to discharge patients into the community'.

RISK ASSESSMENT AND MANAGEMENT FOR COMMUNITY PATIENTS

Providing care in the community means to a certain extent managing risk in the community. Risk assessment and management are covered elsewhere in this volume and will only be addressed briefly here. It has been noted above that particular strategies of managing patients in the community lead to improvements in symptoms, increased contact with services and adherence to treatment regimes. It would be simplistic to imagine that this will lead directly to a decrease in risk behaviour but where previous risk has been associated with relapse of illness such a decrease in risk behaviour can be expected. The contextual and relationship elements of dangerous behaviour, however, are more difficult to control. The awareness of these factors in the patient's previous offending is therefore important in arriving at a working assessment of the risk the person presents. Assessment and management of risk should also take into account the risk the client may present to themselves and the risk of neglect.

CONCLUSIONS

Clearly there is a balance to be drawn between the care of forensic patients and the management of risk they may present. Research which aims to clarify whether coercive treatment schedules are likely to reduce risk may be worthwhile. Up-to-date research on patients on section 41 and whether they are more or less likely to reoffend would be useful. Comparison with the supervised discharge legislation and the effects on the therapeutic relationships of community supervision again would be illuminating. Research into the use of assertive case management across various sites with forensic patients which investigates if it indeed reduces risk or influences it in any way could provide evidence for the clinical effectiveness of this approach. The combination of this and the use of psychotherapeutic interventions versus traditional methods may be useful in developing our understanding of outcomes for forensic patients.

Burrow (1996) suggests that there is a need for research on outcomes for relatives of mentally disordered offenders who live in the community, and notes that this may highlight a need for respite care in the community. Indeed initiatives with relatives and patients in terms of offering respite and crisis beds in the community are notable by their absence in the forensic literature. There is also a notable lack of research literature on providing appropriate community-based accommodation and daytime activities for this patient group.

Given recent concerns the monitoring and development of practice are required to ensure that problems identified in special hospitals in regard to more coercive treatment being used on ethnic minorities are not repeated in community practice.

In designing FCMHN services it may be advisable to establish specialist areas of interest for each nurse. Most services have clinicians who spend a number of sessions per week engaged in work which is not strictly community follow-up of discharged patients. Examples are nurses working in diversion from court or custody projects or those nurses who work in sex offender treatment services or prison liaison. The development of specialist knowledge and expertise in other areas such as substance abuse, family work, specific cognitive-behavioural treatments and victim awareness would be a logical progression. It is of course difficult to imagine one nurse being knowledgeable in all these areas to the extent of being able to offer treatment advice to others. Identifying nurses within teams with special interest areas could assist in developing expertise and practice.

Problems in providing case management services have been identified. Shepherd (1993) acknowledges that resistance to case managers due to inter-agency rivalries may make their job impossible to do. The presence of good quality supervision and support is essential for keeping staff motivated and engaged in work with patients who present challenging behaviours. Dvoskin & Steadman (1994, p. 684) acknowledge that working in high crime areas with patients who are violent, unusual hours, strain on personal relation-ships and lack of career mobility can increase job stress and lead to high turnover. Shepherd (1993, p. 171) also notes that mentally disordered offenders are unattractive to ambitious young therapists. Thus the devel-opment of clinical supervision structure together with academic opportu-nities may assist in attracting the clinicians whom forensic services require.

For forensic community mental health nurses, like many of our patients, the future holds many challenges. Whether this future is bright with innova-tion remains to be seen. What is certain is that community management and treatment are now possible for this group of patients. The time may be right for FCMHNs to assert themselves by providing innovative and research-based practices for this group of patients.

REFERENCES

Bailey, J. & MacCulloch, M. (1992) Patterns of reconviction in patients discharged directly to the community from a special hospital: implications for aftercare. *Journal of Forensic Psychiatry* 3(3), 445–61.

Bennett, J., Done, J. & Hunt, B. (1995) Assessing the side effects of anti-psychotic drugs: a survey of CPN practice. *Journal of Psychiatric and Mental Health Nursing* 2, 177–82.

Birchwood, M., Smith, J., MacMillan, F., Hogg, B., Prasad, R., Harvey, C. & Bering, S. (1989) Predicting relapse in schizophrenia: the development and implementation of an early signs monitoring system using patients and families as observers, a preliminary investigation. *Psychological Medicine* 19, 649–56.

Brooker, C. & White, E. (1997) *The Fourth Quinquennial National Com-munity Mental Health Nursing Census of England and Wales*. University of Manchester.

Buchanan, A. (1992) A two-year prospective study of treatment compliance in patients with schizophrenia. *Psychological Medicine* 22, 787–97.

Burrow, S. (1993) An outline of the forensic nursing role. *British Journal of Nursing* 2(18), 899–904.

Burrow, S. (1996) Community reforms: Do they improve the mental health of clients? *British Journal of Nursing* 5(15), 918–19.

Chaplin, R. & Potter, M. (1996) Tardive dyskinesia: screening and risk disclosure. *Psychiatric Bulletin* 20, 714–16.

Clinical Standards Advisory Group (1995) *Schizophrenia*. Vol. 1. Report of a CSAG Committee on Schizophrenia. HMSO, London.

Coffey, M. (1998a) Occupational stress and burnout: forensic community mental health nurses. How are they faring? Unpublished MSc dissertation, Middlesex University, Enfield.

Coffey, M. (1998b) Provision of out-of-hours support to a forensic population: strategies and research potential. *Journal of Psychiatric and Mental Health Nursing* **5**(5), 367–78.

Coffey, M. & Chaloner, C. (1997) Out-of-hours working: a survey. *Mental Health Nursing* **17**(7), 6–9.

Cooke, A., Ford, R., Thompson, T., Wharne, S. and Haynes, P. (1994) 'Something to lose': Case management for mentally disordered offenders. *Journal of Mental Health* **3**, 59–67.

Cooper, J. E. (1979) Crisis admission units and emergency psychiatric services. *Public Health in Europe* No. 2. World Health Organisation, Copenhagen.

Day, J. C., Wood, G., Dewey, M. & Bentall, R. P. (1995) A self-rating scale for measuring neuroleptic side-effects: validation in a group of schizophrenic patients. *British Journal of Psychiatry* **166**, 650–53.

Department of Health (1990) *Caring for People: the Care Programme Approach.* HMSO, London.

Department of Health (1994) HSG(94)5. *Introduction of Supervision Registers for Mentally Ill People from 1 April 1994.* NHS Management Executive/HMSO, London.

Department of Health (1995) *The Mental Health (Patients in the Community) Act 1995.* HMSO, London.

Department of Health (1998) *Modernising Mental Health Services: Safe, Sound and Supportive.* HMSO, London.

Department of Health-/-Home Office (1992) *Review of Health and Social Services for Mentally Disordered Offenders and Others Requiring Similar Services* (the Reed Report). HMSO, London.

Dvoskin, J. A. and Steadman, H. J. (1994) Using intensive case management to reduce violence by mentally ill persons in the community. *Hospital and Community Psychiatry* **45**(7), pp. 679–84.

Estroff, S., Zimmer, C., Lachicotte, W. & Benoit, J. (1994) The influence of social networks and social support on violence by persons with serious mental illness. *Hospital and Community Psychiatry* **45**, 669–79.

Evans, N. (1996) Defining the role of the forensic community mental health nurse. *Nursing Standard* **10**(49), 35–7.

Ford, R., Ryan, P., Norton, P., Beadsmore, A., Craig, T. & Muijen, M. (1996) Does intensive case management work? Clinical, social and quality of life outcomes from a controlled study. *Journal of Mental Health* **5**(4), 361–8.

Fulop, N. (1995) Supervised discharge: lessons from the U.S. experience. *Mental Health Nursing* **15**(3), 16–20.

Gibbens, T. C. N. & Robertson, G. (1983) A survey of the criminal careers of hospital order patients. *British Journal of Psychiatry* **143**, 362–9.

Gournay, K. (1995) Mental health nurses working purposefully with people with serious and enduring mental illness – an international perspective. *International Journal of Nursing Studies* **32**(4), 341–52.

Gournay, K. & Gray, R. (1998) The role of new drugs in the treatment of schizophrenia. *Mental Health Nursing* **18**(2), 21–4.

Gupta, N. (1995) Keyworkers and the care programme approach: the role and responsibilities of community workers. *Psychiatric Care* **1**(6), 239–42.

Harris, M. & Bergman, H. C. (1988) Misconceptions about the use of case management services by the chronically mentally ill: a utilization analysis. *Hospital and Community Psychiatry* **39**, 1276–80.

Hiday, V. A. & Scheid-Cook T. (1987) The North Carolina experience in outpatient commitment: a critical appraisal. *International Journal of Law and Psychiatry* **10**, 215–32.

Hogan, T. P., Awad, A. G. & Eastwood, R. (1983) A self-report scale predictive of drug compliance in schizophrenics: reliability and discriminative validity. *Psychological Medicine* **13**, 177–83.

Hogarty, G. E., Anderson, C. M., Reiss, D. J., Kornblith, S. J., Greenwald, D. P., Ulrich, R. F. & Carter, M. (1991) Family psychoeducation, social skills training, and maintenance chemotherapy in the aftercare treatment of schizophrenia: two-year effects of a controlled study on relapse and adjustment. *Archives of General Psychiatry* **48**, 340–7.

Holloway, F., Murray, M., Squire, C. & Carson, J. (1996) Intensive case management: putting it into practice. *Psychiatric Bulletin* **20**, 395–7.

Hornung, W. P., Klingberg, S., Feldman, R., Schonauer, K. & Schulze Monking, H. (1998) Collaboration with drug treatment by schizophrenic patients with and without psychoeducational training: results of a 1-year follow-up. *Acta Psychiatrica Scandinavica* **97**, 213–19.

Hoult, J. (1993) Comprehensive services for the mentally ill. *Current Opinion in Psychiatry* **6**, 238–45.

Hughes, I., Hill, B. & Budd, R. (1997) Compliance with anti-psychotic medication: from theory to practice. *Journal of Mental Health* **6**(5), 473–89.

Johnson, S. & Thornicroft, G. (1995) Service models in emergency psychiatry: an international review. In *Emergency Mental Health Services in the Community* (Phelan, M., Strathdee, G. & Thornicroft, G., eds). Cambridge University Press, Cambridge.

Keilitz, I. (1990) Empirical studies of involuntary outpatient commitment: is it working? *Mental and Physical Disability Law Reporter* **14**(4), 368–72.

Kennedy, M. & Jones, E. (1996) Violence from patients in the community: will UK courts impose a duty of care on mental health professionals? *Criminal Behaviour and Mental Health* **9**, 209–17.

MacPherson, R., Jerrom, B. & Hughes, A. (1996) A controlled study of education about drug treatment in schizophrenia. *British Journal of Psychiatry* **168**, 709–17.

Merson, S., Tyrer, P., Onyett, S., Lack, S., Birkett, P. & Johnson, T. (1992) Early intervention in psychiatric emergencies: a controlled clinical trial. *Lancet* **339**, 1311–14.

Miller, R. & Fiddleman, P. (1984) Outpatient commitment: treatment in the least restrictive environment? *Hospital and Community Psychiatry* **35**(2), 147–51.

MIND (1995) *Care not Coercion.* MIND Publications, London.

Mortimer, A. (1994) Newer and older anti-psychotics: A comparative review of appropriate use. *CNS Drugs* **2**(5), 381–96.

Muijen, M., Marks, I., Connolly, J. & Audini, B. (1992) Home based care and standard hospital care for patients with severe mental illness: a randomised controlled trial. *British Medical Journal* **304**, 749–54.

Onyett, S. (1992) *Case Management in Mental Health*. Chapman & Hall, London.

Petch, E. & Bradley, C. (1997) Learning the lessons from homicide inquiries: adding insult to injury? *Journal of Forensic Psychiatry* 8(1), 161–84.

Primm, A. B. (1996) Assertive community treatment. In *Integrated Mental Health Services* (Breakey, W. R., ed.). Oxford University Press, New York.

Pullar, T., Kumar, S. & Peaker, S. (1990) Patterns of compliance in hypertension. *British Journal of Clinical Pharmacology* 30, 381.

Repper, J., Ford, R., & Cooke, A. (1994) How can nurses build trusting relationships with people who have severe and long term mental health problems? Experiences of case managers and their clients. *Journal of Advanced Nursing* 19, 1096–104.

Robertson, G. (1988) Arrest patterns among mentally disordered offenders. *British Journal of Psychiatry* 153, 313–16.

Rollnick, S., Heather, N. & Bell, A. (1992) Negotiating behaviour change in medical settings: The development of brief motivational interviewing. *Journal of Mental Health* 1, 25–37.

Rose, N. (1998) Living dangerously – Risk thinking and risk management. *Mental Health Care* 1(8), 263–6.

Sensky, T., Hughes, T. & Hirsch, S. (1991a) Compulsory psychiatric treatment in the community I. A controlled study of compulsory community treatment with extended leave under the Mental Health Act: Special characteristics of patients treated and impact of treatment. *British Journal of Psychiatry* 158, 792–9.

Sensky, T., Hughes, T. & Hirsch, S. (1991b) Compulsory psychiatric treatment in the community II. A controlled study of patients whom psychiatrists would recommend for compulsory treatment in the community. *British Journal of Psychiatry* 158, 799–804.

Shepherd, G. (1993) Case management. In *The Mentally Disordered Offender in an Era of Community Care: New Directions in Provision* (Watson, W. & Grounds, A., eds). Cambridge University Press, Cambridge.

Sheppard, D. (1996) *Learning the Lessons*, 2nd edn. Zito Trust, London.

Stein, L. I. & Test, M. A. (1980) Alternatives to mental hospital treatment. 1. Conceptual model, treatment program, and clinical evaluation. *Archives of General Psychiatry* 37, 392–7.

Swanson, J. W., Borum, R., Swartz, M. S. & Monohan, J. (1996) Psychotic symptoms and disorders and the risk of violent behaviour in the community. *Criminal Behaviour and Mental Health* 6, 309–29.

Wells, J. S. G. (1998) Severe mental illness, statutory supervision and mental health nursing in the United Kingdom: meeting the challenge. *Journal of Advanced Nursing* 27(4), 698–706.

Withington, J. & Renoden, M. (1997) Sharing medication information with patients. *Mental Health Care* 1(1), 22–4.

Chapter 10
Diversion from the Criminal Justice System

Gina Hillis

INTRODUCTION

People whose mental health problems culminate in their becoming entangled in the criminal justice system should, as a matter of principle, be diverted into appropriate health care services. Where this is not possible there should be provision for appropriate mental health care and for treatment if required, whilst in police custody, during transition through the courts and when in custody in prison, whether remanded or convicted.

Apart from the obvious duty of psychiatric agencies to ensure that this service is provided, it is economical in financial as well as human terms both for the individual and the community in general.

Ethical and legal dilemmas often arise when decisions need to be made which both demonstrate regard for the rights of the individual whilst considering the safety of the general public. These issues require a collaborative approach within the multi-agency setting of police stations, courts and prisons. Inter-agency training is seen as the way forward in order to achieve greater understanding of decision-making processes and to facilitate appropriate interventions.

DEFINITION

'Diversion' occurs when a defendant has been removed from the criminal justice system and placed in the care of health or social services as an alternative to custody. It also takes place if a defendant is referred to psychiatric services and a case is discontinued when it is not in the interests of the general public to pursue it.

'Diversion' does not occur when a defendant receives psychiatric care whilst on bail while the case continues. This occurs in many cases and the term 'diversion' can often be somewhat misleading. For this reason many 'diversion' services are referred to as 'liaison' or 'assessment' services.

The term 'diversion', however, is used in this chapter to cover all aspects of assessment and liaison as well as diversion, whether the defendant's case is pursued by the Criminal Justice System or otherwise. The Home Office (1990a) made recommendations for the diversion of mentally disordered offenders subsequently reflected in the Reed Report (Department of Health/ Home Office, 1992) which advocated the development of diversion services within the broader sense of its meaning.

MIND (1997) advocates changing the term 'mentally disordered offenders' as many individuals have not even been charged or convicted of an offence. This has been further discussed by Kennedy *et al.* (1997) who prefer the term 'mentally vulnerable defendants' as many are not classified as mentally 'disordered' but still have mental health problems. This chapter will use the term 'mentally vulnerable defendants'.

HISTORICAL PERSPECTIVE

The concept of 'diversion' is not a new one and the disposal of mentally disordered offenders is documented as far back as the eighth century. At that time the church dispensed justice because church leaders were the only people who had sufficient understanding of the law and applied it 'in the name of God' and in the name of the current king or queen.

Murder or 'slaying' was punishable according to the status of the victim. The more important the victim, the more severe the punishment. Compensation to the victim's family was also imposed. The punishment for most ordinary people was one year's fasting for accidental murder and five years' fasting for premeditated murder. The reasons behind this form of punishment are questionable considering just how long one could survive in those times with no food when water was often contaminated with diseases such as cholera and typhoid.

Egbert was the Archbishop of York in the eighth century and he appeared to have some notion of the need for compassion towards mentally vulnerable defendants, particularly where the offence was related to mental illness. Egbert said:

> 'If a man fall out of his senses or wits, and it came to pass that he kill someone, let his kinsman pay for the victim, and preserve the slayer against ought else of that kind. If anyone kill him before it is made known whether his friends are willing to intercede for him, those who kill must pay for him to his kin' (Egbert in Walker, 1968, p. 15).

There are many examples documented in English legal history pertaining to the mentally ill. Bracton was the first medieval judge to write on the Laws and Customs of England in the middle of the 13th century. Bracton's principles were really ethical considerations where a mentally ill person was decreed 'in the King's mercy' and a 'Royal Pardon' was to be given to those of 'unsound mind'. He also introduced the notion of *mens rea* as we know it today in terms of proving the intent to commit murder.

'For a crime is not committed unless the will to harm be present. Misdeeds are distinguishable by will and by intention, and then there is what can be said about the child and the madman. For the one is protected by his innocence of design, the other by the misfortune of his deed. In misdeeds we look to the will and not the outcome' (Bracton in Walker, 1968, p. 26).

In Bracton's time responsibility for mentally vulnerable defendants was taken out of the legal system and became the responsibility of the family who were held accountable for any further misdeeds of the offender.

The Mental Health Act 1959 recognised the need for dealing compassionately with mentally vulnerable people who came to the attention of the police. Section 136 gave police power to remove a person to a place of safety in order to be assessed for any subsequent need for treatment. This act also gave powers to approved social workers to assess the suitability for admission to hospital whilst having due regard for the 'least restrictive' option available for the patient. This provision is still inherent in the Mental Health Act 1983.

The Home Office Circular 66/90 (Home Office, 1990a) identified the urgent need for services to be established within the criminal justice system and recommended a complete review of the situation in order to implement radical changes. This report stated that a mentally disordered person should never be remanded to prison simply to receive medical treatment or assessment.

The Reed Report (Department of Health/Home Office, 1992) directed that there should be collaboration between all agencies involved and laid down guidelines as to what was required in order to achieve this. Both reports also scrutinised the possibilities of early intervention and diversion where appropriate as a preventative measure against deterioration in custody. This had previously been studied by Judge Tumin in a report (Home Office, 1990b) which investigated the extent of suicide and self-harm within prisons. Judge Tumin along with Lord Woolf (Home Office, 1990c) continued to study causes and effects of disturbances in prisons following the riots at HMP Strangeways in Manchester.

The *Health of the Nation* (Department of Health, 1992) targets to reduce the number of suicides in custody reflects the concerns raised by these reports. Further concerns engendered at the time created an opportunity for raising awareness, securing funding and setting up services. It was hoped that the 1990s would become the age of enlightenment. This is reflected in the revised Criminal Justice Act 1991 which gives credence to the role of the probation service who not only address the needs of offenders following prosecution, but also provide pre-sentence reports to the courts. These reports enquire into an offender's social circumstances and take account of the potential for diversion into appropriate health and social care options due to the presence of mental health problems.

Diversion is only successful when adequate resources are available to refer to, such as patient beds, accommodation and various community services. More research is currently being undertaken to evaluate services, and the main lesson to be learned is that resources should be provided before embarking upon diversion services as described by James *et al.* (1997). They examined the reduction in remands to prison for psychiatric reports by utilising in-patient facilities offering varying degrees of security. They provided the court with a comprehensive multi-disciplinary assessment on the day of appearance to determine the need for hospital admission. They also provided the psychiatric report following admission to an in-patients unit. This considerably reduced the need for a remand in custody and enabled a more rapid response in reporting back to the court.

James *et al.* (1997) suggest that this model would support one of the Reed Report (Department of Health/Home Office, 1992) recommendations to alter legislation affecting magistrates' power to remand into custody for the sole purpose of providing a psychiatric report. Joseph (1992) highlighted the fact that some defendants are disadvantaged in not being granted bail purely because a remand in custody is sought for the purpose of a psychiatric report.

Birmingham (1998, p. 44) aroused further concern in his comment, 'These are very vulnerable people who are unlikely to maintain contact with services outside prison and whose chaotic behaviour leads them to be put on remand time and time again!'

Exworthy & Parrott (1993) also sought to address the problem of lengthy remands in custody by providing psychiatric reports following successful diversion to hospital or whilst on bail in the community. They substantially reduced the duration and frequency of remands into custody as well as providing appropriate psychiatric follow-up.

Holloway & Shaw (1994) investigated outcomes of patients over an 18-month period following diversion. They found that whilst a small minority reoffended during this time, overall contact with the criminal justice system was much reduced. The majority, however, did not reoffend and also remained in contact with services. They suggest that this may be due to the fact that these patients had a home with some stability and therefore were not vulnerable to the problems that occur to homeless people. This is borne out by Joseph & Potter (1993) who found that homeless offenders generally have poorer outcomes and are more vulnerable to mental illness as well as reoffending behaviour.

Having a home address is an important issue in the decision-making process for defendants applying for bail as discussed by Morgan & Pearce (1989). If defendants are homeless this will reduce the likelihood of being granted bail and hence is an important factor when contemplating diversion. If suitable supported and supervised accommodation is found, in conjunction with referral to appropriate services, this increases the chance of being granted bail. This would appear to support Jones (1992) who advocates the need for specialist bail provision for mentally vulnerable defendants.

Bail hostels form an integral part of the diversion process providing support with supervision and helping to ameliorate the problems associated with homelessness. Kennedy *et al.* (1997) set out to examine the need for psychiatric bail provision and found that one-fifth of defendants with mental health problems benefit from some form of psychiatric bail provision as an alternative to custody.

A study by the mentally disordered offenders project (MENDOP, 1991) also demonstrated this need and was instrumental in the setting up of a specialist bail hostel in Birmingham called Elliott House. It is situated in south Birmingham close to local services and courts and has facilities for 20 male residents. Whilst at Elliott House, clients undergo psychiatric assessment as well as receiving care and treatment from the probation service in conjunction with a visiting multi-disciplinary team from the local medium secure unit. This forms an integral part of Birmingham Diversion Services.

Blumanthal & Wessely (1992) have described court diversion services, some of which are often limited initiatives with incomplete staffing or support and lack involvement of mainstream services. More recently this trend is changing, with involvement from both forensic and mainstream services working together. Often models incorporate mainstream services as discussed by Strong (1996) who advocates multi-agency input and improved liaison between agencies. Bail hostel settings provide the ideal opportunity for collaborative working to occur, particularly in complying with bail packages and in 'moving on' plans for mentally vulnerable defendants.

PRINCIPLES AND PRACTICE

The principles and practice of successful diversion are based on the stages at which diversion can occur, as follows:

(1) Diversion at point of arrest.
(2) Diversion from court.
(3) Diversion from prison.

Access points in the criminal justice system at which liaison/ diversion services can operate

- Community
  - Police station (local services involved)
  - Section 136 Mental Health Act 1983 (to local psychiatric hospital)
- Police station
  - local health and social services
  - community services – psychiatric
  - learning disabilities
  - substance and alcohol abuse
  - hospital admission
  - psychiatric and learning disability
- Magistrates' court
  - as above plus psychiatric input to bail hostels
- Crown Court
  - hospital admission – psychiatric
  - hospital admission – medium secure unit
  - hospital admission – special hospital
  - psychiatric care in prison
- Prison
  - as above plus psychiatric input to bail hostels

People with mental health problems often find themselves in the criminal justice system through no direct fault of their own. The earliest stage at which intervention can occur is usually at the point of arrest when a person is conveyed from an incident to the police station for questioning. Being arrested is an extremely traumatic time for a healthy person but for a person with mental health problems it is likely to be even more bewildering and frightening. The need for experienced mental health professionals to be actively involved in this process has been shown by the many schemes that have mushroomed in recent years.

Liaison and collaboration occur between various disciplines such as the police, defence solicitors, forensic medical examiners, health-care workers and social workers, particularly at the first stage of diversion, i.e. diversion at the point of arrest. The next stage takes place at court prior to appearance before the magistrates. Joseph (1992) observed the 'yawning gap' between diversion of the mentally disordered person from the police station and the next available opportunity during remand in custody. It has now become a possibility to fill this gap at the stage of court appearance.

Awaiting court appearance whilst in overnight custody and the anxiety that this provokes require sensitive and efficient intervention by experienced staff who have the appropriate knowledge of both the criminal justice system and local health-care facilities. At this second stage the list of disciplines involved increases to include the Crown Prosecution Service, custody officers, court clerks, probation and bail information officers.

A further stage at which intervention and diversion can occur is at the commencement of a custodial remand. There are a number of people with mental health problems who are remanded into prison custody in spite of attempts at diversion. This can occur for many reasons but usually happens because the appropriate health care option is unavailable or the gravity of the offence will not allow diversion to take place at an earlier stage. At this third stage the prison staff will inevitably become involved as well.

Key elements in comprehensive provision include the mechanisms set up for efficient liaison between the wide range of disciplines leading to collaboration and prompt decision making resulting in delivery of appropriate care at the earliest opportunity.

MODELS OF DIVERSION

In the early 1990s the United Kingdom had approximately 60 diversion schemes in operation (Backer-Holst, 1994). This figure is arbitrary as many of these were funded for a specific duration and were unable to continue when the funding ceased. There are also many such services in the USA, Australia and New Zealand. All schemes operate differently according to demographic factors such as population, social structure, service provision including availability of regional secure units and the number of police stations and courts within a catchment area.

A different response is required for a highly populated city with many police stations feeding into a busy central court and a rural area with smaller police stations and courts sitting for only a few sessions each week. A tailor-made approach is required for each area and some have developed on-call services with a nurse or psychiatrist serving one or more police stations and often one or more courts. These schemes offer a visiting service, at a designated time each week, to assess those persons thought to have a mental health problem.

CASE STUDY

The subject was a 21-year-old male charged with wounding following an attack on his father with a hammer. He presented as irritable, thought disordered, perplexed, oblivious to his circumstances and unable to comprehend the seriousness of the offence. He was vulnerable in that he could not instruct his solicitor and suggestible in that he agreed with any prospect put before him, and in terms of risk assessment he constituted a high risk. The assault was unprovoked, delusionally led (he perceived his father had killed other people and was evil) and serious in that he had used a weapon.

No alcohol or illicit substance use was elicited. There was no history of self-harm but he expressed ideas that, if the evil were passed down to him, he would have to strangle himself to 'kill the evil'. Whilst he denied auditory hallucinations he appeared to be responding to psychotic stimuli and this was provoking emotional lability with spontaneous laughter and bouts of tearfulness. He agreed to go to hospital until he realised it would mean admission for some weeks which caused him much anxiety.

When assessment was completed, the liaison process with the probation service, the Crown Prosecution Service and the defence solicitor concluded that he required psychiatric assessment and treatment in a hospital setting. As well as his presenting mental illness he was deemed to be potentially suicidal and unpredictable in his capability of making decisions. It was therefore appropriate to request that the court allow him to be bailed to the local psychiatric hospital under Section 2 (Mental Health Act 1983) with the bail being conditional that he reside at the hospital for a period of 28 days. This would allow sufficient time for psychiatric assessments to be completed whilst also ensuring close observation regarding potential suicidal thoughts. The court agreed to this arrangement as it also allowed protection of the general public but stipulated that the admission should be to a locked facility, i.e. the intensive care unit of the local hospital.

He accepted treatment whilst subject to compulsory assessment in hospital, and responded well to medication. When he returned to court 28 days later, he was able to instruct his solicitor to apply for bail. He was bailed to the local bail hostel with arrangements to continue the psychiatric care and subsequently remained there. He was eventually given a 2-year probation order with a condition of treatment.

BIRMINGHAM DIVERSION SERVICES

Diversion services have been operating in Birmingham in the West Midlands since 1991. Birmingham has a population of approximately 2 146 000 and like any large city has its share of deprived areas and high unemployment with all its associated problems, as well as areas of relative wealth.

Diversion at point of arrest

There are twelve main police stations in the Birmingham conurbation, and one such police station in south Birmingham was selected to pilot a scheme for one year in 1992. One forensic community mental health nurse (FCMHN) from the local medium secure unit (MSU) visited the station cells on a daily basis in order to screen all those arrested for mental health problems. When it was realised that many of the arrests occurred during late evening and throughout the night, the scheme responded by providing an additional on-call service.

The first year provided an opportunity for the police to become familiar with recognising mental health problems and the process of diversion at point of arrest (Wix, 1993). Over 700 people were screened and assessed and 7% were found to have a mental health problem; half of the latter were diverted at this point. Most required further assessment and treatment in the community but some required admission to the local psychiatric hospital. Most were not charged following successful arrangements for diversion but a small number could not be diverted at this point as they were required by law to appear before the magistrates in view of the seriousness of the offence.

Court diversion

The Birmingham Magistrates' Courts are situated in the city centre and each day all of the surrounding police stations feed into the main central custody cells. Under the Magistrates' Court Act 1980 a defendant must be brought to the next available court (usually within 24 hours). One of the 24 available courts is allocated to deal with all those arrested and held over-night and sits every day except Sundays, Good Friday and Christmas Day.

The diversion service in the Magistrates' Court commenced as a pilot scheme at the beginning of 1991 and early results proved the need for such a service. The main aim is to provide a proactive approach to screening and identifying mental health problems as opposed to reactively responding to referrals from others (Hillis, 1993).

An FCMHN from the local MSU screens the prosecution files and assesses those defendants thought to have mental health problems prior to their court appearance. Of an average number of 25 overnight defendants approximately three are thought to have mental health problems and are therefore selected for assessment using specific criteria as follows:

(1) Past psychiatric history (if known) and previous recorded convictions with a hospital order.
(2) History of use of alcohol and illicit substances with mental health problems.
(3) Social problems such as homelessness and associated problems.
(4) History of self-harm or suicide attempts.
(5) Behaviour which may be considered as 'bizarre or odd' by arresting officers, custody sergeants or defence solicitors.
(6) Serious offending where custodial remand may be imminent and suicidal behaviour is a potential issue.

These criteria are by no means definitive but seek to give guidelines as to those offenders who require further assessment.

The main reason for input by community forensic nursing as opposed to other staff is their connection with forensic psychiatry, as well as a knowledge of local facilities and their availability to be called to courts and police stations to undertake psychiatric assessments.

Assessment procedure

Assessments are preceded by an explanation to the defendant who is given the choice not to speak or be assessed. In practice very few refuse. The issue of guilt or innocence has no relevance to this assessment and the issue of confidentiality is addressed by UKCC (1998) policy and NHS Trust Procedures which are explained to the defendant. The interview is semi-structured and revolves around basic data collection. It seeks to establish if there is some form of mental illness present. Approximately 50% have an identified mental health problem where recommendations are made to the courts.

When an identified mental health problem is established, the interviewer seeks to examine past history, presenting behaviour, social support networks and abuse of substances, drugs or alcohol. The FCMHN will assess the person's mood, thoughts, perceptual experiences, cognitive functioning and level of understanding. The reaction to their present situation also often provides indicators about mental state. Account is taken of age, sex, physical health and any prescribed medication and also recent changes in sleep, appetite and habits or circumstances.

Psychiatric phenomena may include thought disorder, delusionary or hallucinatory experiences, ideas of reference or connection to events. There may be grandiose ideas, feelings of control by others or unusual and bizarre experiences. Particular attention is paid to the presence of suicidal thoughts, past self-harm and parasuicide. The presence of a plan, a thought-out method and a level of significant intent are considered to be indicators of a serious and high risk. As well as known suicide risk factors in the general population, account must be taken of the feelings of possible guilt and shame connected with the present predicament.

This assessment attempts to define a collection of presenting symptoms in order to aid diagnosis as part of the decision-making process. All assessments are documented and remain confidential. A brief written résumé is provided and liaison takes place with the necessary professionals involved such as Crown Prosecution Service and court probation officer in order to decide on the appropriate course of action. Under the Prosecution of Offences Act 1985 section 23(3) the prosecuting officer can discontinue a case if it is felt to be in the interest of the defendant and not in the public interest to proceed if appropriate care is arranged.

Given that the courts have a public gallery, the utmost discretion has to be observed as breach of confidence must be avoided. If a defendant divulges material of a sensitive nature during assessment, such as other criminal activities, threatened suicide or incriminating evidence, then the nurse must obtain advice immediately and discuss if a breach of confidence is felt necessary to protect the defendant or others. Should a defendant confess to other offences the nurse has a duty by law to inform the police.

During the first seven years of the Birmingham service over 3500 people were assessed from a total population of over 21 000 defendants. Over half of those assessed were found to have a mental health problem. This is roughly 8% or so of those reaching the magistrates' overnight court. Approximately one-fifth of those required admission to hospital either by informal or compulsory means. Civil sections such as Sections 2 and 3 of the Mental Health Act 1983 were most commonly used. Over three-fifths required out-patient treatment or follow-up in the community and the remainder were those requiring admission to the secure settings. In the case of dangerous offending behaviour, urgent psychiatric assessments were arranged at the health-care centre during initial remand into custody.

Gender breakdown showed 90% males assessed. The ethnic breakdown showed an over-representation of African Caribbean and Asian people but was, however, representative of the ethnic breakdown of those arrested. There were occasions when diversion was not successful at this point, usually due to lack of hospital beds, dispute over catchment areas (particularly if the person was of no fixed abode), and inability to find suitable accommodation for bail purposes. Bail is often denied due to lack of community ties and often when further reports are required for the court. It will also be refused if the person has no fixed abode and is deemed likely to abscond and not reappear.

Prison diversion

A forensic nurse from the MSU visits Birmingham Prison each day to screen and assess all prisoners received within the last 24 hours. These prisoners come not only from Birmingham courts but also from surrounding courts and all are filtered by the screening nurse. An assessment takes place and the health-care centre is used when a prisoner is found to have a mental health problem or mental illness. Following discussion with staff in the health-care centre the visiting psychiatrist is requested to assess the prisoner with a view to hospital admission. Application may then be made to the court for hospital admission as a condition of bail. This service has been operational now since March 1993. The population of Birmingham Prison is male only and as yet there is no such service for females, many of whom are remanded to prisons outside the West Midlands.

Approximately 850 newly remanded prisoners are assessed each year, of which just under half have a mental health problem and a quarter of these require immediate admission to the health-care centre. The remaining three-quarters require various interventions such as a recommendation to reside in a multi-cell as suicidal views are expressed. Others are referred to drugs counselling, alcohol groups and anxiety management groups. Some in a normal prison location are referred to the visiting health-care nurses who visit other locations within the prison.

Diversion from prison is achieved for approximately 3.5% of prisoners, some of whom are bailed on second court appearance and some of whom are admitted to hospitals using Mental Health Act transfer sections (47/48). This service has been extended to assess sentenced prisoners as well as those on remand.

DIVERSION SERVICES COMMUNITY SUPPORT

Short-term community follow-up for those persons requiring psychiatric care but for whom links have not yet been forged with local services is often required. It is an interim measure to prevent a breakdown in communications and to maintain contact until local services are able to offer community support. This caseload is generated from successful diversions from police stations, courts and prison. The defendant is visited frequently for some 3 to 10 weeks before being transferred to local services. Some of the community follow-up involves visiting local bail hostels.

LEGAL AND ETHICAL ISSUES

A registered nurse will adhere to the Guidelines for Professional Practice (UKCC, 1998) as well as to policy dictated by local services. When involved in the assessment of a mentally disordered offender there are other considerations to be taken into account such as the Home Office Code of Practice (Home Office, 1995) for the Police and Criminal Evidence Act of 1984, as well as the Prosecution of Offences Act 1985, which are all enshrined in the Criminal Justice Act 1991. Each profession has to base decisions according to the law relating to their field such as probation, the Crown Prosecution Service, defence solicitors and prison services to name a few, and in the case of mentally disordered offenders the Mental Health Act 1983.

Whilst each profession is subject to their own legislation there are also rules, regulations and guidelines to follow in order to preserve a nationally consistent approach and ensure the highest standards are maintained in terms of European Law under the Convention of Human Rights and Fundamental Freedoms (European Convention, 1996).

Nurses working in diversion services need to be cognisant of the codes of conduct of other disciplines, for example approved social workers as well as other advocacy roles such as appropriate adults.

A common theme which instils anxiety in most professions and disciplines alike is the decision-making process where there is an element of risk to the general public as well as the defendant. Whilst adherence to the law is paramount, this situation often poses many ethical dilemmas for nurses who are often asked advice following assessment.

Given the relatively short period of time in which to reach a decision regarding the potential risk of dangerousness to the public it is not possible to perform a comprehensive risk assessment. It is not surprising that the courts will err on the side of safety in terms of protecting the public and may prefer a short remand in custody pending further assessment. In cases where bail is granted they may wish to apply strict conditions to the bail, for example with regard to compulsory hospital admission rather than informal admission. Pollock & Webster (1990, p. 489) argue that the scientific theories about human behaviour used for assessment of clinical dangerousness are at odds with the legal idea of dangerousness and warn clinicians against losing sight of this fact by 'becoming trapped in a web of conceptual confusions, struggling with unanswerable questions and impossible demands'. This statement illustrates clearly the situation in which nurses working in diversion services often find themselves.

Mentally vulnerable defendants often find themselves under tighter constraints by the criminal justice system possibly as a result of fears regarding the unpredictability of mental illness largely due to media sensationalism. There has been a plethora of inquiries, the most famous of which is the Clunis inquiry (Ritchie *et al.*, 1994). This report highlighted many issues including the need for more inter-agency collaboration and the introduction of supervision registers in order to effectively highlight areas of risk with the aim of preventing further tragedies.

The information gained from the initial assessment and also from records of previous offending can contribute to risk assessment and management strategies which will be compiled by the clinical team who undertake further psychiatric care. Walker (1996) and Grounds (1995) emphasise that it is imperative to gather all information known about a mentally disordered offender, and Prins (1991) advocates multi-disciplinary assessments. This entails sharing of information which can on occasions compromise the issue of confidentiality. If a defendant confesses to criminal activities during assessment the course of action is clear in that it must be reported to the police. In the case of dangerous behaviour or risk to others, confidentiality is often breached in good faith in terms of protecting others or, indeed, the defendant themselves (particularly where ideas of suicide or self-harm have been expressed), providing this decision can be justified. In taking decisions regarding a breach of confidentiality it is wise to examine past behaviour as a measure of possible future behaviours; as stated by Gunn (1993, p. 627), 'the best predictor of future violence is previous violence'.

Whatever choices or decisions are made both by the individual defendant and the agencies or professions involved the primary aim must be for common sense to prevail. If each agency or profession involved had some common training as a multi-disciplinary group this would enhance working relationships with a greater understanding of the differing roles and responsibilities.

EDUCATION AND TRAINING

In order for services to achieve and maintain high standards, training and experiential placements should be initiated. Some services provide training in diversion but at present this is largely on an *ad hoc* basis. With the services currently provided in Birmingham it has been possible to develop an English National Board (ENB) course in conjunction with a local university regarding comprehensive care of mentally disordered offenders in diversion services. This course contributes to studies at degree level but has a substantial clinical emphasis as it is offered to a wide variety of disciplines in both health and non-health-care agencies. Such courses encourage research not only into clinical outcomes but also to evaluate the effectiveness of the services being provided.

CONCLUSION

Diversion is the term generally used to describe a range of assessment and liaison services in police stations, courts and prisons for mentally vulnerable defendants. It is not, in fact, a new concept but one which has historically been accepted as a compassionate method of disposal for mentally disordered defendants where psychiatric illness was pronounced enough to be detected and had a relationship with offending behaviour. It was not common practice however, as treatment was less sophisticated than current psychiatry offers.

Various models of diversion services have been developed which reflect the demography and services in any given locality. Rural areas favour reactive service provision taking referrals from local police stations and courts with nurses covering large catchment areas with lower populations. Many have opted to provide a multi-agency panel, meeting and assessing defendants at pre-arranged times and undertaking further follow-up often in the community during the bail period. City and urban areas often favour proactive service provision by attending police stations, courts and prisons daily in order to screen out defendants for assessment and facilitate referrals to local psychiatric and social services. Both models often offer an on-call service in addition, which assists in early resolution and intervention where necessary.

It has been demonstrated that a large number of agencies and disciplines are involved, and successful diversion can only be achieved when all agencies pull together in collaboration. There are differing opinions as to which agencies such as probation, health or social services should take the lead role. The training, skills and versatility of forensic nurses, however, render them ideally suitable to take a lead role in actively co-ordinating the input from other agencies once the initial mental health problem has been assessed.

A national picture is emerging that diverting people is a sound practice as it relieves the criminal justice system of people with mental health problems which they are not equipped to deal with and places those primarily in need of health care in the appropriate place. Diversion is, however, only as successful as the resources which can be utilised and made available.

From the individual's point of view it is their right to receive health care when required and people with mental health problems are often unable to avail themselves of help. Thus, the emphasis is upon the need for a proactive service where this is possible. This takes the care directly to the person in police stations, courts and prisons as reactive services leave the screening to non-health-care employees who have no psychiatric background and are less equipped to detect mental illness.

The services in Birmingham address the need to divert people with mental health problems at several stages of progression through the criminal justice system such as diversion at the point of arrest, and in the courts and prison. As well as the established links between the forensic medium secure unit and the local psychiatric hospitals the diversion services have developed short-term follow-up in the community whilst establishing local referrals. The specialised bail hostel for mentally disordered defendants is also an integral part of this service.

There are many legal and ethical implications involved in diversion services which require a collaborative approach from all agencies involved. Each agency has different aims and objectives during the decision-making process, and in order to work effectively together there must be a common 'language' between them. This enhances a common-sense approach to address ethical dilemmas and legal requirements.

For inter-agency and multi-disciplinary cohesion to occur, opportunities should be available to participate in joint training and educational opportunities. The established services in Birmingham have been able to offer such training at an academic level as well as a clinical experiential level to all agencies involved in the diversion process. Such courses highlight the need for further academic research to be undertaken into both service provision for and clinical progress of those defendants who have been diverted.

Perhaps further progress will be made towards meeting the needs of some of the most seriously ill and disadvantaged group of people who are entitled to and deserve the best possible care and treatment available.

REFERENCES

Backer-Holst, T. (1994) A new window of opportunity. *Psychiatric Care* 1(1), 15–18.

Birmingham, L. (1998) Remand prisons miss mental illness. *Psychiatric Care* 5(2), 44.

Blumanthal, S. & Wessely, S. (1992) National survey of current arrangements for diversion from custody in England and Wales. *British Medical Journal* 305, 1322–5.

Department of Health (1992) *Health of the Nation*. HMSO, London.

Department of Health/Home Office (1992) *Review of Health and Social Services for Mentally Disordered Offenders and Others Requiring Similar Services* (The Reed Report). HMSO, London.

European Convention (1996) European Convention of Human Rights and Fundamental Freedoms (Intergovernmental Report), Brussels.

Exworthy, T. & Parrott, J. (1993) Evaluation of a diversion from custody scheme at magistrates courts. *Journal of Forensic Psychiatry* 4(3), 497–505.

Grounds, A. (1995) Risk assessment and management in clinical context. In *Psychiatric Patient Violence: Risk and Response* (Crichton, J., ed.). Duckworth, London.

Gunn, J. (1993) Dangerousness. In *Forensic Psychiatry, Clinical, Legal and Ethical Issues* (Gunn, J. & Taylor, P., eds). Butterworth Heinemann, London.

Hillis, G. (1993) Diverting tactics. *Nursing Times* 89(1), 24.

Holloway, J. & Shaw J. (1994) Providing a forensic psychiatry service to a magistrates court: a follow-up study. *Journal of Forensic Psychiatry* 4(3), 575–81.

Home Office (1990a) Provision for mentally disordered offenders. Circular 66/90. HMSO, London.

Home Office (1990b) *The Report of a Review by Her Majesty's Chief Inspector of Prisons of Suicide and Self Harm in Prison Service Establishments*. HMSO, London.

Home Office (1990c) *Prison disturbances, April 1990* (The Woolf Report). HMSO, London.

Home Office (1995) Police and Criminal Evidence Act 1984. Code of Practice (Revised Edition). HMSO, London.

James, D., Cripps, J., Gilluley, P. & Harlow, P. (1997) Court focused model of forensic psychiatry provision to Central London: abolishing remands to prison. *Journal of Forensic Psychiatry* 8(2), 390–405.

Jones, H. (1992) Report of the Telethon Inquiry into the relationship between mental health, homelessness and the Criminal Justice System. NACRO, London.

Joseph, P. (1992) *Psychiatric Assessment at the Magistrates Court*. Home Office & Department of Health, London.

Joseph, P. & Potter, M. (1993) Diversion from custody 1: Psychiatric assessment at the magistrates court. *British Journal of Psychiatry* 162, 325–30.

Kennedy, M., Truman, C., Keyes, S. & Cameron, A. (1997) Supported bail for mentally vulnerable defendants. *The Howard Journal* **36**(2), May 1997.

MENDOP (1991) A proposal for a bail hostel for the mentally disordered offender in the West Midlands (unpublished). Birmingham MDO Project. West Midlands Probation Service.

MIND (1997) *MIND's policy on people with mental health problems and the Criminal Justice System*. MIND, London.

Morgan, P. & Pearce, R. (1989) Remand decisions in Brighton and Bournemouth. (Home Office Research and Planning Unit paper No. 53). HMSO, London.

Pollock, N. & Webster, C. (1990) The clinical assessment of dangerousness. In *Principles and Practice of Forensic Psychiatry* (Bluglass, R. & Bowker, P., eds). Churchill Livingstone, Edinburgh.

Prins, H. (1991) Dangerous people or dangerous situations – some further thoughts. *Medicine, Science & Law* **31**(1), 25–37.

Ritchie, J. H, Dick, D. & Lingham, R. (1994) *The Report of the Inquiry into the Care and Treatment of Christopher Clunis*. HMSO, London.

Strong, S. (1996) Diversionary tactics. *Community Care* June, 13–19.

UKCC (1998) *Guidelines for Mental Health and Learning Disabilities Nursing*. UKCC, London.

Walker, N. (1968) *Crime and Insanity in England. 1 The Historical Perspective*. Edinburgh University Press, Edinburgh.

Walker, N., ed. (1996) *Dangerous People*. Blackstone Press, London.

Wix, S. (1993) Diversion at the point of arrest. *Psychiatric Care* **1**(3), 102–4.

Chapter 11
Relatives and Informal Caregivers

Doug MacInnes

CAREGIVING

Within this chapter the term 'caregiver' will be used, which is inclusive of family members and close friends of the mentally disordered offender. Schene (1990) defines caregiving as the relationship between individuals who are typically related through kinship. The caregiver assumes an unpaid and unanticipated responsibility for another, the care recipient, whose mental health problems are disabling and of a long-term nature, with no curative treatment available. The care recipient is unable to fulfil the reciprocal obligations associated with normative adult relationships. In addition, mental health problems are often serious enough to require substantial amounts of care. The situation becomes burdensome for the caregiver through the addition of a caring role, as well as the normal family/friendship role.

Research and clinical literature on family experiences of caring have mainly focused on caregivers of people who require personal tending because of physical disability or cognitive incapacity (Lefley, 1996). This has led to a limited amount of literature being published in relation to caregivers of persons with long-term illness (Perring *et al.*, 1990). Caregiving in mental illness does not involve tending to physical ailments, but may involve hours devoted to activities of daily living. Lefley (1996) maintained that it may also involve time and effort in attempting to access mental health services, and interactions with the criminal justice system.

CASE STUDY

Michael Adams is a 24-year-old man with a five-year history of admissions to psychiatric units for schizophrenia. The most common reason for him to be admitted was his accusatory behaviour to his mother (Brenda) and brother (Robin) with whom he lived, which often resulted in his assaulting them.

Three months ago he started to refuse to take his medication, and despite concerns expressed by his mother to the health services, no action was taken to assess Michael's mental state. Michael awoke early one morning and without warning went into his brother's bedroom and stabbed him with a knife. His brother managed to run out of the family home and get assistance. Michael was subsequently arrested and found to be suffering from paranoid delusions, which had precipitated the attack.

Initially, Michael's mother was unable to get any information either from the police or the health services as to what was happening to Michael, and it was ten days before she was informed that he was being transferred to a psychiatric hospital. He was eventually placed on Section 37/41 of the Mental Health Act 1983 and admitted to a forensic mental health unit.

As part of Michael's treatment programme it was decided to involve the family. However, his brother stated he did not want anything to do with him, and refused to talk to any services except to remark that, when the family had requested help, no one had bothered and now it was too late. Michael's mother was also angry with the health services, stating that she had pleaded with both the police and local psychiatric services to help Michael on numerous occasions as she was aware he was 'getting out of control', but that the common response from the health services was that he was not ill enough to be admitted and the best course of action was to contact the police, with the police response being the opposing view (that is, he was the health services' responsibility). This was compounded by the fact that the local consultant psychiatrist had refused to see Michael's mother on her own, as it would breach the rules of confidentiality with Michael.

Work with the family was further complicated by the fact that Michael's brother told his mother that if she spoke with Michael, he (Robin) would never talk to her again. This subsequently occurred. It also transpired that during the period of Michael's illness, other friends and family members had systematically stopped contact with Michael and his mother. The only support available to Michael's mother came from a distant aunt and from the health services. His mother also told the forensic mental health team of other occasions, which had hitherto been unknown, when Michael had threatened her and Robin with knives.

Other problems had included Michael demanding money from her, which she had given him to prevent confrontation, with the result that she was constantly in debt. Michael would also play his music in his room until five o'clock in the morning which would frequently result in neighbours complaining to her and the police. He would stay in bed for most of the day and often refuse to wash or change his clothes. Mrs Adams felt embarrassed as she felt that Michael's state reflected badly on her. She felt scared of Michael, and thought that the only way for both Michael and herself to be safe was for him to be detained in a secure environment for the foreseeable future.

CAREGIVERS OF THE MENTALLY ILL: A HISTORICAL OVERVIEW

Prior to the establishment of mental institutions in the mid to late 1800s, the main caregiving role of a mentally ill person was undertaken by the family (Grob, 1994). However, with the development of asylums, the patient became isolated from the family. Terkelson (1990) noted that this was not because the family was viewed as contributing to the development of the mental illness, but because the family lived in the community and was unable to shield the patient from the pressures of community life. The consequences of this were that the patient and family were distanced, and the skills the family and community had in dealing with the difficulties presented by the patient were eroded. Long years spent in institutions created psychological separation and abandonment.

Contemporary policy has attempted to reunite patients and their families as a part of the community care philosophy. In the report which provided the basis for the present community care legislation, Griffiths (1988) commented that community care should build first on the availability of informal carers and neighbourhood support. The policy has placed friends and family into a caregiving role for which they are untrained and unprepared. Furthermore, as Lefley (1996) has noted, health professionals have failed to prepare families for the caregiving role in dealing with the severely mentally ill.

CAREGIVERS AND MENTALLY DISORDERED OFFENDERS

There have been few studies that have examined the family environments of clients with mental illness, and the ways in which caregivers cope with the difficulties they face. However, there is an even greater scarcity of reports examining the caregiving role within forensic mental health.

The caregiving role in published investigations focuses on the caregiving environments in relation to violence and mental illness. There is little exploration of other types of offending or the specific stressors that caregivers face (Wessely *et al.*, 1994).

Robinson *et al.* (1991) stated that approximately 50% of the victims of homicides within Great Britain are family members. When examining mentally disordered offenders Robertson (1988) found in a study of remand prisoners in South London that 39% of homicide victims by schizophrenic offenders were family members or close friends. More recently, the Confidential Inquiry into Homicides and Suicides by Mentally Ill People (Royal College of Psychiatrists, 1996) concluded that 64% of homicide victims of mentally disordered offenders were family members. However, during the two-year time-scale of the study only 39 homicides were committed by people with mental illness.

A cohort of 167 mentally ill individuals were followed up by Estroff & Zimmer (1994) over an 18-month period. The study assessed the threats of violence made by the cohort, and violent acts during this time-scale. The sample were all in the 'early stages of their psychiatric history'. They found that 35.6% of the cohort either threatened violence or committed a violent act within the period of the study. Twice as many threatened violence than carried out attacks. Those with schizophrenia were more likely to threaten or commit a violent act. The targets for violence were known to the client in 77% of the cases, with violence directed against relatives in 53% of the cases. Parents, and more significantly mothers, were most at risk of being targets of violence, and of being the repeated targets of violence. Within the relative group, mothers are predominantly the targets, with 28% of assaults being against the mother in the family. There was an increased likelihood of violence occurring in households where the adult mentally ill offender and the mother resided together, especially if no father was present in the household. This was also found by Steinwachs *et al.* (1992) who added that over 33% of female parents alter their behaviour to avoid upsetting the client. Lawson (1986) found that relatives, and especially parents, tolerated a large degree of threatening behaviour and violence from clients, over an extended period. Estroff & Zimmer (1994) asserted that adult child to parent violence is a pattern of violence that is unique to the caregivers of the mentally ill.

There was a disproportionately high number of attacks on spouses, with the risk being twice as high as for other family members (Estroff & Zimmer, 1994). This figure is supported by the findings of Hafner & Boker (1973) who found that 39% of homicides committed by the mentally disordered are on spouses, as opposed to 23% of homicides within the normal criminal population. Estroff & Zimmer (1994) also examined the relationship between gender and violence within the social environment. Most violence was committed by men on women (60%), whilst men to men violence accounted for only 10% of the violent attacks. Men and women threatened their relatives and non-relatives in equal proportions, but actual assaults on relatives accounted for 56% of male violence and 75% of female violence. In the inquiry into homicides and suicides by mentally ill people (Royal College of Psychiatrists, 1996), the number of homicides on family members by female mentally disordered offenders was higher than the male group, with 82% of victims being a family member.

A study by Klassen & O'Connor (1988) concluded that people who lived with others who were not relatives are more likely to threaten violence. The sample may have had a longer psychiatric history, with consequently greater stress on caregivers. Therefore, they would have been more likely to have been excluded from the caregiving household, thus explaining the result of the study (Estroff & Zimmer 1994).

The group who were violent perceived their main caregiver as more threatening and hostile than did the non-violent group. The mentally disordered clients identified in the Estroff & Zimmer (1994) study state that there are few services for the mentally ill and this contributed to onset of violent behaviour. The client's financial dependence on relatives was perceived to be a factor for increasing the risk of violent threats or acts.

THE SOCIAL RELATIONSHIP BETWEEN MENTAL ILLNESS AND THE FAMILY

The relationships between family members seems to have an influence on the course and development of the illness (Atkinson & Coia, 1995). The most recognised area in research has been the concept of expressed emotion (EE). This has been defined as a measure of the emotional temperature by Vaughn (1989) and is defined operationally following an assessment interview. It has three parts: critical comments; hostility; and emotional overinvolvement (Vaughn & Leff, 1976). If a family is rated as high on one or more of the scales, they are assessed as being a high EE family. Many studies have confirmed that high EE families pose an increased risk for the patient to relapse. The concept of expressed emotion is a useful measure in the outcome of the course of schizophrenia and a measure of the efficacy of interventions (Lam, 1991). However, there is concern that the description of high expressed emotion families is perceived as a pejorative label (Kavanagh, 1992). In addition, Atkinson & Coia (1995) point out that after nearly 20 years of refining of the concept by Vaughn & Leff (1976), it has still not been generalised to be used within clinical settings. In a similar vein, Lam (1991) notes that one of the theoretical problems associated with expressed emotion is that the concept remains an empirical one which is not understood. Therefore, it is difficult to theorise on the mechanisms that are contributing to effective therapeutic change.

Lam (1991) has pointed out that a common component in all successful intervention packages has been the use of therapeutic techniques to assist the way in which the family deals with problems. The development of these coping skills enables the family to help the client stay well, become aware of their appraisal of the illness, and assess their coping resources.

OFFICIAL REPORTS

Although the number of clinical studies into the caregiver's role and environment in respect of mentally disordered offenders is limited, the importance of the role is acknowledged in a series of government recommendations and official inquiry reports.

The Mental Health Act Code of Practice recommends that when considering after-care for any person with psychiatric problems, the views of any relative, friend or supporter of the patient should be taken into consideration (Department of Health and Welsh Office, 1993). The Department of Health (1990) details principles governing the discharge and after-care of all mentally ill people in the Care Programme Approach. One of the essential elements of the Care Programme Approach is that there is a care plan agreed between the relevant professional staff, the patient and his or her carers, and this is recorded in writing.

In forensic mental health care, the Review of Health and Social Services for Mentally Disordered Offenders (Department of Health/Home Office, 1992) noted that there is an important role for patients and their families. The review stated that families and carers should be involved in the planning of care programmes whenever this is consistent with the patient's wishes. In addition, it recognised that caregivers may have needs of their own and that support is needed for families at an early stage of mental distress (Department of Health/Home Office, 1992, p. 13). The role of caregivers is specifically detailed with the recommendation that families and carers should be regarded as part of the team responsible for a patient with their own needs taken into account.

Official inquiries have examined the care and after-care of individual or groups of mentally ill clients, most of whom could be considered as forensic clients. These reviews have noted that families and informal patients need to be more fully informed about treatment and more closely involved in care planning for patients. Furthermore, consultant psychiatrists should be encouraged to see the families of mental health patients and to use relatives' knowledge of patients. The Ashworth Inquiry report (Blom-Cooper *et al.*, 1992) declared that families should be involved on a regular basis with their relative's treatment. On a more general level, Blom-Cooper *et al.* (1995) asserted that there needs to be local development of good practice standards on working with carers. The Royal College of Psychiatrists (1996, p. 68) noted a need for 'wider provision of family involvement and treatment in the care of seriously mentally ill people'.

SOCIAL AND PROFESSIONAL FACTORS

The process of defining illness representations, coping responses and outcome appraisal, does not occur in a social vacuum (Leventhal *et al.*, 1987). Social, cultural, institutional and personal factors influence the representation of health threats, and the planning and performing of coping responses.

Social support

Cohen & Sokolovsky (1979) stated that social network is a term used to denote individuals linked by social ties. Implicit within the term is the notion that individuals are in communication with one another. Harvey (1996) found that, compared to a 'normal' person who had a social network of approximately 40 people, a person with schizophrenia had on average four to five people within their social network. This social network comprised mainly family members. The size of the social network was negatively correlated to symptomatology and relapse. Harvey *et al.* (1996) noted that first-admission schizophrenics had a larger and more inter-connected social network than did patients with chronic schizophrenia.

In Harvey's (1996) survey of people with schizophrenia living in a London borough, social isolation of patients increased with the increasing severity of psychotic symptoms. The studies found that more frequent social contact is correlated to both a larger social network and to greater satisfaction with the network. Sullivan & Poertner (1989) found that the smaller the network becomes the more it is dominated by family members. The network size lessens the longer the illness, and also with more severe symptomatology. There is evidence to show that when families start to become less involved, the contact with health professionals increases. The reasons for the reduced social networks are not discussed, but it is clear that impaired social networks are related to poor prognosis.

Estroff *et al.*'s (1994) study of the carers of people with severe mental illness concluded that mothers are the main individual who cares for the majority of patients, and are at high risk of violence by the patient. The study also ascertained that fathers are rarely attacked. In Judge's (1994) research it was found that lack of friends for caregivers may be a major problem as it deprives them of respite from the duties of care. Social isolation and stigmatisation may also occur due to the behaviour of the mentally ill family member. Lefley (1996) also noted that caregivers often suffer social withdrawal from friends and other family members.

PROFESSIONAL SUPPORT

The relationship between health professionals and lay people is an important one. Leventhal *et al.* (1987) noted that illness representations often emerge from individuals' interpretations of the information to which they are exposed during encounters with health professionals. In addition, Horne (1997) found that patients and carers often have representations different from those of health professionals and this can play a significant part in whether individuals accept the professional role in combating the illness.

In the past, the relationship between professional groups and caregivers has been uneasy. Francell *et al.* (1988) stated that families experience profound burdens as a result of their interactions with the health services. The beneficial effect of having good relationships between health professionals and families was asserted by Karanci (1995) who found that families perceive as helpful the interest and support given to them by health professionals. Tessler *et al.* (1991) found that of a group of 409 respondents in three US cities, 274 (70%) had been in contact with mental health professionals. Of those who had no contact, 43% had stated that they wished to have some form of contact. Social workers (31%) were the professional groups with whom caregivers stated they had most contact, psychiatrists having contact with 27% of the sample. The study also found that parents were significantly more likely to be in contact with professionals than other family members. Nurses had formal contact with only 5% of the caregivers.

In a National Schizophrenia Fellowship survey of 345 carers by Hogman & Pearson (1996) only 21% of the respondents interviewed had been in contact with a health service professional within the last six months. Within the previous three months, psychiatrists had been in contact with 46% of the sample, whilst 42% stated they had been in contact with a psychiatric nurse, and 32% with a social worker. However, the latter two were either community psychiatric nurses and/or keyworkers, so contact may have been mandatory. The respondents were also asked for their views as to whom they would contact in the event of a crisis. The respondents chose the GP in 55% of cases; the hospital 33%; CPN 30%; police 25%; psychiatrist 24%; other family members 22%; and social workers 14%.

In Tessler *et al.*'s study (1991) there were consistent complaints about the relationship between mental health professionals and families. These are families not being given information about the patient and their illness and who are not being involved in treatment planning. This has been found in other studies (Perring, 1991; Hatfield, 1994; Shepherd *et al.*, 1994; Hogman & Pearson, 1996; Lefley, 1996). Lefley (1996) further commented that professionals often give ambiguous and contradictory information, and have no facility for training or giving information to caregivers on how to deal with the difficulties they face. Caregivers also complained that they only have contact with staff when the patient's history is required, or when families are catapulted into family therapy regardless of their wishes with the implicit or explicit message that the patient's illness is symptomatic of a greater family problem. Atkinson & Coia (1995) suggest that services in Great Britain are patient orientated and that confidentiality is a major concern. Therefore, caregivers' needs are ignored, and they perceive services as uncaring. They further resent the expectation that they are expected to care for the patient once the acute episode had passed. Shepherd *et al.* (1994) examined the views of service users, carers and service providers. The conclusions reached were that carers are far more critical of all aspects of care as opposed to service users and providers. Specific concerns included access to services, having regular updates from professionals, receiving specific carer education about schizophrenia, the availability of a wider range of day-care services, receiving respite care, and better public awareness and education.

Not all studies of carers have found them to be dissatisfied with services (McCarthy *et al.*, 1989). Wray (1994), in a small-scale study, found most carers were happy with the service received. The study also found that satisfaction with services was correlated with their access to services. Grella & Grusky (1989) found that families were more likely to be satisfied with services if they had contact with a specified case manager. Another factor in reducing dissatisfaction in families is regular contact with mental health professionals. Tessler *et al.* (1991) found more satisfaction with those caregivers who had been in contact with a health professional within the last six months.

One criticism of the studies reported here is that the issues were predetermined by the researchers, and so it is difficult to assess the strength of caregivers' feelings. A number of the caregivers contacted were members of pressure groups which may have made the responses unrepresentative of caregivers overall. This was noted by Tessler *et al.* (1991) who added that little effort had been made to survey caregivers who had no contact with professionals.

Within the study carried out by the author, the caregivers of mentally disordered offenders expressed anger towards services. Many caregivers stated that they were not included in any decisions about the patient's future and were not given information by professionals. The level of anger was statistically significantly higher for the caregivers of mentally disordered offenders as opposed to those who cared for non-offenders. In addition, caregivers of mentally disordered offenders received less contact with health service professionals. In terms of nursing contact, the differences can be seen in Box 11.1. This shows that the caregivers of mentally disordered offenders

Box 11.1   Contact with nursing staff (MacInnes, 1999)

	Forensic caregivers	Non-forensic caregivers
CPN contact	55.7%	78.6%
CPN contact In last month	29.1%	60.7%
Helpfulness of contact	45.4%	72.61%
Ward nurse contact	84.8%	60.7%
Ward nurse contact In last month	39.2%	53.57%
Helpfulness of ward nurse contact	32.8%	76.4%

have less regular contact with nursing staff, even though more caregivers of mentally disordered offenders have had contact with ward nursing staff. More importantly, the levels of satisfaction with the contact are markedly lower in the forensic group.

BURDEN

The caregivers of people with mental illness encounter stressors that are either directly or indirectly related to the illness. These difficulties have been described as family burden (Atkinson & Coia, 1995).

The adverse consequences of psychiatric disorders for caregivers have been known since the 1950s (Schene *et al.*, 1994). The initial studies examined the feasibility of discharging patients from institutions and into the community, with subsequent studies refining the concept of caregiving, its content and underlying structure. Burden was measured as an outcome variable in programme evaluations and controlled clinical trials. The effect was noted by McCreadie *et al.* (1987), with 75% of individuals caring for a family member with schizophrenia having high levels of psychological distress. Lefley (1987) also noted that the severity of disturbance or disability was generally correlated with levels of burden. McCarthy *et al.* (1989) identified three consistent themes in the early studies. These are as follows:

- caregivers are subject to considerable, even severe, emotional and material hardship, as a result of their caring role
- caregivers complain very little
- better contact with services is needed.

Fadden *et al.* (1987) found that the most distressing symptoms for relatives were disturbed behaviour, aggression, delusions and hallucinations, while the main symptoms were withdrawal, depression, and hypochondriasis. This has been the main finding in the majority of studies on family burden (Atkinson & Coia, 1995). Other findings include the fact that the more members there are within the household the less is the burden for individual family members; and that there is a relationship between social class, financial burden, and housing conditions.

Burden is related to educational level, and might be responsible for lack of knowledge of services and of the organisation of these services (Lefley, 1996). One of the biggest difficulties in gaining consistent information about caregiver burden has been the lack of agreement between researchers as to which different dimensions of burden should be included in the measures (Szmukler *et al.*, 1996). Both Platt (1985) and Schene *et al.* (1994) have documented the dimensions that have been utilised in different studies, with Schene *et al.* (1994) showing that 20 different dimensions had been used. These are set out in Box 11.2. Szmukler *et al.* (1996) maintain that any valid burden measure should also contain measures to examine caregiver appraisal and coping, for each specific burden.

Box 11.2   Dimensions assessed by caregiver burden instruments (Schene *et al.*, 1994)

- Effect on family interaction
- Effect on family routine
- Effect on leisure
- Effect on work/employment
- Effect on other outside household
- Effect on children
- Financial consequences
- Distress
- Stigma
- Worrying

- Effect on mental health
- Effect on physical health
- Effect on use of psychotropics
- Effect on social network
- Helping the patient with activities of daily living
- Supervising the patient
- Encouraging the patient
- Shame
- Guilt
- Global burden

MacInnes (1999) found that the caregivers of mentally disordered offenders noted burdens in relation to: patient violence either towards the caregiver or to others; anger towards services; and feelings of hopelessness or helplessness about their caregiving role.

COPING RESPONSES

Various theoretical approaches to family stress and coping are found in the literature (Lefley, 1996). Pearlin & Schooler (1978) suggest that coping is the things that people do to avoid life strains. Coping behaviours are used: to eliminate or modify the conditions that give rise to problems; to perceptually control the meaning of the experience in such a way that neutralises its problematic aspects and keeps the emotional consequences within manageable bounds. Lefley (1996) adds that coping behaviours begin with the caregiver's interactions with the mentally ill person for whom they are caring, but often go well beyond that limited involvement.

In the 1980s a number of studies examined the coping responses of caregivers of people with schizophrenia (Birchwood, 1983; Birchwood & Smith, 1987; Birchwood & Cochrane, 1990) based on the concepts of coping devised by Folkman & Lazarus (1980). A number of consistent coping responses were found which are presented in Box 11.3. The studies of behavioural disturbance concluded that initial family burden resulted in the caregivers developing family coping strategies/styles to either modify or exacerbate the burdensome behaviours. In turn, the altered behaviour of the person with schizophrenia is perceived differently by the caregiver depending on the outcome of the coping response. Birchwood (1983) interviewed the close caregivers of people diagnosed as having schizophrenia in relation to their coping responses. Seven broad coping styles were identified which applied to all areas of behaviour, and were validated subsequently by other studies (Atkinson & Coia, 1995).

Two other coping responses were also ascertained which applied to specific burdens. Reassurance occurs in response to positive symptoms and has been measured in other studies. The other response, submission, was not measured in subsequent projects as this applies in response to threats or acts of aggression. This coping response may be more prevalent in the caregivers of mentally disordered offenders. The nine coping responses are shown in Box 11.3.

Box 11.3   Coping styles identified by Birchwood (1983)

(1) Coercion – adopting a punitive approach

(2) Avoidance – includes responses which minimise caregiver's exposure to the behaviour

(3) Ignore/accept – includes indifferent reactions, where caregivers do not perceive the behaviour as problematical

(4) Collusion – actively condoning or supporting the client's behaviour.

(5) Constructive – special action taken by the caregiver in order to ameliorate the behaviour

(6) Resignation – where initial efforts to control the behaviour fail, and caregivers express a sense of powerlessness

(7) Disorganised – expressing feelings of desperation and helplessness

(8) Reassurance – presents a calm and stable exterior to the client, but does not agree with the individual's beliefs. It is reported only in relation to positive symptoms

(9) Submission – acquiesces to the aggressive demands of the patient. This is reported only when aggression or threats of aggression have been reported

---

The studies of Birchwood (1983) and Birchwood & Cochrane (1990) reported that perceived control is associated with ignore/accept, collusion and constructive styles, while less control is associated with avoidance and disorganised styles. In relation to positive symptoms, some caregivers are likely to respond in a disorganised way, while coercion is positively correlated to the patient being withdrawn or inactive. Coercion is more prevalent in caregivers of patients who had higher numbers of relapses or readmissions. Caregivers would, however, tend to use reassurance and disorganised coping responses when they were faced with high levels of behavioural disturbance arising from persistent symptoms.

FAMILY MANAGEMENT AND FAMILY INTERVENTIONS

The greatest influence of expressed emotion (EE) has been in stimulating the development of family interventions. The interventions have been primarily concerned with reducing the relapse rates in schizophrenic patients. In these studies expressed emotion ratings were used as an index of high risk of relapse (Falloon *et al.*, 1982; Hogarty *et al.*, 1986) or as a focus of the intervention to reduce the expressed emotion status from high to low (Leff *et al.*, 1982, Tarrier *et al.*, 1989).

The interventions used were educational groups, caregiver support groups, and individual family therapy (Leff *et al.*, 1982, 1989); behavioural family work (Tarrier *et al.*, 1988); education, problem-solving, and communication training (Falloon *et al.*, 1985); and education and family skills training (Hogarty *et al.*, 1986). The intervention studies maintained differences over the high EE control groups for up to eight years, although two-thirds of the clients where family intervention occurred eventually relapsed.

Client's level of social functioning was higher in low EE families (Falloon *et al.*, 1984; Barrowclough & Tarrier, 1992) and a number of the interventions resulted in significant changes of families from high EE to low EE status (Leff *et al.*, 1982; Hogarty *et al.*, 1986; Tarrier *et al.*, 1988).

Recent research by Birchwood *et al.* (1989) has concentrated on educating caregivers about signs and symptoms that occur when a patient is relapsing, and using the caregivers and patients as observers to monitor the patient's well-being. The results suggest that this led to an increase in the likelihood of effective early intervention procedures, and also offered the client and the caregiver an opportunity to act as partners in the client's care. Another development documented by Brooker *et al.* (1994) described a package of training for community nurses. The aim of the training is to engage with clients and family, assess caregivers, organise household meetings, educate families, teach communication skills, examine family problem-solving, examine drug compliance, be aware of crisis management, give social skills training, and enable the family to undertake cognitive-behavioural strategies for alleviating symptoms. Although the study sample was small, the evidence of the enhanced training suggested that it improved the ability of families to deal with the difficulties they faced.

A major criticism of the clinical applications of the majority of the interventions has been that few mental health services have targeted the most seriously mentally ill people. Most resources are geared to people with less serious psychiatric problems, at the expense of those with more severe illnesses (Brooker & Butterworth, 1993). In addition, most studies have been conducted on small samples with highly skilled professionals (Lam, 1991; Kuipers *et al.*, 1992). This is in contrast to the service allocated to the control groups, and also to what is available within the normal range of services provided by health professionals. The development of training courses (Brooker *et al.*, 1994) has addressed this lack of skills for community mental health nurses (CMHNs), though the numbers who have trained are small. Intervention studies had problems with non-compliance, with potential participants either not wishing to participate or dropping out of the studies. The concern is that the clients who are most at risk of relapse, and the caregivers who are most in need of support, are the families who drop out of intervention studies.

FAMILY INTERVENTIONS WITH CAREGIVERS

There have been few published reports examining family interventions with the caregivers of mentally disordered offenders (McCann & McKeown, 1995a). Certain authors have postulated approaches that clinicians should utilise when working with caregivers. However, the approaches tend to concentrate on violence within the caregiver environment. Bentovim (1990) wrote that, when choosing a family treatment strategy, it is important that the criteria for successful rehabilitation are lasting changes in family structure and relationships. An alternative approach was advocated by Latham (1986) who suggests that the way to reduce violence in families is to develop a non-violent problem intervention programme, using a behavioural approach.

Gasson (1991) surveyed caregivers of clients on a pre-discharge forensic unit to identify types of support and information required. Relatives wanted information about rehabilitation and after-care proposals, but were not concerned about clinics' resources and facilities, the Mental Health Act or the role of the Mental Health Act Tribunal. The caregivers wanted to meet with social workers and CMHNs, but not with ward nursing staff and pharmacists. A monthly relative support group established at a special hospital was studied by McCann (1993). Evaluation was by determining the amount of time spent discussing different issues. In-patient care and treatment took up 26% of the group time, after-care 10%, the role of the group 18%, outside agencies 14%, liaison with staff 13% and education 13%. The benefits reported were that the caregivers receive more information about in-patient care and treatment; they are involved in the care of the client; and anxiety levels are reduced. However, caregivers are in need of more specific information regarding schizophrenia and medication.

A relatives' assessment schedule was developed by McKeown & McCann (1995) with specific reference to the caregivers of forensic clients. It focuses on two areas: relatives' thoughts/beliefs about symptomatology; and the areas of stress which the caregiver experiences in relation to contact with the client or with the hospital. These specific areas are seen by the authors as being important within their clinical area, which is a special hospital. Therefore the focus on the caregiver–hospital contact is more important for the caregivers of this group of clients. McCann *et al.* (1996) reported an examination into the needs of 17 caregivers of people with schizophrenia within a special hospital and the way in which the knowledge held might influence the stresses faced by the caregiver. The findings suggest that caregivers are unaware of environmental factors affecting the course and outcome of schizophrenia and of the role that medication plays in the prevention of relapse. This lack of knowledge led to some caregivers mis-interpreting some of the client's behaviours. In addition, caregivers often detected changes in their client's behaviour prior to admission or offending. This was particularly so when observing communication withdrawal and violence. Services did not react to concerns raised by caregivers when the client was becoming unwell. The studies also provided the first opportunity for many caregivers to discuss their feelings, which the authors judge is an important component for any future work.

The ways in which psychosocial interventions might be implemented within a forensic environment are noted by McCann & McKeown (1995b). They state that it is important to involve family members in the care and management of forensic clients, but that 'in a hospital setting, especially a long term unit, the family becomes the professional network of staff, and fellow patients'. Thus the role of the caregiver is examined firmly within the context of a hospital environment.

Robinson *et al.* (1991) used a family therapy approach within a secure unit. The approach had four stages: acquiring information to fully assess the situation and emphasise dangerousness; increasing and strengthening communication between family members and professionals; facilitating reparation and giving the victims the chance to come to terms with their trauma; and the specific factors within the family system which contributed to the offence. No evaluation of the efficacy of the intervention was discussed though it was acknowledged that much of what is important within family therapy happens outside the sessions in the form of both general and day-to-day interactions and formal home work. In a secure setting this opportunity is restricted to visiting times and periods of leave. Therefore, progress may be slower and the effect on relationships and behaviour within the secure unit is studied rather than that within the context of the family (Robinson *et al.*, 1991).

ILLNESS BELIEFS

The effect that illness beliefs have on an individual's capacity to interpret health-related burdens and consequently the coping responses to these burdens have been studied extensively within the health psychology field (Petrie & Weinman, 1997). Research has shown that people appear to regulate their health behaviour according to a framework which guides interpretations of health events and the coping responses. They also guide the entry and use of treatments and the evaluation of treatment effects.

The self-regulatory model was developed by Leventhal and colleagues in the 1980s. It has an underlying control system that can be divided into three components or stages. These are:

(1) Illness representations. The representation of a problem involves a set of attributes that identify or specify the features of a problem by which the individual identifies the meaning of the illness and goals for action.
(2) Coping plan. The development and implementation of a coping strategy. This consists of a set of specific behaviours and expectations respecting their effectiveness or impact on the defined problem.
(3) Appraisal process. The appraisal process evaluates whether movement has occurred towards or away from the specific goals of the coping plan.

The formation of illness representations (Leventhal & Neretz, 1985) is a fundamental stage in that it drives coping and appraisal and influences behaviour. Five attributes have been identified. These are shown in Box 11.4.

Box 11.4   Illness representations

(1) **Identity**. Variables that identify the presence or absence of the illness. Illnesses can be identified abstractly by labels (schizophrenia) and concretely by signs (hallucinations) and symptoms (withdrawal).
(2) **Consequence**. The perceived physical, social and economic consequences of the disease.
(3) **Causes**. The perceived causes of the disease.
(4) **Time line**. The perceived time frame for the development and duration of the illness threat.
(5) **Cure/control**. The perceived effect of treatment or a return to previous 'wellness'.

ILLNESS BELIEFS AND MENTAL ILLNESS

In terms of the assessment of family mental health beliefs and their correlation with coping responses, only a small amount of research has occurred. Barrowclough & Tarrier (1992, p. 75) note:

> 'lay people develop their own subjective models of illness in order to make sense of ill health and these influence the assimilation of any new information offered to them. The use of lay models of sickness by the patient and caregiver is likely to occur in psychiatric illness where symptoms are seen in terms of changes in behaviour and not as physical signs of pathology.'

Health-care professionals usually hold a disease model of schizophrenia whereas the family have individualised models of illness. Such illness models shape the ways in which caregivers adopt coping responses to the various health threats of the illness. There is evidence to suggest that caregivers engage in a process of trying to find causal explanations for the behaviours and symptoms of the patient, and the answers to these questions play a major role in the coping responses adopted (Barrowclough & Tarrier, 1992). In relation to this Barrowclough *et al.* (1987) developed a Knowledge About Schizophrenia Inventory (KASI) which aimed to assess and evaluate caregivers' beliefs and attitudes in six key areas. These are detailed in Box 11.5. Several of these key areas overlap with the illness representations described by Leventhal and colleagues (Leventhal *et al.*, 1987). In addition Horne (1997) has written of the need for treatment issues to be considered when examining illness representations. When examining caregivers' beliefs it would seem that the issue of treatment efficacy, with special emphasis on medication, would play a major role in determining the burden faced and their coping responses to these burdens.

Box 11.5   The Knowledge About Schizophrenia Inventory

(1) Diagnosis
(2) Symptomatology
(3) Aetiology
(4) Medication
(5) Prognosis
(6) Management

This was the basis of the research by the author (MacInnes, 1999), with the six representations mentioned above being examined in relation to burdens faced and coping responses. The main results show that there was no difference in representations between caregivers and mentally disordered offenders, and also that certain coping styles were predictive of specific illness representations. This gives support to the argument that coping styles are independent of burden once the effect of behavioural disturbance is withdrawn. The study also found that the coping responses to problem-focused burdens were directly affected by the illness representations, though coping responses to emotion-focused burdens were not.

The relationship between illness representations, problem-focused burdens and coping is briefly mentioned in relation to the burden of patient violence. To begin with, the levels of violence reported by caregivers were significantly increased within the forensic caregivers group. There were also significantly higher levels of serious violence, with over a quarter of the caregivers either being the victims of patient violence or seeing the patient perform acts of violence that included use of weapons or hospitalisation with severe injuries. There is a significant association between not agreeing with the diagnosis of mental illness, perceiving the illness as curable, and colluding with the patient. The collusion occurred primarily through either minimising the seriousness of the violence or blaming others for causing the violence.

Alternatively, the coping response of acting constructively through either contacting services or trying to diffuse the situation by calming the patient was associated with the caregiver perceiving the illness as incurable. A constructive approach and the response of avoidance were associated with perceiving the treatment by medication as efficacious. A collusive response was however associated with reservations about medication efficacy. Certain illness representations are important in these findings. To begin with, less than 50% of caregivers were in agreement with the diagnosis that was given to the patient. This was in part due to the fact that approximately one-third of the sample were unable to remember being told or were given incorrect information as to the diagnosis. Therefore there seems to be some need for staff to ensure that caregivers have been given basic information about the patient's condition such as the diagnosis as well as enough time to discuss any concerns or misconceptions about the illness. The effectiveness of treatment is also an important part of the way in which caregivers interpret the extent of the health threat and its effect on themselves.

One major fact emerged from the study. The majority of caregivers only knew about one form of treatment. Medication was known to 98% of the caregivers as a form of treatment compared with only 13% who were aware of any form of counselling approach that was occurring with the patient. This again is an area where involvement by nursing staff can be beneficial. Although the other representations were not significantly associated with coping responses to violence, they were significantly associated with coping responses to other burdens. This finding seems to support

Szmukler *et al.*'s (1996) view that coping responses should be examined in relation to individual burdens.

CONCLUSIONS

There are increased burdens for caregivers of mentally disordered offenders, and these burdens are more severe than those from non-forensic mentally disordered groups. In addition, they receive less support from family, friends and professionals, and although there are a number of official reports detailing the need for family support and information for these caregivers, there is a dearth of research and clinical work. Nurses have most informal contact with caregivers yet have limited formal contact. Mental health nurses are in an ideal position to offer support and to develop methods of interventions that benefit caregivers.

One area for development for forensic mental health nurses may be in the examination of caregivers' illness beliefs and in exploring the relationship between these beliefs and their effect on caregivers' coping responses to the burdens faced. The fact that only 50% of caregivers agree with the diagnosis must affect their views as to the role and approach of health services. A basic educational approach will give caregivers a greater understanding of the nature of the illness and the role of services.

The violence that caregivers face should be acknowledged, and health professionals need to be aware of the increased likelihood of violence to which caregivers of mentally disordered offenders are exposed. This is important when viewing the potential reluctance of caregivers to visit or to attend family meetings and their concerns about the future.

Although there are issues relating to confidentiality, the needs of caregivers in respect of information about the patient need to be addressed. It may require discussion with other professional groups, voluntary groups, government agencies, and patient and carer groups, but there is a necessity for some change in the consistent reluctance of services to give information to caregivers.

REFERENCES

Atkinson, J. & Coia, D. (1995) *Families Coping with Schizophrenia*. John Wiley, Chichester.

Barrowclough, C. & Tarrier, N. (1992) *Families of Schizophrenic Patients: Cognitive Behavioural Interventions*. Chapman & Hall, London.

Barrowclough, C., Tarrier, N., Watts, S., Vaughn, C., Bamrah, J. & Freeman, H. (1987) Assessing the functional value of relatives' knowledge about schizophrenia: a preliminary report. *British Journal of Psychiatry* 151, 1–8.

Bentovim, A. (1990) Family violence: clinical aspects. In *Principles and Practices of Forensic Psychiatry* (Bluglass, R. & Bowden, P., eds), pp. 529–41. Churchill Livingstone, Edinburgh.

Birchwood, M. (1983) Family coping behaviour and the course of schizophrenia. Unpublished PhD thesis, University of Birmingham.

Birchwood, M. & Cochrane, R. (1990) Families coping with schizophrenia – coping styles, their origins and correlates. *Psychological Medicine* 20, 857–65.

Birchwood, M. & Smith, J. (1987) Schizophrenia and the family. In *Coping with Disorder in the Family* (Orford, J., ed.), pp. 7–38. Croom Helm, London.

Birchwood, M., Smith, J., MacMillan, F., Hogg, B., Prasad, R., Harvey, C. & Berings, S. (1989) Predicting relapse in schizophrenia: the development and implementation of an early signs monitoring system using patients and families as observers. A preliminary investigation. *Psychological Medicine* 19, 649–56.

Blom-Cooper, L., Brown, M., Dolan, R. & Murphy, E. (1992) *Report of the Committee of Inquiry into Complaints about Ashworth Hospital*. HMSO, London.

Blom-Cooper, L., Hally, H. & Murphy, E. (1995) *The Falling Shadow*. Duckworth, London.

Brooker, C. & Butterworth, A. (1993) Training in psycho-social intervention: the impact on the role of community psychiatric nurses. *Journal of Advanced Nursing* 18(4), 583–90.

Brooker, C., Falloon, I., Butterworth, A., Goldberg, D., Graham-Hole, V. & Hillier, V. (1994) The outcome of training community psychiatric nurses to deliver psychosocial intervention. *British Journal of Psychiatry* 165, 222–30.

Cohen, C. & Sokolovsky, J. (1979) Clinical use of network analysis for psychiatric and aged populations. *Community Mental Health Journal* 15, 203–13.

Department of Health (1990) HC(90)23/LASSL(90)11. The Care Programme Approach. HMSO, London.

Department of Health/Home Office (1992) *Review of Health and Social Services for Mentally Disordered Offenders and Others Requiring Similar Services* (The Reed Report). HMSO, London.

Department of Health and Welsh Office (1993). *Code of Practice: Mental Health Act 1983*. HMSO, London.

Estroff, S. & Zimmer, C. (1994) Social networks, social support, and violence among people with severe persistent mental illness. In *Violence and Mental Disorder* (Monahan, J. & Steadman, H., eds), pp. 259–95. Chicago University Press, Chicago.

Estroff, S., Zimmer, C., Lachicotte, W. & Benoit, J. (1994) The influence of social networks and social support on violence by persons with serious mental illness. *Hospital and Community Psychiatry* 41, 669–79.

Fadden, G., Bebbington, P. & Kuipers, L. (1987) Burden of care. *British Journal of Psychiatry* 150, 285–92.

Folkman, S. & Lazarus, R. (1980) An analysis of coping in a middle aged community sample. *Journal of Health and Social Behaviour* 21, 219–39.

Falloon, I., Boyd, J. & McGill, C. (1982) Family management in the prevention of exacerbations of schizophrenia: a controlled study. *New England Journal of Medicine* 306, 1437–40.

Falloon, I., Boyd, J. & McGill, C. (1984) *Family Care of Schizophrenia*. Guildford Press, New York.

Falloon, I. Boyd, J., McGill, C., Williamson, M., Razani, J., Moss, H., Gliderman, A. & Simson, G. (1985) Family management in the prevention of morbidity of schizophrenia: clinical outcome of a two year longitudinal study. *Archives of General Psychiatry* **42**, 887–96.

Francell, C., Conn, V. & Gray, P. (1988) Families' perceptions of burden of care for chronic mentally ill relatives. *Hospital & Community Psychiatry* **39**, 1296–300.

Gasson, B. (1991) Relatives support – a preliminary study. *The Tabloid* Issue No. 5.

Grella, C. & Grusky, O. (1989) Families of the seriously mentally ill and their satisfaction with services. *Hospital and Community Psychiatry* **45**, 831–5.

Griffiths, R. (1988) *Community Care: Agenda for Action. A Report to the Secretary of State For Social Services*. HMSO, London.

Grob, G. (1994) *The Mad among Us: A History of the Care of America's Mentally Ill*. Free Press, New York.

Hafner, H. & Boker, W. (1973) Mentally disordered violent offenders. *Social Psychiatry* **8**, 220–9.

Harvey, C. (1996) The Camden schizophrenia surveys. I The psychiatric, behavioural and social characteristics of the severely mentally ill in an Inner London Health District. *British Journal of Psychiatry* **168**, 410–17.

Harvey, C., Pantelis, C., Taylor, J., McCabe, P., Lefevre, K., Campbell, P. & Hirsch, S. (1996) The Camden Schizophrenia Surveys. II High prevalence of schizophrenia in an Inner London Borough and its relationship to sociodemographic factors. *British Journal of Psychiatry* **168**, 418–26.

Hatfield, A. (1994) *Family Interventions in Mental Illness*. Jossey-Bass, San Francisco.

Hogarty, G., Anderson, C., Reiss, D., Kornblith, S., Greenwald, D., Java, C., Madonia, M. & the EPICS Schizophrenia Research Group (1986) Family psychoeducation, social skills training and maintenance chemotherapy in the care and aftercare treatment of schizophrenia. *Archives of General Psychiatry* **43**, 633–42.

Hogman, G. & Pearson, G. (1996) *The Silent Partners*. National Schizophrenia Fellowship.

Horne, R. (1997) Representations of medication and treatment: advances of theory and measurement. In *Perceptions of Health and Illness: Current Research and Applications* (Petrie, K. J. & Weinman, J. A., eds), pp. 155–88). Harwood Academic Publishers, Amsterdam.

Judge, K. (1994) Serving children, siblings and spouses: understanding the needs of other family members. In *Helping Families Cope with Mental Illness* (Lefley, H. & Wasow, M., eds), pp. 161–94. Harwood Academic, Newark, NJ.

Karanci, A. N. (1995) Caregivers of Turkish schizophrenic patients: causal attributions, burdens and attitudes to help from the health professions. *Social Psychiatry & Psychiatric Epidemiology* **30**, 261–8.

Kavanagh, D. (1992) Recent developments in expressed emotion and schizophrenia. *British Journal of Psychiatry* **160**, 601–620.

Klassen, D. & O'Connor, W. (1988) Crime, in-patient admissions and violence among mental patients. *International Journal of Law and Psychiatry* **11**, 305–312.

Kuipers, E., Leff, J. & Lam, D. (1992) *Family Work for Schizophrenia: A Practical Guide.* Gaskell Press, London.

Lam, D. (1991) Psychosocial family intervention in schizophrenia: a review of empirical studies. *Psychological Medicine* 21, 423–41.

Latham, T. (1986) Violence in the family. *Journal of Family Therapy* 8, 125–37.

Lawson, W. (1986) Chronic mental illness and the black family. *American Journal of Social Psychiatry* 6, 57–61.

Leff, J., Kuipers, L., Berkowitz, R., Eberlein-Vries, R. & Sturgeon, D. (1982) A controlled trial of social intervention in the families of schizophrenic patients. *British Journal of Psychiatry* 141, 121–34.

Leff, J., Berkowitz, R., Shavit, N., Strachan, A., Glas, I. & Vaughn, C. (1989) A trial of family therapy vs a relative's group for schizophrenia. *British Journal of Psychiatry* 154, 58–66.

Lefley, H. (1987) The family's response to mental illness in a relative. In *Families of the Mentally Ill: Meeting the Challenges* (Hatfiled, A., ed.), pp. 3–21. Jossey-Bass, San Francisco.

Lefley, H. (1996) *Family Caregiving in Mental Illness.* Sage, Newbury Park, California.

Leventhal, H. & Neretz, D. (1985) The assessment of illness cognition. In *Measurement Strategies in Health Psychology* (Karoly, P., ed.), pp. 517–54). John Wiley, Chichester.

Leventhal, H., Benyamin, Y., Brownlee, S., Diefenbach, M., Leventhal, E., Patrick-Miller, L. & Robitaille, C. (1987) Illness representations: theoretical foundations. In *Perceptions of Health and Illness: Current Research and Applications* (Petrie, K. & Weinman, J., eds). Harwood Academic Publishers, Amsterdam.

MacInnes, D. (1999) The perceptions of the relatives and informal caregivers of schizophrenic offenders. Unpublished PhD thesis, University of London.

McCann, G. (1993) Relatives' support groups in a special hospital: an evaluation study. *Journal of Advanced Nursing* 18, 1883–8.

McCann, G. & McKeown, M. (1995a) Clinical management: a special case. *Journal of Nursing Management* 3, 115–20.

McCann, G & McKeown, M. (1995b) Applying psychosocial interventions: the Thorn initiative in a forensic setting. *Psychiatric Care* 2(4), 133–6.

McCann, G., McKeown, M. & Porter, I. (1996) Understanding the needs of relatives of patients within a special hospital for mentally disordered offenders: a basis for improved services. *Journal of Advanced Nursing* 23, 346–52.

McCarthy, B., Lesage, A., Brewin, C., Brugha, T., Mangan, S. & Wing, J. (1989) Needs for care among the relatives of long term users of day care. *Psychological Medicine* 19, 725–36.

McCreadie, R., Wiles, D., Moore, J. & Grant, S. (1987) The Scottish First Episode Schizophrenia Study: IV. Psychiatric and social impact on relatives. *British Journal of Psychiatry* 150, 340–44.

McKeown, M. & McCann, G. (1995) A schedule for assessing relatives. The relative assessment interview for schizophrenia in a secure environment (RAISSE). *Psychiatric Care* 2, 84–8.

Pearlin, L. & Schooler, C. (1978) The structure of coping. *Journal of Health and Social Behaviour* 19, 2–21.

Perring, C (1991) How do discharged psychiatric patients fare in the community? In *Dependency to Enterprise* (Hutton, J., Hutton, S., Pinch, T. & Shiell, A., eds). Routledge, London.

Perring, C., Twigg, J. & Atkin, K. (1990) *Families Caring for People Diagnosed as Mentally Ill: The Literature Re-examined*. HMSO, London.

Petrie, K. P. & Weinman, J. A. (1997) *Perceptions of Health and Illness: Current Research and Applications*. Harwood Academic Publishers, Amsterdam.

Platt, S. (1985) Measuring the burden of psychiatric illness on the family: an evaluation of some rating scales. *Psychological Medicine* 15, 383–93.

Robertson, G. (1988) Arrest patterns in mentally disordered offenders. *British Journal of Psychiatry* 153, 313–16.

Robinson, S., Vivian-Byrne, S., Driscoll, R. & Cordess, C. (1991) Family work with victims and offenders in a secure unit. *Journal of Family Therapy* 13(1), 105–16.

Royal College of Psychiatrists (1996) *Report of the Confidential Inquiry into Homicides and Suicides by Mentally Ill People*. Royal College of Psychiatrists, London.

Schene, A. (1990) Objective and subjective dimensions of family burden. *Social Psychiatry & Psychiatric Epidemiology* 25, 289–97.

Schene, A., Tessler, R. & Gamache, G. (1994) Instruments measuring family or caregiver burden in severe mental illness. *Social Psychiatry & Psychiatric Epidemiology* 29, 228–40.

Shepherd, G., Murray, A. & Muijen, M. (1994) *Relative Values: The Differing Views of Carers and Professionals on Services for People with Schizophrenia in the Community*. Sainsbury Centre, London.

Steinwachs, D., Kasper, J. & Skinner, E. (1992) *Family Perspectives on Meeting the Needs for Care of Severely Mentally Ill Relatives*. Johns Hopkins University, Baltimore.

Sullivan, W. & Poertner, J. (1989) Social support and life stress: a mental health consumers perspective. *Community Mental Health Journal* 25, 21–32.

Szmukler, G., Burgess, P., Herrman, H., Benson, A., Colusa, S. & Bloch, S. (1996) Caring for relatives with serious mental illness: the development of the experience of caregiving inventory. *Social Psychiatry and Psychiatric Epidemiology* 31, 137–48.

Tarrier, N., Barrowclough, C., Vaughn, C., Bamrah, J., Porceddu, K., Watts, S. & Freeman, H. (1988) The community management of schizophrenia: a controlled trial of behavioural intervention with families to reduce relapse. *British Journal of Psychiatry* 153, 532–42.

Tarrier, N., Barrowclough, C., Vaughn, C., Bamrah, J., Porceddu, K., Watts, S. & Freeman, H. (1989) The community management of schizophrenia: a two year follow-up of a behavioural intervention with families. *British Journal of Psychiatry* 154, 625–8.

Terkelson, K. (1990) A historical perspective on family–provider relationships. In *Families as Allies in Treatment of the Mentally Ill; New Directions for Mental Health Professionals* (Lefley, H. & Johnson, D., eds), pp. 3–21. American Psychiatric Press, Washington, DC.

Tessler, R., Gamache, G. & Fisher, G. (1991) Patterns of contact of patients' families with mental health professionals and attitudes towards professionals. *Hospital and Community Psychiatry* 42, 929–35.

Vaughn, C. (1989) Expressed emotion in family relationships. *Journal of Child Psychology and Psychiatry* **30**, 13–32.

Vaughn, C. & Leff, J. (1976) The influence of family and social factors in the course of mental illness. *British Journal of Psychiatry* **129**, 125–37.

Wessely, S., Castle, D., Douglas, A. & Taylor, P. (1994) The criminal careers of incident cases of schizophrenia. *Psychological Medicine* **24**, 483–502.

Wray, S. (1994) Schizophrenia sufferers and their carers: a survey of understanding of the condition and its treatment and of satisfaction with services. *Journal of Psychiatric and Mental Health Nursing* **1**, 115–24.

Chapter 12

Psychosocial Interventions

Mick McKeown and Ged McCann

INTRODUCTION

This chapter will review psychosocial interventions and the research which underpins them. It will subsequently explore how recent policy and research evidence support the introduction of psychosocial interventions to the care of mentally disordered offenders. A case exists for their introduction not only in community services but within in-patient secure forensic services. Finally, a vision of future services for this client group and the necessary structural and training requirements to enable its realisation will be described.

Psychosocial interventions refers to a number of largely behavioural or cognitive-behavioural psychological techniques geared towards the management of psychosis. The approach is problem-centred, sidestepping philosophical debates about diagnostic specificity or labelling, and places a particular emphasis upon the importance of stress in the course of psychotic problems. Psychosocial interventions attempt to include, wherever possible, significant people in the social network of the patient in the treatment process, and usually involve family members in structured family therapy. Within forensic care environments, however, especially in conditions of high security, we may also need to contemplate the important role assumed by professional staff in patients' social networks.

CASE STUDY

Bill had been in a special hospital for 13 years after killing his mother whilst suffering from auditory hallucinations and paranoid delusions. Previously he had a history of mental illness and had been living rough, travelling across the country, and frequently returning home to his mother. This behaviour coupled with alcoholism resulted in his alienation from the rest of his family, comprising four married brothers, none of whom had a history of mental illness.

Throughout his in-patient stay Bill continued to experience auditory hallucinations and paranoid delusions. The hallucinations took the form of his brothers continually shouting abuse at him, or describing him in negative ways. These voices were usually worse at night and resulted in Bill remaining socially isolated, preoccupied, and with little motivation or interest in himself. His most notable delusion was the belief that others were talking about him and passing comments about him being homosexual or 'queer'. These beliefs often led to assaults against other patients or staff, resulting in seclusion or other restrictive regimes. He had not met or spoken to any of his brothers since his court case.

Applying psychosocial interventions with Bill resulted firstly in a focused assessment of his symptoms. His delusions and hallucinations were assessed in depth and indicated not only the frequency and levels of distress associated with the voices, but also the content and what meaning Bill attached to them. Cognitive-behavioural intervention then focused on his feelings and beliefs regarding his brothers and what view of him they, and others, might hold. Work also began on grief counselling in relation to his mother, which had not been undertaken since the offence.

At the same time each of Bill's brothers was contacted and two agreed to meet with him at the hospital. Support was provided to all of the brothers, but structured educational work relating to schizophrenia was undertaken with the two visiting brothers. This involved detailed assessments of the needs of the brothers and a series of group psycho-educational sessions. Emotional support was also provided and sessional work was undertaken with one brother and Bill. This resulted in an increase in contact between Bill and his family which, together with the cognitive sessions, produced a reduction in the frequency of the voices and associated distress. Eighteen months later Bill was transferred out of the special hospital to a local medium secure unit where this family-based, psychosocial work was continued, and focused more on Bill's and his family's future needs.

BACKGROUND TO PSYCHOSOCIAL INTERVENTIONS

There is a large body of research which has demonstrated the efficacy of a range of psychosocial interventions in the management of schizophrenia. Controlled studies have demonstrated improved outcomes for patients with serious mental illness when specific packages of interventions are delivered in a structured way. These psychosocial intervention packages typically involve detailed assessments of clients and their carers, education about schizophrenia, the utilisation of communication and problem-solving strategies to reduce stress and specific cognitive-behavioural treatments designed to ameliorate symptoms. These psychosocial interventions are underpinned by conceptual models of psychosis which view symptoms in terms of the interaction between exposure to environmental stress and individual vulnerability factors (Zubin & Spring, 1977; Neuchterlain & Dawson, 1984).

Much of this research has focused on the influence of family interactions and the concept of expressed emotion (EE) as an especially important source of psychosocial stress. EE is a term used to describe certain domestic environments where relationships exhibit a significant degree of hostility, criticism or emotional over-involvement (Brown *et al.*, 1962). EE levels are measured in families using a semi-structured assessment tool, the Camberwell Family Interview (CFI). This instrument elicits relatives' comments about living with a person with schizophrenia, what sort of problems the sufferer has, and whether these are thought to result in any problems within the family. Examples of critical comments might include negative remarks about a person's behaviour, such as lying in bed or self-neglect. Hostile comments may be recognised from tone of voice, and often attribute negative behaviour to a personal trait, such as laziness. Emotional over-involvement can encompass a number of reported behaviours such as attempting to do everything for a person, keeping a very close eye on them all the time, or self-sacrificing behaviour such as giving up employment or socialising to spend more time in a caring role at home. Identifying these factors during interviews with relatives results in a rating of high EE whereas an absence of these factors results in a rating of low EE.

Replication studies (Brown *et al.*, 1972; Vaughn & Leff, 1976) have consistently demonstrated a strong relationship between high EE and an increased probability of relapse, usually indicating readmission to hospital. A series of intervention studies therefore targeted a reduction in EE in identified families in order to reduce relapse rates. The most beneficial have involved therapies which include the whole family, viewing them as therapeutic allies, working towards achieving coping and stress reduction through the employment of effective communication and problem-solving skills learnt in a behavioural framework. Controlled evaluations of structured family therapy have been carried out by a number of clinical research teams resulting in significant reductions in relapse rates. In some cases this continues at two-year follow-up (Falloon *et al.*, 1985; Leff *et al.*, 1985, 1990; Hogarty *et al.*, 1986; Tarrier *et al.*, 1989).

Recent studies have successfully evaluated the therapeutic benefit of cognitive-behavioural interventions aimed at the reduction of the symptoms of serious mental illness, and their associated distress (Sellwood *et al.*, 1994). These have included the use of focusing and other strategies in the management of auditory hallucinations (Bentall *et al.*, 1994; Chadwick & Birchwood, 1994), and belief modification techniques for delusions (Chadwick & Lowe, 1990). A number of small-scale randomised controlled trials demonstrating the value of this approach have been reported (Kingdon &

Turkington, 1991; Tarrier *et al.*, 1993; Garety *et al.*, 1994), the most recent of which has demonstrated the value of adding cognitive-behaviour therapy to the routine care given to acute in-patients (Drury *et al.*, 1996). Other important work has been in the field of early warning signs monitoring to avoid relapse (Birchwood *et al.*, 1997) and in using psychological strategies to enhance compliance with neuroleptic medication (Kemp *et al.*, 1996).

POLICY TRENDS

In the wider National Health Service there is a welcome policy shift towards a lead role for primary care services (Department of Health, 1997, 1998) accompanied by a more general trend for the delivery of care to be based upon the best quality research evidence available. The shift to a primary-care-led NHS is in one sense a natural, if overdue, progression from the founding principles of establishing health as a cornerstone of the fledgling post-war welfare state. Other progressive ideological and clinical forces have coalesced over the last half century or so, driving the process of deinstitutionalisation and culminating in the notion of care in the community. More recently, academic and political scrutiny of psychiatric services and professional training has given rise to a number of policy guidelines concerning the care of people with severe and enduring problems (Department of Health, 1995). All of these developments have implications for practitioners interested in the care of mentally disordered offenders.

Despite much that is laudable about the idea of community care, a pernicious lack of funding has been just one of a number of problems which have beset the implementation of this policy goal. Of particular concern has been the care of people who present varying degrees of risk of dangerousness or vulnerability. Latterly, such concerns have been acutely focused upon tragic failings of community care exemplified in high-profile cases of self-harm, assault or murder, ushering in new legislative devices for professional surveillance and control. These developments create further problems and can be seen in one sense as an inevitable consequence of contemplating the risk management issues implicit in the guiding principles of the Reed Report (Department of Health/Home Office, 1992; McCann, 1998).

The Reed review of services for mentally disordered offenders argued for a service philosophy based on minimum levels of security appropriate to degree of risk and care provision as close as possible to one's home or family, in the community if possible (Department of Health/Home Office, 1992). Clearly the establishment of services on this basis presents challenges for practitioners charged with the responsibility of delivering them. Even if such systems are actualised, a sizeable portion of service provision will remain configured around some sort of secure in-patient setting.

People suffering from severe and enduring problems also exercise the greatest potential demand upon mental health services and this is reflected proportionally in forensic services. However, services across the board have been criticised for failing to give the needs of this client group sufficient priority (Gournay, 1994). Some of this critique arises from the inquiry into service failings (Ritchie *et al.*, 1994; Blom-Cooper *et al.*, 1992; Davies, 1995) and allegations of systematic abuse and neglect (Blom-Cooper *et al.*, 1992). More generic criticisms are to be found in a number of government-sponsored reviews (Mental Health Nursing Review Team, 1994; Reed, 1994; Clinical Standards Advisory Group, 1995). In-patient services too have attracted their own examination, for example in the report of The National Visit to acute psychiatric wards carried out by the Mental Health Act Commission and the Sainsbury Centre (MHAC/Sainsbury Centre, 1997).

The overwhelming recommendation to be found in these reports is that services must become more systematic and focused in their delivery of care. There is a consensus that appropriate assessment and treatment are of paramount concern and should include the delivery of a range of evidence-based psychosocial interventions under the aegis of sound case management principles. To this end, meeting the needs of the severely mentally ill has become a national priority for both purchasers and providers.

A major plank of complying with this agenda is the need to provide relevant practitioner training. The National Visit quality audit highlights this point, remarking upon the lack of an appropriate therapeutic environment within in-patient settings, with the perception that this was at least partly due to inadequate preparation of mental health nurses to meet the needs of this client group.

'Many nurses were trained at a time when a number of patients on acute wards had less severe forms of illness. As the patients on acute wards now have more severe forms of illness, such as schizophrenia and manic-depressive psychosis, different interventions are required. Nurses will therefore need to have skills in communication with people who have thought disorders, and they will need to learn some of the more recent therapeutic psychological interventions for these problems' (MHAC/ Sainsbury Centre, 1997).

Thus wider policy developments and their impact upon services for mentally disordered offenders, and the contemplation of objective scrutiny of general psychiatric services and their failings, make a persuasive case for the systematic implementation of services which can effectively meet the needs of the severely mentally ill. The proposed vehicle for delivering such a system is the implementation of well organised and individualised packages of psychosocial interventions associated with staff training.

In recommending this approach the policy brokers have relied upon scientific evaluation of psychotic pathology and psychosocial interventions in practice.

Most of this research which has evaluated clinical practice and training initiatives in psychosocial interventions has, however, been geared towards improving community-based services. Little research has been undertaken which has evaluated the efficacy of applying psychosocial interventions within in-patient settings. There is a real need to adapt this body of research and apply it not only within general wards, but also within secure settings. Despite care in the community policies and the retraction of continuing institutional care for this client group, some patients spend appreciable amounts of time within residential facilities staffed by professional carers. There are no grounds for assuming that this picture will alter significantly in the future. As indicated above, systematic psychological interventions are rarely provided within in-patient settings, so clients frequently complain about the poverty of the therapeutic environment (Rogers *et al.*, 1993). Moreover, studies have examined EE as exhibited by staff in institutional settings indicating that staff–patient relationships influence the course of schizophrenia (Moore *et al.*, 1992). Benefits to patients, staff and the organisation might therefore be realised if interventions were implemented to improve staff–patient relationships and reduce environmental stress. Further, a trial of cognitive-behavioural interventions with acute psychotic in-patients has demonstrated the value of this approach in terms of rapid and more complete recovery from psychotic episodes and a sustained reduction of symptomatology (Drury *et al.*, 1996).

APPLYING PSYCHOSOCIAL INTERVENTIONS

The abundance of quality research, together with a number of important policy imperatives, constitutes a powerful rationale for incorporating such work into the care and management of mentally disordered offenders (McCann & McKeown, 1995a). Most mentally disordered offenders have been primarily diagnosed as having some form of psychotic disorder. Many of the concerns which drive government thinking arise from a conceptualisation of this client group which focuses upon public safety, and result from official scrutiny of failings in the forensic system. A substantial portion of the care of mentally disordered offenders takes place in in-patient environments, with many spending at least some of their patient career in a secure ward setting. A strong case can be made for adapting the psychosocial model so that it better fits the contingencies and practicalities of institutional care. Conversely, the trend towards care in the community encompasses services for mentally disordered offenders, and it would seem to make sense to provide such care within a tried and tested framework.

ASSESSMENT

Regardless of a person's position within the overall health-care system the assessment and management of dangerousness and vulnerability are paramount concerns. The psychosocial approach is essentially concerned with systematising care and is closely associated with models of multi-disciplinary case management and the goal of achieving seamless services. As such, the specific interventions employed are predicated upon the regular use of systematic and reliable assessment tools addressing various important outcomes. Accurate and reliable assessments can be undertaken of general mental health needs, positive and negative psychotic symptoms, anxiety, depression, suicidality, social functioning, side-effects of medication and specific behavioural problems. Traditionally, nurses in particular have rarely got involved with the use of systematic assessment tools, perhaps viewing them as reductionist. A consequence of this has been a difficulty in prioritising and planning care, possibly arising from the lack of precision in assessment that hampers the formulation of particular problems and goals. The use of formal assessment tools enables a comprehensive evaluation of a person's problems, which the skilled practitioner can then contextualise by exploring them further with the individual patient and others in the care team.

An immediate benefit of systematising the assessment of psychotic symptomatology in the context of multi-disciplinary care planning would be to enable practitioners to explore links between an individual's psychosis and their offending behaviour. This would be compatible with the call for the disaggregation of component factors in patient risk when making risk management decisions (Steadman *et al.*, 1994).

As a considerable focus of psychosocial working is about the engagement and involvement of families, we must recognise that they will have their own needs, some of which will directly or indirectly arise from their relative's offending history. Similarly, our ability to work constructively with a particular patient may depend upon gathering useful assessment material from relatives, carers or close friends. This is particularly important if structured family therapy or other work with carers is intended. Therefore, it is important when considering the issue of assessment to attempt to elicit valuable information from significant people in the social network of the patient. We devised an assessment schedule for identifying the problems and needs of the carers of mentally disordered offenders detained in a secure environment. The Relative Assessment Interview for Schizophrenia in a Secure Environment (RAISSE) is a semi-structured interview developed from previous general instruments to take into account the special circumstances pertaining to the experience of having a relationship with a forensic patient within a secure setting (McKeown & McCann, 1995).

The assessment covers three broad areas: information about the patient's schizophrenia, family stresses and coping, the events leading to the patient's contact with forensic services and admission to a secure setting, current relationships, visiting and other contact. Of particular interest are the relative's thoughts and feelings about the offence and the admission to forensic care. Carers may have experienced the stigmatising effects of intrusive media coverage or negative reactions from neighbours or colleagues. They may have formed particular views about any link between illness and the offence, influencing how they cope. Relationships can be adversely affected, especially if the offence has been committed within the family, resulting in possible feelings of rejection, hostility, anger, shame or guilt, denial or even depression similar to bereavement. How family members react can have long-term consequences for their continued relationships. For instance, contact time or the quality of communications between family members can be affected. The trappings of security in forensic environments can compound the stresses which a relative may feel, as can a lack of involvement or communication with care team members.

FAMILY WORK

It is thought that high EE family environments are sources of chronic stress which negatively impact upon the symptoms of the psychotic family member. This may be exhibited in tensions and arguments at home, commonly around the effects of negative symptoms – a person not getting out of bed, for instance. Importantly, high EE needs to be viewed as an understandable coping style when faced with what can seem inexplicable behaviour on the part of a relative with schizophrenia. Families can struggle to make sense of a person's changed behaviour, or to know how to handle changed expectations and aspirations for that person. It is not uncommon for families to misattribute as wilful actions behaviour which is at least partly understandable in terms of pathology. This sort of response may lie behind feelings of criticism or hostility. Similarly, emotional over-involvement may be understood as the normal, indeed socially approved, response towards a relative apparently in need of support and protection.

Behavioural family therapy progresses through stages of psycho-education, communication skills training, and problem-solving skills training (Falloon *et al.*, 1988). Psycho-education is targeted upon deficits in family knowledge about schizophrenia which are likely to result in increased stress if acted upon. The Knowledge About Schizophrenia Interview [KASI] (Barrowclough *et al.*, 1987) is a useful structured assessment tool for addressing functional knowledge. Communication skills training attempts to address certain key skills which, if practised by everyone, ought to make an impact upon overall stress levels. Falloon and colleagues (1988) suggest that this can be accomplished by achieving competence in the four skills of expressing positive feelings, making a positive request, expressing negative feelings and active listening. These communication skills are also seen as the necessary prerequisites for the family as a group to be able to effectively solve problems among themselves. A six-stage problem-solving method is taught which involves agreeing a definition of the problem, generating possible solutions, evaluating each potential solution, choosing the best option, planning how best to carry out this solution, carrying out the plan and reviewing its effectiveness.

In order to explore how this family-based approach needed to be modified and adapted for a forensic in-patient setting, research was undertaken at Ashworth Special Hospital. The project illustrated how services can be developed which involve families and can address some of the particular needs that arise within forensic environments (McCann, 1993; McKeown & McCann, 1995; McCann *et al.*, 1995, 1996; McCann & Clancy, 1996). The project had a number of strands which included research aimed at identifying and understanding the needs of relatives of special hospital patients, evaluating the functional knowledge of relatives, the provision of psycho-education groups for relatives and evaluation of their impact. The overall aim was to provide a basis for improved services for relatives which had come in for particular criticism from the Public Inquiry of 1992:

> 'Regrettably the regime at Ashworth ... seems to have been designed to deter rather than encourage relatives to participate in their relative's care' (Blom-Cooper *et al.*, 1992)

Such observations were borne out by the comments of relatives attending the first support group of its kind in the hospital (McCann, 1993). These relatives had numerous concerns which they felt were not being addressed. Relatives were largely ignorant of the workings of hospital and care teams and had other information needs about mental illness and treatment. They had particular anxieties about medication and seclusion, often fuelled by adverse media coverage of the hospital. Having a relationship to a serious offender can raise quite specific problems for relatives who are often treated as if 'guilty by association, suffering ostracism, abuse and sometimes physical violence ... they are in their own prison cells' (Groocock, 1989).

A systematic content analysis of tape-recorded RAISSE interviews with 17 Ashworth relatives yielded an illuminating insight into their thoughts and feelings, highlighting a stressful scenario of feeling unsupported, and frustrated at their lack of involvement or contribution in day-to-day care (McCann *et al.*, 1996). The scrutiny of the interviews revealed six recurrent themes. Relatives experienced stress arising from specific life events surrounding the patient. Though these refer to specific incidents, such as the offence itself, the court case, police involvement, or admission to secure hospital care, it is worth noting that the stress is not necessarily short-lived. Other, continual stress caused chronic anxiety and worries which had little to do with events surrounding the offence. For instance, relatives experienced persistent stress in contemplating the general welfare of the patient. Some stress related to anticipation of, or reflection on, visits which were characteristically stressful or unsatisfying experiences. Adaptive self-coping strategies were adopted by many of the relatives. Three core strategies emerged: attribution of the patient's offence to his illness, reliance upon their social network to reduce stress, and maintaining contact with the patient through visiting. Maladaptive self-coping strategies were also described. These included: bottling up feelings, social withdrawal because of the offence, and hostile reactions to stress with feelings of revenge against the patient or others. Relatives commented in even numbers about both positive and negative aspects of their contact with the hospital. Such observations focused upon the staff and their abilities, hospital facilities, or the general atmosphere being either relaxing or anxiety provoking. Signs of illness were a theme in most of the relatives' recounting of their experiences. Almost all had witnessed, and often reported to services, changes in their relative's behaviour or appearance prior to committing the offence. Such observations were in some cases accompanied by expressed concerns about risk of dangerousness which were not given credence by services until it was too late.

A number of key implications arise from this research for forensic practitioners and services. There is an immediate need for the provision of information and support for relatives of forensic patients and, crucially, they need to be more closely involved in their relative's care. A lack of knowledge about psychotic illness can lead to misattributions about behaviour, which can affect the quality of continuing relationships or, worse, result in estrangement. This is particularly important in contemplation of offending behaviour. When visiting a secure hospital, relatives face numerous difficulties which can be exacerbated by anxieties about what the person will be like when they get there. Pressure on all parties to have a pleasant visit can preclude discussion of sensitive issues, such as the offence, leading to continuing worries, for example about future discharge plans.

It is apparent that relatives' initial experiences of the psychiatric and criminal justice systems can have damaging and enduring effects, at a time when they have pressing personal needs. Services which do not make efforts to support and engage relatives at these distressing times lose an excellent opportunity to forge lasting, mutually beneficial therapeutic alliances. More disturbing is the frequency with which relatives report their own informal assessments of risk falling on the deaf ears of disinterested professionals. It would appear that the early engagement and involvement of relatives offer potential avenues toward preventative health work in the forensic field.

Following this review of relatives' needs at Ashworth an attempt was made to establish some innovations in service provision to address some of the issues raised. One initiative involved expanding a small network of ward-based relatives' support groups where visitors to the hospital could meet and discuss issues of common concern or could be briefed on matters of general interest. The philosophy driving the groups was one of developing independence from professional staff input, so that the groups could eventually become self-sustaining with professional contributions only arising on invitation. These groups serve a number of functions for relatives, bringing them into closer contact with the hospital, enabling engagement with appropriate channels for raising concerns, and providing mutual support and advice and the opportunity for airing knowledge and information.

Another initiative was specifically focused upon meeting the information needs of groups of relatives (McCann & Clancy, 1996). This involved the delivery of targeted psycho-education packages in a group work format and evaluating the effectiveness in this particular context using repeat measures of functional knowledge elicited by the KASI. Four two-hour sessions were spread over a two-month period and timetabled so that relatives could attend before normal visiting times. The groups were kept small to enable engagement with individuals' needs. The psycho-education work undertaken in the sessions was supported by two specially produced information booklets which adapted previously available materials (Smith & Birchwood, 1991) for use in forensic settings.

The evaluation compared pre- and post-KASI scores for relatives who completed the group against a control group who were waiting to attend the programme. Many of the relatives already had quite high KASI scores prior to the intervention, yet significant knowledge gain was demonstrated in relation to the important KASI sections of course and prognosis and management. This reflected the emphasis given to these topics in the sessions, partly guided by the relatives' own preferences relating to current and future concerns around 'what to do'. An interesting aspect of this group was the group members' subjective reflections on the value of attending. Though the focus of the work was intended to be education, many of the participants reported emotional support as an important benefit. Relatives reported appreciating the opportunity to mix and share feelings with similarly situated others.

PROBLEM-CENTRED WORK WITH INDIVIDUALS

The lack of precision in psychiatric delineation of distinct disease categorisations or taxonomies has led some academics and researchers to question the validity of diagnostic terms such as schizophrenia, and to call for a focus instead upon the specific problems identified in therapeutic alliance with patients (Bentall, 1990). Such a focus, with an emphasis upon collaborative and participative work towards the resolution of agreed problems, is central to applying psychosocial interventions.

Once problems have been identified and realisable goals have been planned, a number of psychological management strategies can be employed in their resolution. The most effective of these are cognitive-behavioural in orientation and include tactics for coping strategy enhancement, modification of delusional beliefs, minimising hallucinations or attendant distress, aiding communication in thought disorder, minimising the social disability from negative symptoms, avoiding relapse by monitoring early signs (prodromes), promoting effective compliance with neuroleptic medication and working with other problematic behaviours such as substance use or self-harm. This work is underpinned by a normalising philosophy of psychotic experiences where what is important is the meaningfulness of symptoms and the roles they play in people's lives. This therapeutic stance challenges certain conventional views of hallucinations and delusions, emphasising that people can begin to take control over symptoms and problems which are essentially amenable to reasoning. Coping strategy enhancement builds upon the recognition that most people who have psychotic problems will have developed some coping strategies of their own to minimise the effects of certain symptoms. For instance, a person who hears voices may find that listening to music, perhaps via a personal stereo, distracts from the content of the voices, and hence reduces distress. Other therapeutic approaches involve developing individualised packages of training, which aim to supplement and advance a person's chosen coping strategies. People with delusions can be helped to shift the degree of conviction with which they hold irrational beliefs by a number of techniques. These approaches rely on a cognitive model of belief acquisition and maintenance in which a person's beliefs act as an interpretational filter on the world and in which selective attention is paid to events, furnishing evidence which confirms and supports those beliefs already in place. Chadwick & Lowe (1990) successfully modified the delusional beliefs of their clients by verbally challenging the evidence which was provided by the clients in support of their belief, or by subjecting this to reality testing.

Research has been undertaken into a variety of strategies for dealing with hallucinations, mainly hearing voices. The range of therapies includes operant procedures (Nydegger, 1972), systematic desensitisation (Slade, 1972), thought-stopping (Johnson *et al.*, 1983), distraction therapies (Margo *et al.*, 1981; Nelson *et al.*, 1991; Gallagher *et al.*, 1994), ear plugs (James, 1983), first person singular therapy (Greene, 1978) and focusing/reattribution (Bentall *et al.*, 1994). Slade & Bentall (1988) reviewed the numerous psychological approaches to treating voices and suggested that they could be divided into three categories of approach: those that emphasise distraction, those that invite people to focus on their voices, and those that entail anxiety reduction.

Distraction techniques by definition attempt to divert people's attention away from their voices. This can involve passive strategies, like listening to music, or active strategies like doing mental arithmetic or reading. Sometimes it can be more helpful to practise active distraction vocally, such as reading aloud, humming or whistling. It is not really clear why any of these methods should work, but they undoubtedly do for some people. One theory is that voices are essentially misperceptions of the sort of internal voices that everyone has. Observations of sub-vocal speech (physiological activity in the region of the vocal chords) in subjects thinking to themselves are replicated in people actively hearing voices. Active distractions like reading aloud can be thought of as effective because they present an alternative use for the voice mechanism; for this reason they are sometimes referred to as counter-stimulation.

Reattribution therapy works with the notion of helping people to change possible misattributions they may have regarding the source of their voices, or other beliefs they may hold about the voices. People can be taught to attend to qualitative dimensions of the voice-hearing experience, such as the varying characteristics of the voice, tone, pitch or loudness or whether the voice is recognisable. Special attention is given to helping the person examine what the voice or voices actually say, what this means for the voice hearer, and what they believe about the experience. These beliefs can then be modified to reduce distress or the frequency of the voices.

Anxiety reduction techniques can help to reduce subjective feelings of stress and minimise the frequency or intensity of hallucinatory experiences. Clearly, many of the strategies described here as employed by therapists will have been arrived at by individual voice hearers themselves in attempts at self-coping. The international self-help group the Hearing Voices Network brings together many of these themes under a philosophy of accepting voices as real and meaningful phenomena, only promoting effective therapies if the experience of voice hearing is distressing (Romme & Escher, 1993).

Thought disorder is often referred to as speech disorder because the disturbance to a person's cognitive faculties is witnessed in the consequential disruption to forms and patterns of speech. At its most extreme, thought disorder can result in seemingly incomprehensible talk which can appear to defy any attempts at meaningful communication on the part of carers or professionals. However, innovative approaches of thought linkage and clarification have been utilised to make sense of illogical and incoherent speech (Kingdon & Turkington, 1994). These strategies involve patience and perseverance on the part of the therapist, moving through stages of listening, stopping, rephrasing, and checking and agreeing accuracy of meaning, in an attempt to focus upon fragments of speech which make some sense amongst the jumble.

Because serious psychotic illness can result in periods of relative wellness, separated by episodes of relapse, it has been observed that prior to each relapse individuals may experience a number of problems which constitute 'early warning signs' of impending relapse. This pre-relapse period has been referred to as a prodrome. It is possible to help people and their carers to describe their own prodromal signature of early warning signs in an attempt to recognise their future reappearance in time to seek remedial treatment and avoid relapse (Birchwood *et al.*, 1997).

A major problem with any long-term maintenance therapy, including anti-psychotic drugs, is the degree of non-compliance with treatment regimens. Compliance therapy aims to promote understanding of the value of neuroleptic medication in avoiding relapse and hence acceptance of the need to adhere to prescribed regimes. Previous studies have highlighted factors adversely affecting treatment adherence, notably distressing side effects, and have found that simple didactic approaches to education are not effective. Kemp and colleagues (1997) have produced a handbook which presents a three-stage approach derived from cognitive-behavioural elements and the principles of motivational interviewing (Miller & Rollnick 1991). A controlled evaluation demonstrated improved attitudes to treatment and compliance which were maintained at six-month follow-up (Kemp *et al.*, 1996).

The problem-centred approach is also amenable for targeting other behaviours which can cause difficulties for psychotic patients. An example is problematic substance use, which has led to the coining of the term dual diagnosis to incorporate those seen to have co-morbid problems. Various authors have argued for integrated services for people with both severe mental health problems and problematic drug use, in this context arguing for the appropriateness of the psychosocial model in identifying specific problems and how they might be linked (McKeown & Derricott, 1996). For example, substance use can involve attempts to self-medicate symptoms or adverse side effects of prescribed medication, or the expansion of a person's social network. In such circumstances practitioners operating a problem-centred approach have the opportunity, in a non-judgmental manner, to engage clients in discussions of the impact of drug use on other aspects of their lives and work towards maximising positive outcomes and minimising harm.

MULTI-DISCIPLINARY TEAMWORKING

For psychosocial interventions to be successful they need to be implemented within an appropriate system of case management and multi-disciplinary team working. Organisational models in the context of case managing rehabilitation services in a special hospital (McCann & McKeown,

1995b) and multi-disciplinary care planning in a high dependency unit (Savage & McKeown, 1997) have been described. Such models essentially involve systems which enable thorough and reliable assessment, and multi-disciplinary management of care. They also allow for the clear recording of a range of effective interventions, making accountability explicit and subject to regular review, and involve the service user and significant others in its construction. The interplay between professionals from varying philosophical perspectives and training backgrounds is a reflection of the family's role in the overall management of a complex problem. Research has clearly indicated the strain family members are under when living with a person with a severe mental illness. This strain is exacerbated when the relatives involved have no clear understanding of the illness, have difficulty in communicating effectively and have no clear process of dealing with problems when they arise. Within professional teams there is a clear need to ensure that professionals understand and agree on the presenting problems, have an effective method of communication and are organisationally competent to deal with problems in a structured, systematic way.

Consideration must also be given to the potentially damaging role of individual interactions with patients. Often the social networks of mentally disordered offenders are limited, with family relationships strained or non-existent. Professionals can assume a significant role in any patient's network of contacts. This is particularly so within in-patient settings where most patients will spend more time in close contact with professional carers than they will with their families or friends. Research in a variety of institutional settings has described high EE relationships between staff and patients (Moore *et al.*, 1992), where similar examples of criticism, hostility and emotional over-involvement have been identified. Other potential sources of stress will arise from the physical environment and routines of security which are often imposed.

Thus in forensic in-patient settings we can begin to view individual staff members as significant persons within a patient's social network, and in many ways as analogous to family members in their interactions. The implications of such a scenario are twofold. First, practitioners will need to understand and be able to identify how their interactions may have an impact on the course of schizophrenia and have the skills to modify those interactions. Secondly, within the context of the ward environment staff must identify those policies and procedures which may act as potential sources of stress and mediate these stressors in their day-to-day interactions with patients. This might involve consistently modelling the key communication skills and problem-solving approaches seen to minimise interrelationship stress in social networks; and working to resolve any apparent tensions or stresses through small patient/staff group meetings and in individual or group clinical supervision sessions where staff interactions can be discussed and improved. Such an approach would be compatible with collaborative models of therapeutic alliance and would mimic the process of family therapy.

FUTURE DIRECTIONS

Services for mentally disordered offenders could be greatly enhanced by incorporating a range of psychosocial interventions into the routine practice of staff working in diverse forensic settings, from the community to conditions of high security. In many senses the care and management of psychotic problems ought not to be appreciably different between general psychiatric services and forensic care. Across the board symptom reduction, enhancement of social functioning, medication compliance and relapse prevention are required. Yet the implementation of novel psychological management approaches to the exploration and treatment of hallucinations and delusions may realise fruitful avenues of engagement with individuals' propensity for dangerousness. Similarly, a strong case can be made for involving families in the full gamut of forensic services, not least because of their potential role as allies in assessment and therapy.

The systematic implementation of psychosocial interventions also raises the possibility of achieving new levels of interdisciplinary cooperation and democracy within shared decision making. Psychosocial interventions cannot be delivered without a system for effective team working. In turn, this necessitates a coordinated approach to practitioner training which prepares staff to practise the appropriate competencies and enables them to adopt such skills in their routine practice. To date, despite the undoubted quality of current training initiatives, there has been a woeful inability to translate this into service level change. New models of training are required which do not just focus upon changing individual practitioners, but also focus upon organisational change in the setting in which the taught knowledge and skills are to be applied.

Lessons from the field of organisational psychology suggest that the best way to achieve such enduring changes in practice and systems is to concentrate upon training whole teams, rather than isolated practitioners, in the context of the workplace environment where they will be expected to practise new methods (Corrigan & McCracken, 1997; McKeown *et al.*, 1998). Such an approach would build on the skills of practitioners and assist them to modify and adapt the psychosocial model to suit the contingencies and practicalities of the particular setting in which it is to be applied. As such the training process would involve a symbiotic interplay between grassroots practitioners and the trainers so that the delivery of psychosocial care can endure in the real world of forensic practice.

A long-term developmental project at an inner-city high dependency unit involving ward-based teaching and adaptation of psychosocial working has been evaluated recently (McKeown *et al.*, 1997). This initiative resulted in the incorporation of a range of systematic assessment tools into routine practice and a new format for multi-disciplinary care planning and documentation (Savage & McKeown, 1997). After 18 months of continued input significant changes were measured in the acquisition of staff knowledge, the quality of care plans, and reductions in staff stress.

The project described above represents an interesting but modest attempt to translate the psychosocial model, developed in community settings, to the context of ward environments. A strong case can be made for revolutionising multi-disciplinary practitioner training, moving it away from classrooms back into real world environments. Furthermore, for substantial changes to be made to the practices of teams, the trainers themselves must become embedded in the team for an appreciable amount of time. We believe that it is only by such an approach that psychosocial interventions can become organisationally embedded in routine practice in a way that will endure on cessation of the training initiative (McKeown *et al.*, 1998). Services for mentally disordered offenders could be the ideal place to start.

REFERENCES

Barrowclough, C., Tarrier, N., Watts, S., Vaughn, C., Bamrah, J. & Freeman, H. (1987) Assessing the functional value of relatives' reported knowledge about schizophrenia. *British Journal of Psychiatry* **151**, 1–8

Bentall, R. (ed.) (1990) *Reconstructing Schizophrenia.* Routledge, London.

Bentall, R. P., Haddock, G. & Slade, P. D. (1994) Cognitive behavior therapy for persistent auditory hallucinations: from theory to therapy. *Behavior Therapy* **25**, 51–66.

Birchwood, M., McGorry, P. & Jackson, H. (1997) Early intervention in schizophrenia. *British Journal of Psychiatry* **170**, 2–5.

Blom-Cooper, L., Brown, M., Dolan, R. & Murphy, E. (1992) *Report of the Committee of Inquiry into Complaints about Ashworth Hospital.* HMSO, London.

Brown, G. W., Birley, J. L. T. & Wing, J. K. (1972) Influence of family life on the course of schizophrenia disorders: replication. *British Journal of Psychiatry* **121**, 241–58.

Brown, G. W., Monck, E. M., Carstairs, G. M. & Wing, J. K. (1962) Influence of family life on the course of schizophrenia disorders. *British Journal of Preventative and Social Medicine* **16**, 55–68.

Chadwick, P. & Birchwood, M. (1994) The omnipotence of voices: a cognitive approach to auditory hallucinations. *British Journal of Psychiatry* **164**, 190–201.

Chadwick, P. & Lowe, C. (1990) The measurement and modification of delusional beliefs. *Journal of Consulting and Clinical Psychology* **58**, 225–32.

Clinical Standards Advisory Group Report on Schizophrenia (1995) *Clinical Standards Advisory Group: Schizophrenia. Volume 1. Report of a CSAG Committee on Schizophrenia.* HMSO, London.

Corrigan, P. & McCracken, S. (1997) Psychiatric rehabilitation and staff development: educational and organisational models. *Clinical Psychology Review* **15**, 699–719.

Davies, N. (1995) *Report of the Inquiry into the Circumstances Leading to the Death of Jonathan Newby.* HMSO, London.

Department of Health (1995) *Building Bridges – A Guide to Arrangements for Interagency Working for the Care and Protection of Severely Mentally Ill People.* HMSO, London.

Department of Health (1997) *NHS (Primary Care) Act.* HMSO, London.

Department of Health (1998) *Our Healthier Nation.* HMSO, London.

Department of Health/Home Office (1992) *Review of Health and Social Services for Mentally Disordered Offenders and Others Requiring Similar Services* (The Reed Report). HMSO, London.

Drury, V., Birchwood, M., Cochrane, R. & MacMillan, F. (1996) Cognitive-behaviour therapy for acute psychosis. *British Journal of Psychiatry* **169**, 593–607.

Falloon, I., Boyd, J., McGill, C., Williamson, M., Razani, J., Moss, H., Gilderman, A. & Simson, G. (1985) Family management in the prevention of morbidity of schizophrenia: clinical outcome of a two year longitudinal study. *Archives of General Psychiatry* **42**, 887–96.

Falloon, I., Meuser, K., Gingerich, S., Rappaport, S., McGill, C. & Hole, V. (1988) *Behavioural Family Therapy: A Workbook.* Buckingham Mental Health Service, Buckingham.

Gallagher, A., Dinan, T. & Baker, L. (1994) The effects of varying auditory input on schizophrenic hallucinations: a replication. *British Journal of Medical Psychology* **67**, 67–76.

Garety, P. A., Kuipers, L., Fowler, D., Chamberlain, F. & Dunn, G. (1994) Cognitive behavioural therapy for drug-resistant psychosis. *British Journal of Medical Psychology* **67**, 259–71.

Gournay, K. (1994) Redirecting the emphasis to serious mental illness. *Nursing Times* **90**(25), 40–41.

Greene, R. (1978) Auditory hallucination reduction: first person singular therapy. *Journal of Contemporary Psychotherapy* **9**, 167–70.

Groocock, V. (1989) The sins of the children visited on the parents. *The Independent* 16 March, p. 6.

Hogarty, G., Anderson, C., Reiss, D., Kornblith, S., Greenwald, D., Jarvna, C. & Madonia, M. (1986) Family psychoeducation, social skills training, and maintenance chemotherapy in the aftercare treatment of schizophrenia. *Archives of General Psychiatry* **43**, 633–42.

James, D. (1983) The experimental treatment of two cases of auditory hallucinations. *British Journal of Psychiatry* **143**, 515–16.

Johnson, C., Gilmore, J. & Shenoy, R. (1983) Thought stopping and anger induction in the treatment of hallucinations and obsessional ruminations. *Psychotherapy: Theory, Research, Practice* **20**, 445–8.

Kemp, R., Hayward, P., Applewhaite, G., Everitt, B. & David, A. (1996) Compliance therapy in psychotic patients: a randomised controlled trial. *British Medical Journal* **312**, 345–9.

Kemp, R., Hayward, P. & David, A. (1997) *Compliance Therapy Manual*. The Maudsley, London.

Kingdon, D. G. & Turkington, D. (1991) Preliminary report: the use of cognitive behaviour therapy and a normalizing rationale in schizophrenia. *Journal of Nervous and Mental Disease* **179**, 207–11.

Kingdon, D. & Turkington, D. (1994) *Cognitive Behavioural Therapy of Schizophrenia*. Guildford Press, New York.

Leff, J., Berkowitz, R., Shavit, A., Strachan, A. & Vaughn, C. (1990) A trial of family therapy v. a relatives group for schizophrenia: two year follow-up. *British Journal of Psychiatry* **157**, 571–7.

Leff, J., Kuipers, L., Berkowitz, R. & Sturgeon, D. (1985) A controlled trial of social intervention in the families of schizophrenic patients: two year follow-up. *British Journal of Psychiatry* **146**, 594–600.

McCann, G. (1993) Relatives' support groups in a special hospital: an evaluation study. *Journal of Advanced Nursing* **18**, 1883–8.

McCann, G. (1998) Control in the community. In *Critical Perspectives in Forensic Care: Inside Out* (Mason, T. & Mercer, D., eds). Macmillan, London.

McCann, G. & Clancy, B. (1996) Family matters. *Nursing Times* **92**(7), 46–8.

McCann, G. & McKeown, M. (1995a) Applying psychosocial interventions within a forensic environment. *Psychiatric Care* **2**, 133–6.

McCann, G. & McKeown, M. (1995b) Clinical management: a special case. *Journal of Nursing Management* **3**, 115–20.

McCann, G., McKeown, M. & Porter, I. (1995) Identifying the needs of the relatives of forensic patients. *Nursing Times* **91**(24), 35–7.

McCann, G., McKeown, M. & Porter, I. (1996) Understanding the needs of relatives of patients within a special hospital for mentally disordered offenders: a basis for improved services. *Journal of Advanced Nursing* **23**, 346–52.

McKeown, M. & Derricott, J. (1996) Muddy waters. *Nursing Times* **92**(28), 30–31.

McKeown, M. & McCann, G. (1995) A schedule for assessing relatives: the Relative Assessment Interview for Schizophrenia in a Secure Environment. *Psychiatric Care* **2**(3), 84–8.

McKeown, M., Finlayson, S. & Roberts, K. (1997) Implementing a psychosocial model of practice within a ward environment. Paper presented to the Second International Conference on Psychological Treatments for Schizophrenia, Oxford, 2 and 3 October.

McKeown, M., McCann, G. & Bentall, R. (1998) Time for action: a new system of training mental health practitioners. *Mental Health Care* **1**(5), 158.

Margo, A., Hemsley, D. & Slade P. (1981) The effects of varying auditory input on schizophrenic hallucinations. *British Journal of Psychiatry* **139**, 122–7.

Mental Health Act Commission and the Sainsbury Centre (1997). *The National Visit*. Sainsbury Centre for Mental Health, London.

Mental Health Nursing Review Team (1994) *Working in Partnership: A Collaborative Approach to Care. Report of the Mental Health Nursing Review Team* [Butterworth Report]. HMSO, London.

Miller, W. & Rollnick, S. (1991) *Motivational Interviewing: Preparing People to Change*. Guildford Press, New York.

Moore, E., Ball, R. & Kuipers, L. (1992) Expressed emotion in staff working with the long-term adult mentally ill. *British Journal of Psychiatry* **161**, 802–808.

Nelson, H., Thrasher, S. & Barnes, T. (1991) Practical ways of relieving auditory hallucinations. *British Medical Journal* **302**, 307.

Neuchterlain, K. & Dawson, M. (1984) A heuristic vulnerability-stress model of schizophrenic episodes. *Schizophrenia Bulletin* **10**, 300–312.

Nydegger, R. (1972) The elimination of hallucinatory and delusional behaviour by verbal conditioning and assertive training: a case study. *Journal of Behaviour Therapy and Experimental Psychiatry* **3**, 225–7.

Reed, J. (1994) *Report of the Working Group on High Security and Related Psychiatric Provision*. Department of Health, London.

Ritchie, J., Dick, D. & Lingham, R. (1994) Report of the Inquiry into the Care and Treatment of Christopher Clunis. HMSO, London.

Rogers, A., Pilgrim, D. & Lacey, R. (1993) *Experiencing Psychiatry: Users' Views of Services*. Macmillan in association with MIND Publications, London.

Romme, M. & Escher, S. (1993) *Accepting Voices*. MIND Publications, London.

Savage, L. & McKeown, M. (1997) Towards a new model for practice in a HDU. *Psychiatric Care* **4**, 182–6.

Sellwood, W., Haddock, G., Tarrier, N. & Yusupoff, L. (1994) Advances in the psychological management of positive symptoms of schizophrenia. *International Review of Psychiatry* **6**, 201–15.

Slade, P. (1972) The effects of systematic desensitisation on auditory hallucinations. *Behaviour Research and Therapy* **10**, 85–91.

Slade, P. & Bentall, R. (1988) *Sensory Deception: A Scientific Analysis of Hallucinations*. Croom Helm, London.

Smith, J. & Birchwood, M. (1991) *Understanding Schizophrenia* [series of booklets]. Bromsgrove and Redditch Health Authority.

Steadman, J., Monahan, J., Applebaum, P., Grisso, T., Mulvey, E., Roth, L., Robbins, P. & Klassen, D. (1994) Designing a new generation of risk assessment in research. In *Violence and Mental Disorder* (Monahan, J. & Steadman, J., eds). University of Chicago Press, Chicago.

Tarrier, N., Barrowclough, C., Vaughn, C., Bamrah, J., Porceddu, K., Watts, S. & Freeman, H. (1989) The community management of schizophrenia: two year follow-up of a behavioural intervention with families. *British Journal of Psychiatry* **154**, 625–8.

Tarrier, N., Beckett, R., Harwood, S., Baker, A., Yusupoff, L. & Ugarteburu, I. (1993) A trial of two cognitive-behavioural methods of treating drug-resistant residual psychotic symptoms in schizophrenic patients I: Outcome. *British Journal of Psychiatry* **162**, 524–32.

Vaughn, C. E. & Leff, J. (1976) The influence of family and social factors on the course of psychiatric illness: A comparison of schizophrenic and depressed neurotic patients. *British Journal of Psychiatry* **129**, 125–37.

Zubin, J. & Spring, B. (1977) Vulnerability: a new view of schizophrenia. *Journal of Abnormal Psychology* **86**, 260–266.

Chapter 13
Addressing Issues of Sexuality

Nicola Evans and Jenifer Clarke

INTRODUCTION

Sexuality is a fundamental aspect of human existence and the promotion of sexual health is considered to be an essential nursing function (Fogel, 1990).

In recent years, there has been great progress in our understanding of human sexuality, both normal and disordered. A key publication has been the Royal College of Nursing document *Sexual Health – Key Issues within Mental Health Services* (RCN, 1996) which acknowledged that users of mental health have sexual needs. There are as yet no specific guidelines for forensic mental health settings. The result of this may be that forensic nurses attempt to adapt existing guidelines for their patient group in order to shape and develop their practice.

Forensic mental health nurses are confronted with unique, complex challenges when working with patients' sexuality, sexual expressions and emerging relationships. Whilst forensic nurses need to champion the patients' sexual rights (Topping-Morris, 1996) they must equally '...act in such a manner to promote and safeguard the interest of individual patients and serve the interests of society' (UKCC, 1992).

Interwoven within sexual activity are the complicated issues of how therapeutic relationships function, and how the boundary of these relationships is determined, demanding that the forensic nurse has a level of self-awareness that they understand their own feelings about the patient's offending behaviour (Scales *et al.*, 1993). Often with this group of patients, sexuality, sexual expression, sexual offending or having experienced abusive relationships can be connected with both their mental health problem and the formulation of the risk they present to both self and others. As the main focus of forensic nursing is working with this connection of risk and health, it is essential that sexual health be addressed within a holistic approach.

This chapter will explore the dilemmas confronting forensic nurses, and suggest possible routes for addressing issues of sexuality. The authors have attempted to limit any gender bias although we acknowledge that our female gender may have adversely affected the perspective presented here and acknowledge the importance of securing 'both gender' agreement on these contentious issues.

CURRENT LITERATURE

What is sexuality?

The recent interest within nursing literature concerning sexual health and the expression of sexual needs has promoted healthy discussion and debate around the delicate matter of sexuality and performance of sexual acts linked by Rowan (1989) to a person's interpersonal domain.

The concept of sexuality may be interpreted differently depending on a person's theoretical, cultural or professional background. Hogan (1980) refined the idea that sexuality was more than concerned with relationships but that it is 'a basic need and an aspect of humanness that cannot be divorced from life events. It influences our thoughts, actions and interactions and is involved in aspects of physical and mental health'.

Sexuality and nursing

Nursing models acknowledge the need for the primary nurse to assess the patient's ability to express his or her sexuality in a manner that is neither exploitative nor abusive, within the context of their cultural or societal norm (Roy, 1980; Peplau, 1988). However, the predominance of studies within the nursing literature focuses upon scenarios which do not consider the need for nursing care plans to address sexual needs.

Despite nurses' own beliefs that they are addressing sexuality, Sharkey (1997) argues that patients themselves are not even being asked these important questions, or that nurses are insensitive to sexual feelings and will ignore relevant clinical needs as a consequence of incomplete sexual history-taking (Smith, 1992). Lewis & Bor's study (1994) identified that nurses rarely find the opportunity within the ward schedule for discussing sexual issues. One hypothesis offered by Waterhouse & Metcalfe (1991) is that nurses do not consider discussion of sexual concerns because they feel anxious or embarrassed. Nurses assume that patients are heterosexual (Brogan, 1997), and focus their questioning on this assumption, possibly due to the ignorance or prejudice that nurses feel when faced with gay or lesbian patients (Platzer & James, 1997; Wells, 1997).

It has been recognised however that the sexual needs of mental health service users have been long overlooked (Royal College of Nursing, 1996), and that gender-specific and gender-sensitive systems need to be developed within this clinical field (Department of Health, 1994). It might even be perceived that omission of this act is comparable to the re-abuse of a patient who was abused previously (Doob, 1992). It is widely recognised that a high percentage of people with mental health problems have suffered childhood sexual abuse (Beitchman *et al.*, 1992). Sayce (1993) cited studies suggesting one in two females seeking psychiatric help and one in five males seeking psychiatric help have previously been abused. Hence the dilemma posed for nurses when introducing sexual health as a topic within the initial nursing assessment is that there needs to be balance between empowering patients to talk about their sexual development and allowing patients' privacy (Carr, 1996). Aiyegbusi (1992) stresses the importance of exploring possible links with previous abusive experiences and the patient's symptoms of mental illness.

In forensic mental health nursing, patients are often treated with high-dose anti-psychotic medication, resulting in loss of libido, galactorrhoea, amenorrhoea and sexual dysfunction (Woolfe & Jackson, 1996). Nurses need to work in a sensitive manner to establish normal patterns of sexual expression for the patient and to determine what effect both treatment and detention have on the patient and his expression of sexuality rather than interpret any sexual behaviour by the patient as either asexual or hypersexed (Purdie, 1996).

THEORETICAL PERSPECTIVE

Sexuality is an integral part of every human being and encompasses the way one looks, behaves and relates to others as well as intimate sexual activity. The context for understanding sexuality is therefore complex and involves a number of biological, psychological and sociological elements.

The genes and chromosomes that direct the creation and evolution of anatomic structure are the beginnings of the biological development of sexuality (Levine, 1992). These physiological factors are responsible for the physical state of gender and may partly influence the psychological dimensions of both gender and sexuality.

Psychoanalytic view

Sigmund Freud theorised extensively about the nature of sexuality and sexual development. Freud (1905) demonstrated that sensual behaviours and levels of libidinal gratification were connected to the phases of psychosexual development, and believed that a person's choice of sexual expression was influenced from an interplay of heredity and biological and sociological factors.

One of Freud's most significant contributions was the recognition that children have sexual feelings and sexual sensations. He termed the sex drive 'libido' and believed that the child's libido focused upon a series of bodily parts in a developmental manner. The psychosexual stages that Freud described are:

(1) The oral stage, from birth to 18 months. The infant derives pleasure from stimulating the mouth, lips, tongue and other organs related to the oral zone.

(2) The anal stage, from 1 to 3 years. The child's attention is focused on the acquisition of sphincter control. The child is striving for independence although he is also threatened by the anxieties of separation and intensification of his powerful dependency wishes.

(3) The phallic stage, from 3 to 5 years. The phallic stage is characterised by the child's focusing on the genital area, and by sexual interest and sexual arousal.

   The foundation for a sense of a specific gender identity develops as the child integrates instinctual drives whilst in the phallic stage. The oedipal situation and its conflicts are essential to integrate psychosexual functioning and to consolidate sexual identity.

(4) The latency stage, from 5 years to adolescence. The child enters a prolonged stage where sexual impulses are repressed. Latency is often considered to be a stage of inactivity during which sexual interest is thought to be quiescent. A further integration of oedipal identification and consolidation of gender identity continues during latency.

Freud has been criticised in recent years because of the lack of scientific evidence underpinning his work. The psychoanalytic understanding of psychosexual development continues to be revised and expanded upon. The analytic understanding of the process by which sexual identity is established and its interplay with other complex factors contribute to the critical internal integration and organisation of the child's emerging personality (Erikson, 1963; Kernberg, 1974).

Behavioural view

Behaviourists view sexual behaviour as a measurable response, with both physiological and psychological components, to a learned stimulus or reinforcement event. Intrapsychic dynamics are often considered irrelevant as behaviourists are concerned with the maintenance rather than the origins of sexual disorders. Kernberg (1974) considered how social learning and cognitive learning apply to sexual development. He described how behaviours are either rewarded or punished with impacts on one's self-concept. Stereotypical behaviour is thought to influence a person's sexual identity; doing 'boy's things' will positively shape the concept 'I am a boy'.

SEXUAL EXPRESSION

A person expresses their sexuality as determined by their sexual preference. Sexual arousal and interest are most likely to be provoked by a specific type of person and/or type of activity with that person (Bancroft, 1992).

Heterosexuality

Heterosexuality implies a person is sexually attracted to a person of the opposite sex. The 'chemistry' of sexual attraction is difficult to explain. Whilst physical attractiveness plays an important part in personality development and enhancing self-esteem, it does not necessarily imply sexual attractiveness. There is a suggestion that women are more reliant on their physical attraction than their male counterparts. Whilst women are more interested in what a man does, a man is more interested in how a woman looks (Dion, 1981). Physical attractiveness may be a crucial factor in identifying a prospective sexual partner in the short term. In the longer term, the way a couple deal with on-going challenges may determine whether sexual desire is maintained or fades away (Levine, 1992).

Homosexuality

Sandford & Platzer (1998) portrayed a disturbing account of attempts to treat homosexuality as a psychiatric disorder. Psychiatry developed a spectrum of treatment responses as a way of coping with people who transgress society's norms. Homosexual patients were subjected to an array of interventions, ranging from a type of electric shock treatment to aversion therapy. Misunderstandings about homosexuality stem from stereotyping and a failure to recognise that 'homosexuals are no less heterogeneous than heterosexuals' (Bancroft, 1992).

Bisexuality

Bisexuality is defined as sexual attraction to persons of both sexes and engagement in both heterosexual and homosexual activity (Thomas, 1980). Bisexuality is thought to be more common amongst females than males (Levine, 1992). The same misunderstanding as described for homosexuality can be applied to bisexuality. The heterosexual component is overlooked in favour of penalising the homosexual component. Psychoanalytical theory of bisexualism implies that a bisexual tendency lurks within all people covertly if not overtly.

Trans-sexualism

A trans-sexual is a genetically anatomised male or female who expresses with strong conviction that he or she has the mind of the opposite sex. He or she may live as a member of the opposite sex either part time or full time and may seek to change his or her original gender through medical or surgical gender reassignment. Trans-sexuality differs from homosexuality in that the trans-sexual does not want a relationship with a person of the same sex, but wishes his or her own gender to be changed.

Transvestism

Transvestism is defined as dressing in the clothes of the opposite sex, or cross-dressing, within specific situations or environments. Bancroft (1992) describes three variations of the cross-dressing experience.

(1) The fetishistic transvestite who is more commonly of male gender. The fetish is the wearing of female clothes, which is found to be sexually arousing and usually leads to masturbation.

(2) The double-role transvestite who spends part of his time as a hetero-sexual male and the other part attempting to pass as a female. Unlike trans-sexuality, the double-role transvestite does not request medical or surgical intervention for gender reassignment.

Table 13.1 Examples of paraphilias

Paedophilia	Sexual interest in children
Exhibitionism	Exposure of one's genitals to an unsuspecting stranger
Fetishism	Sexual arousal from handling, possessing or wearing certain articles
Sexual sadism	Inflicting psychological or physical suffering and humiliation to become sexually aroused
Sexual masochism	Suffering by being humiliated, beaten or bound for sexual arousal
Frotteurism	Touching and rubbing against a non-consenting person
Necrophilia	Sexual arousal from contact with corpses
Voyeurism	Spying on unsuspecting people who are either naked, in the act of undressing or engaged in sexual activity
Uralagina	Sexual arousal from spraying urine
Bestiality	Sexual activity with animals

(3)   The homosexual transvestite is attracted to members of the same sex and is not attempting to impersonate members of the opposite sex.

Paraphilias

Nurses within secure environments frequently care for patients who have a history of disordered and offensive sexual behaviour. This group of deviant sexual behaviours such as paedophilia, bestiality and sado-masochistic behaviours frequently present as contributory factors in the offending profile of mentally disordered offenders (see Table 13.1).

MANAGEMENT OF SEXUAL ACTIVITY

The following (fictional) case examples will be used to demonstrate the process of decision making about how to manage sexual expression and activity in forensic settings. This will demonstrate the complexities of such decision making, the importance of thorough assessments and the nurse's role in attempting to balance empowerment and protection of the individual patient.

Niskala (1986) suggests that this will ensure that the containment offered promotes a therapeutic relationship in which the patient feels safe, trusted and trustful, and valued, and one from which they can grow.

Case study 1

John and Rita are both in-patients on the pre-discharge ward of a medium secure unit. Rita has a history of being in relationships with men who have been physically abusive towards her. In the context of her most recent relationship, she became increasingly frightened, fearful that her partner would one day kill her and her children. She started to believe that her partner was poisoning her and her children's food, was having her followed and was going to kill her while she was asleep. For these reasons, she began hiding a kitchen knife in her bedside drawer. One night, Rita killed her partner by stabbing him repeatedly in the chest.

John was recently transferred from a special hospital on trial leave to the medium secure unit. He has a relapsing-remitting psychotic illness which is currently well maintained. John's offence was armed robbery.

Rita and John have been mentally well for some months. John, particularly, has a high level of insight into his illness, including knowledge of relapse indicators and strategies to prevent relapse.

It has been noticed that John and Rita have been spending increasing amounts of time together. John approached his primary nurse to say that he and Rita had started a relationship and wanted to have some time in either of their bedrooms so that they could develop their relationship to an intimate level with dignity.

The medium secure unit that John and Rita are in has mixed sex wards. Each patient has an individual room, with their own key for their room. Within the guidelines offered by the unit it is advocated that patients should not go into each other's bedrooms without agreement beforehand by the respective clinical teams.

The relevant issues raised by this case are:

- confidentiality
- recognising and protecting John and Rita's vulnerabilities
- their individual ability to give consent
- their individual rights to have relationships
- the importance of risk assessment within the clinical decision-making
- the nurse's role in health promotion
- their individual rights to sexually express themselves

John and Rita each had separate care teams. The initial challenge was to allow a discussion including relevant personnel from each of the care teams, with the patient's individual opinions and wishes represented within that.

As John was new to the service, little was understood about how he would cope with the increased challenges of living on a mixed sex ward, in a less secure environment, with increased family and other social contact, but with a relatively controlled psychosis. Some of the difficulties with working with this group of patients include the fact that the illness component of their presentation is understood and usually stable, but factors such as the context in which they are living, the familial relationships, and significantly absent relationships have not been fully tested out until these patients have moved on to less secure environments (Burrows, 1993). Although some work may have been done with patients' sexuality whilst they have been in special provision, the introduction of that patient to a more stimulating, challenging, less secure environment allows for clarification, contradiction or refinement of previously held hypotheses on this patient's sexual behavioural patterns.

Rita had previously been involved in abusive relationships. Part of her multi-disciplinary treatment package included exploration of her previous patterns of relationship forming, self-esteem building and assertiveness. This combination was specifically aimed at empowering Rita to form relationships in which there was a more equal power balance. It was suggested that the interest with this particular relationship may have been Rita's attempts at testing out her newly acquired perspective and interpersonal skills, especially assertion.

In order to fully explore all the issues, two main processes were suggested. The first was for a joint team meeting to discuss specifically this relationship and how information may be shared and a decision reached. The second suggestion was that Rita and John could talk together about their relationship with a skilled facilitator that would allow the respective clinical teams to understand more about the relationship and patterns of communication themselves. Such additional information would provide rich detail to empower nurses and other disciplines to make decisions resulting in the least restrictive practices (Bates, 1995). This would allow John and Rita their rights for sexual expression in a safe manner (Royal College of Psychiatrists, 1996) whilst ensuring the safe management of known risks.

The additional information gained from four couple sessions allowed the respective clinical teams to understand how John and Rita interacted as a partnership. Following a second joint clinical team meeting, it was agreed for John and Rita to have a time-limited period in their bedrooms for privacy. They initially used this time for private discussions, but as their relationship developed, John and Rita were able to become more intimate and retain their dignity. John and Rita were invited individually to talk with their respective primary nurses about safer sex and contraception, and to determine whether either Rita or John had any learning needs about sexual health. John and Rita later decided that they would like to talk to a practitioner from the sexual health clinic. A practitioner from the sexual health clinic arranged to see them both and discuss their needs in private.

Ongoing evaluation of the couple's relationship was made possible through the use of the couple sessions, which John and Rita began to value as a productive and supportive intervention.

Case study 2

Lucy was a young woman who had three pre-school-age children, cared for by foster parents. She had been admitted to the medium secure unit following a psychotic episode, during which she had assaulted a police officer. When the overt psychosis had subsided, Lucy continued to declare her intense wish to have a fourth child. Lucy herself had had difficulty bonding with her three children for various reasons. Enquiries with Lucy's extended family discovered that Lucy had loved her children very much, but at times of mental distress neglected them. Lucy felt that she had failed as a mother to her three existing children. She hoped that this fourth child would allow her to 'be a proper mother', to stay well and to look after her new baby.

At this time Lucy was not in a steady relationship. Neither were there any plans for her discharge. She was still undergoing a process of in-patient treatment which was expected to last a further few months. Lucy's plans were to have a sexual relationship with a man who was willing on the ward, with the intention of becoming pregnant.

At this time, Lucy was on a high dose of neuroleptic medication, which resulted in her having amenorrhoea and galactorrhoea. These symptoms convinced Lucy that she was indeed pregnant, although she did deny having had any sexual encounter at that time. Lucy agreed to a pregnancy test which proved to be negative.

The relevant issues raised in this case are:

- how to protect Lucy from a pregnancy that would, from previous history, result in her child being taken into care, considering the lack of adequate facilities for mothers and their children within secure provision (Devi, 1992)
- how to protect Lucy from sexual exploitation by men on the mixed sex ward
- how to protect sexually vulnerable men from Lucy's exploitation
- how to determine at what point Lucy was able to give informed consent to engage in sexual activity

At clinical team level, it was discussed and agreed that, from Lucy's history of sexual abuse, having had her three children cared for by social services and her current sexual vulnerability, she needed to be protected from exploitation. There was a realisation that preventing Lucy from having a sexual relationship could only be a temporary intervention. This itself was achieved by ensuring Lucy was placed on an observational level that ensured her protection but allowed her as much freedom as possible without compromising her.

Due to Lucy's sexual disinhibition, the observing nurse was female. There were times when Lucy would dress in very revealing clothes, which the female nurse was then able to talk with her about, with a reduced risk of these comments being misinterpreted.

The primary nurse worked with Lucy on her self-concept and self-esteem. A working hypothesis was that Lucy could not identify any strengths that were unrelated to her childbearing ability. Therefore, Lucy was encouraged to take part in activities such as art and pottery that allowed her to achieve something herself unrelated to childbearing. Alongside the work of the primary nurse, the clinical nurse specialist worked with Lucy through a programme which built on and developed Lucy's sexual awareness, including contraception, prevention of sexually transmitted diseases and how to access 'well woman' services in the community setting.

Following comprehensive negotiations with social services, Lucy was able to visit her children at infrequent periods initially.

The whole package as well as development of her social skills seemed to shift Lucy's thinking about the possibility of having another child. Lucy consequently became less interested in pursuing sexual liaison with other patients, and at a later point decided to start using contraception.

Observation levels were adjusted accordingly in a graduated process which reflected Lucy's ability to think through her options instead of acting impulsively.

MASTURBATION

'Masturbation is a common if not universal behaviour' (Bancroft, 1992). Bancroft further described how masturbation is usually regarded as undesirable and is an aspect of sexuality that causes embarrassment.

Mentally disordered offenders are often detained in secure environments which determine with whom they will live, how much privacy they will be afforded and with whom they may develop intimate relationships (Topping-Morris, 1992). Within such restrictive conditions, masturbation may be the only available option for relieving sexual frustration. This in itself may be compromised by the nature of nursing observations prescribed.

Case study

Stephen is a 24-year-old heterosexual male who is considered to be a high suicide risk. As a consequence of Stephen's risk to himself, he was being nursed on 1:1 special observations. Stephen masturbated once or twice daily whilst either in the bedroom or bathroom. On occasions, the observing nurse was female; the feelings described by these female nurses were that they felt uncomfortable and embarrassed about being in his presence at these times

Exploring and understanding a patient's masturbatory habits is as essential as knowing about a patient's sleep or dietary needs. Sexuality is integral within our concept of holism. Specifically with mentally disordered offenders, formulating an understanding of the patient's sexuality is an important part of the forensic nurse's role within the risk assessment.

In the case example, Stephen was encouraged to ask for a male observing nurse, although he was reluctant to do so. The male nurses reported that Stephen would turn his back on the escorting nurse when he was masturbating. Alternatively, when female nurses were observing, Stephen would masturbate facing the nurses, and staring them directly in the face.

In discussion about this behaviour, it emerged that Stephen described himself as having a 'high sex drive'. He said he usually masturbated twice daily if he was not able to fulfil his sexual needs with his partner. Stephen sometimes forced his girlfriend to have sex with him, feeling that it was his right to have sex whenever he felt the need. He spoke about masturbating to fantasies of 'power and control' which he also attempted to act out with his girlfriend. His girlfriend confirmed this to be the case, stating that although she was unhappy about this she did not know what to do about it. Although sexual offending had not been recorded in his history, from this discovery it became important to include sexual threat within his risk assessment and management strategy.

Whilst it is a fundamental right of every patient to have their sexual needs met, the connections between the patient's sexual needs and offending behaviour need to be understood.

THERAPEUTIC RELATIONSHIPS

Boundaries between nurses and patients

Forensic nurses care for vulnerable people who may be thought disordered, may have relationship difficulties or may be emotionally fragile. Whilst there is a need to develop a trusting, therapeutic relationship with the patient, there is also a need to ensure that patients and individual staff members are protected.

In the same way as paedophiles seek out employment opportunities to work with children, a very small number of abusive individuals will choose to work as nurses with this vulnerable group of patients. Detained patients can be especially vulnerable as there is a clear power imbalance between the nurse and the patient. In this case the patient may be dependent upon the nurse writing a supportive report for a Mental Health Review Tribunal advocating discharge, or is dependent upon the nurse for basic needs to be met. In these circumstances where the patient feels this power imbalance, this may result in the patient being compliant and unassertive and possibly repeating patterns of earlier life events when they had been abused by people in a dominant or caring role.

The following example hypothetically illustrates the difficulty in identifying a determined and secretive female employee who could possibly groom a well regulated organisation to sexually exploit a patient.

Scenario 1

Helen, a 25-year-old single woman with a diagnosis of schizophrenia, was admitted to a regional secure unit. Having been both sexually and physically abused during her previous hospital admissions, it was recognised that Helen was vulnerable to potential exploitation by other patients. It had been assumed that nurses employed on the unit held beneficence as their primary motivating factor for wanting to work in the caring profession.

Helen was allocated a female primary nurse with whom she was reluctant to engage therapeutically. As Helen's presenting problem and risk area was that she was actively suicidal, there was great relief amongst the nursing team that she finally was beginning to disclose to one particular staff nurse, Susan. Susan and Helen appeared to have developed a trusting relationship, but it was noticed that, when Susan was on leave, Helen would become hostile and would make comments that she could not talk to other staff.

It later became apparent that Susan had suggested to Helen which staff to talk to and which to avoid; as Finklehor (1984) suggested, Susan groomed both Helen and the nursing team to avoid one another.

Susan resigned from her post as a staff nurse abruptly. Following this, despite having made steady progress, Helen's mood lowered dramatically with an increased incidence of deliberate self-harm attempts. One afternoon, following an emotional family visit, Helen disclosed to her female primary nurse that she and Susan had been having a sexual relationship, but that Susan had warned Helen not to ever talk to anyone about it. As it was not known where Susan had gone, the inquiry following Helen's disclosure was limited and the complaint was passed on to both the police and the UKCC.

Scenario 2

While the last scenario demonstrated a clear betrayal of trust, there are people who become perpetrators without having premeditated the act, but who as a result of their own vulnerabilities and unpreparedness to deal with others' emotions, drift into a position where they form abusive relationships (Gallop, 1998).

Claire was transferred from a remand centre to hospital following her committal to crown court on a charge of homicide. She was a 20-year-old divorced woman with a bipolar affective illness and was reported as being promiscuous and sexually orientated to both men and women.

Andrew, Claire's primary nurse, developed what appeared to be a good therapeutic relationship with Claire, spending long periods of time with her on a one-to-one basis. Claire frequently became distressed and at such times asked Andrew to hold her hand because it was comforting. This hand holding later progressed to cuddling at Claire's request. On several occasions, Andrew massaged Claire's neck and shoulders because this seemed to reduce Claire's physical symptoms of stress. Andrew did not document or disclose these interventions to other staff.

The clinical team considered some weeks later that Claire's illness had responded well enough to treatment that she could stand trial. Following this, she was given a non-custodial sentence and returned home. Claire asked Andrew to visit her at home but Andrew refused. Claire then made a complaint that Andrew had used inappropriate touch with her. Andrew was suspended pending an inquiry.

Attachments that patients form with nurses may be described as transference phenomena. Claire's history of sexual abuse made her vulnerable and fearful of being in a caring environment. The eroticisation or sexual-isation of her relationship with the nurse may have been a re-enactment of an earlier relationship (Welldon, 1997). Similarly, Andrew's counter-transference responses may have resulted in him violating his own pro-fessional boundaries to meet his own needs through this relationship. Transference and counter-transference phenomena need to be explored in both clinical supervision and in multi-professional risk assessment to safeguard against ambiguous, confusing relationships. The nurse, as the professional, has the responsibility to maintain boundaries. Gallop (1993) states that boundary violations often start with excessive self-disclosure that develops into a special relationship that may include secrecy and fantasies of saving the patient in order for the professional to feel successful or needed.

Appropriateness of touch

Some nursing activities require physical contact, such as administration of depot medication. Every individual has different needs and wishes in terms of how they like to touch others and how they themselves like to be touched. It should not be assumed that what comforts one patient will automatically comfort another. Patients who have previously been sexually or physically abused may in particular not wish to be touched as this may act as a trigger for distressing memories of the past abuse. Therefore a prerequisite for good practice is to include in the preliminary assessment with patients an understanding of the implications of using touch therapeutically with that patient.

RECOMMENDATIONS FOR FUTURE RESEARCH AND PRACTICE

To assist our development of awareness of sexual issues and nursing prac-tice, further research into patients' lived experiences of forensic mental health care and how that affects their expression of sexuality is essential. During our researching of this topic area, it was apparent that there is little available literature that discusses abuse and harassment in same-sex set-tings. In order to generate such literature, it is imperative that such research be undertaken. Local guidelines and protocols should be developed that advise appropriate courses of action to promote sexual health. These proto-cols should recommend procedures for inter-agency working, for example with sexual health clinics, and for the development of facilities that enable conjugal visits, for example family visiting rooms.

CONCLUSIONS

Each forensic patient has individual healthcare needs and the same can be said regarding the patient's sexuality. As much as the literature attempts to address this complex clinical puzzle, there can be no doubt that it is through reflecting on our work with patients that nurses continue to understand sexual issues and develop their knowledge and skills base.

Part of rehabilitation programmes for people who have sexually offended is to test out their responses to mixing with their victim group. Within forensic settings, there is potentially a mix of people who have been victims of sexual abuse and others who have been perpetrators of sexual offences, although these two states frequently exist within one person. It is being suggested that we acknowledge both patients' vulnerabilities and also the risks they present in terms of sexual expression.

Whilst Department of Health plans for wards to revert to single-sex accommodation are a recognition of the need to protect some of these vulnerable patients, this alone cannot be assumed to be the strategy that will eliminate the risk of abusive relationships developing. Female patients are as much at risk from other females, either staff or patients, and likewise male patients. Therefore segregation of genders will not necessarily reduce frequency or severity of abusive relationships.

More importantly, the patient's vulnerability or potential for sexual offending should be proactively assessed, monitored and addressed within their whole treatment plan. Whilst the forensic nurse is in the prime position to observe and intervene at a ward-based level, the responsibility for including this within both the risk assessment and risk management plan falls on the entire clinical team.

The ultimate goal is to enable the patient to safely achieve optimum sexual health with the resource and support needed. The forensic patient's sexual health must be an integral part of care planning with the primary nurse taking the leading role in promoting healthy sexual functioning.

Ultimately, the factor that will allow us to provide the care that is deserved by patients in forensic settings is to encourage patients to voice their needs either individually or collectively, and for the users of the service to fundamentally shape that service.

REFERENCES

Aiyegbusi, A. (1992) Self harm in secure environments. In *Aspects of Forensic Psychiatric Nursing* (Morrison, P. & Burnard, P., eds). Avebury, Aldershot.
Bancroft, J. (1992) *Human Sexuality and Its Problems*, 2nd edn. Churchilll Livingstone, Edinburgh.

Bates, A. (1995) Mental disorder and criminal behaviour: the assessment and management of those at risk of re-offending. *Psychiatric Care* **2**(3), 96–100.

Beitchman, J. H., Zucker, K. J., Hood, J. E., da Costa, G. A., Akman, D. & Cassavia, E. (1992) A review of the long term effects of child sexual abuse. *Child Abuse and Neglect* **16**(1), 101–18.

Brogan, M. (1997) Healthcare for lesbians: attitudes and experiences. *Nursing Standard* **11**(45), 39–42.

Burrows, S. (1993) An outline of the forensic nurse's role. *British Journal of Nursing* **2**, 18.

Carr, G. (1996) Themes relating to sexuality that emerged from a discourse analysis of the *Nursing Times* between 1980–1990. *Journal of Advanced Nursing* **24**(1), 196–212.

Department of Health (1994) *Working in Partnership: Report of the Review of Mental Health Nursing*. HMSO, London.

Devi, S. (1992) Caring for mothers and babies in secure settings. In *Aspects of Forensic Psychiatric Nursing* (Morrison, P. & Burnard, P., eds). Avebury, Aldershot.

Dion, K. (1981) Physical attractiveness, sex roles and heterosexual attraction. In *The Basis of Human Sexual Attraction* (Cook, M., ed.), pp. 3–22. Academic Press, London.

Doob, D. (1992) Female sexual abuse survivors as patients: avoiding re-traumatisation. *Archives of Psychiatric Nursing* **6**(4), 245–51.

Erikson, E. H. (1963) *Childhood and Society*. Norton, New York.

Finkelhor, D. (1984) *Child Sexual Abuse: New Theory and Research*. Free Press, New York.

Fogel, C. I. (1990) *Sexual Health Promotion*. W. B. Saunders, Philadelphia.

Freud, S. (1905) *Three Essays on the Theory of Sexuality*, standard edn, Vol. 7, pp. 123–245. Hogarth Press, London.

Gallop, R. (1993) Sexual contact between nurses and patients. *Canadian Nurse* **89**(2), 28–31.

Gallop, R. (1998) Abuse of power in the nurse/client relationship: definition, research and organisational response *Nursing Standard* **12**(37), 43–7.

Hogan, R. M. (1980) *Human Sexuality: A Nursing Perspective*. Appleton Century Crofts, New York.

Kernberg, O. F. (1974) Barriers to falling and remaining in love. *Journal of the American Psychoanalytic Association* **22**, 486–511.

Levine, S. B. (1992) *Sexual Life. A Clinician's Guide*. Plenum Press, New York.

Lewis, S. & Bor, R. (1994) Nurses' knowledge of and attitudes towards sexuality and the relationship of these with nursing practice. *Journal of Advanced Nursing* **20**, 251–9.

Niskala, H. (1986) Competencies and skills required by nurses working in forensic areas. *Western Journal of Nursing Research* **8**(4), 400–13.

Peplau, H. (1988) *Interpersonal Relations in Nursing*, 2nd edn. Macmillan, London.

Platzer, H. & James, T. (1997) Methodological issues conducting sensitive research on lesbian and gay men's experience of nursing care. *Journal of Advanced Nursing* **25**(3), 626–33.

Purdie, H. (1996) Management of sexuality in a mental health setting. *Nursing Standard* **11**(12), 47–50.

Rowan, J. (1989) *The Hemed God. Feminism and Health as Wounding and Healing*. Routledge, London.

Roy, C. (1980) The Roy Adaptation Model. In *Conceptual Models for Nursing Practice* (Reihl, J. P. & Roy, C., eds). Appleton Century Crofts, Norwalk.

Royal College of Nursing (1996) *Sexual Health – Key Issues within Mental Health Services*. RCN, London.

Royal College of Psychiatrists (1996) *Sexual Abuse and Harrassment in Psychiatric Settings*. RCP, London.

Sandford, T. & Platzer, H. (1998) A shocking legacy in mental health practice. *Mental Health Practice* 1(5), 6–7.

Sayce, L. (1993) Given a voice. *Nursing Times* 89(36), 48–50.

Scales, C. J., Mitchell, J. L. and Smith, R. D. (1993) Survey report on forensic nursing. *Journal of Psychosocial Nursing* 31(11), 39–44.

Sharkey, V. B. (1997) Sexuality, sexual abuse. Omissions in admissions. *Journal of Advanced Nursing* 25(5), 1025–32.

Smith, G. B. (1992) Nursing care challenges: homosexual psychiatric patients. *Journal of Psychosocial Nursing* 30(12), 15–21.

Thomas, S. P. (1980) Bisexuality: a sexual orientation of great diversity. *Psychosocial Nursing Mental Health Service* 18(4), 19.

Topping-Morris, B. (1992) An historical and personal view of forensic nursing services. In *Aspects of Forensic Psychiatric Nursing* (Morrison, P. & Burnard, P., eds). Avebury, Aldershot.

Topping-Morris, B. (1996) Promoting the sexual health of users of mental health services: a time for action. *Psychiatric Care* 3(2), 70–73.

United Kingdom Central Council for Nursing, Midwifery and Health Visiting (1992) *Code of Professional Conduct*. UKCC, London.

Waterhouse, J. & Metcalfe, M. (1991) Attitudes towards nurses discussing sexual concern with patients. *Journal of Advanced Nursing* 16, 1048–54.

Welldon, E. (1997) The practical approach. In *A Practical Guide to Forensic Psychotherapy* (Welldon, E. & Van Velsen, C., eds). Jessica Kingsley, London.

Wells, A. (1997) Homophobia and nursing care. *Nursing Standard* 12(6), 41–2.

Woolfe, L. & Jackson, B. (1996) Coffee and condoms: the implementation of a sexual health programme in acute psychiatry in an inner city area. *Psychiatric Care* 23(2), 299–304.

Chapter 14
Ethics and Morality

Chris Chaloner

INTRODUCTION

Forensic mental health nursing is associated with a breadth of issues demanding ethical reflection, and the unique challenges of clinical practice create many potential 'moral dilemmas'. Nursing and the care and management of mentally disordered offender patients demand constant reflection on the morality of practice.

The care of the mentally disordered has long been related to various aspects of social and personal morality. Prior to its domination by medicine and psychiatry, the affinity of 'madness' with 'immorality' was one of the defining characteristics of varied approaches to the care and treatment of the mentally ill. Those regarded as 'mad' may also have been considered unwilling or incapable of according with the moral rules of society. Thus, the unfortunate stigma of mental illness was constructed. To suffer from a mental illness was socially unacceptable, and working with such people was regarded as '... degrading and odious employment, and seldom accepted but by idle and disorderly persons.' (Haslam, 1809).

Today, although approaches to mental illness remain far from ideal, it is possible to perceive a more positive social attitude both to those with a mental disorder and to individuals professionally involved in their care. However, the more negative associations may persist for mentally disordered offenders and forensic mental health professionals.

As a result of their offending behaviour a small proportion of mentally disordered offenders generate an inordinate amount of negative social comment, and forensic mental health services are regularly subjected to public scrutiny and criticism. Central to any moral inquiry regarding forensic mental health services lie questions regarding the care and management of patients and the nature of those who choose to work within such a unique area of health care.

This chapter explores some of the ethical issues relevant to forensic health practice. Following a brief introduction to ethics, its relationship to forensic mental health nursing is discussed. The resolution of 'ethical dilemmas' is considered and two primary ethical aspects of the forensic specialism are examined: the ethical context of practice and the ethical issues which may arise within clinical practice. Finally, the 'ethical nature' of forensic mental health nurses is explored and suggestions for future moral inquiry are made.

ETHICS

Ethics is a branch of philosophy which, in its simplest sense, helps to inform us about the rights and wrongs of a particular issue, situation, action or decision. But this elementary conception frequently leads to misperceptions about what ethics can and can't achieve.

> 'It might be thought that an understanding of ethics can resolve the moral dilemmas encountered in practice. However, an awareness of ethics can only guide effective practice and assist in finding informed responses to ethical questions' (Chaloner, 1998, p. 28).

Ethics is about more than simply identifying the right or wrong action, decision, etc. Such normative ethics (Beauchamp & Childress, 1994, p. 4) represent only one aspect of ethical thinking. Ethical deliberation may also require reflection on the values, beliefs and emotions relevant to a particular issue. Ethics encompasses many interrelated components and provides a framework for examining the morality of human behaviour in a much broader manner than 'right' and 'wrong'. 'A well-developed ethical theory provides a framework within which agents can reflect on the acceptability of actions and can evaluate moral judgements and moral character' (Beauchamp & Childress, 1994, p. 44).

For some, the requirements of ethical deliberation may be a deterrent to the exploration of the moral aspects of a situation. Ethics may be claimed to be of academic interest only and not connected to the realities of practice. However, as Singer observes: '... ethics is not an ideal system that is noble in theory but no good in practice. The reverse of this is closer to the truth ... for the whole point of ethical judgements is to guide practice' (Singer, 1993, p. 2).

The considered application of ethical theory and principles can assist in the process of ethical deliberation. Theories such as *consequentialism* (the moral worth of a particular action being judged by its outcome or 'consequences'), and *deontology* (undertaking one's inherent moral duty, regardless of its consequences – for example, a duty to always tell the truth) are frequently cited within ethical teaching as means by which the ethical aspects of a situation may be most effectively addressed. The use of ethical principles such as beneficence, non-maleficence, respect for autonomy, and justice (Beauchamp & Childress, 1994; Gillon & Lloyd, 1994) can also contribute to an understanding of ethics and to answering important questions such as 'What should I do?'.

RESOLVING 'ETHICAL DILEMMAS'

Obviously, a 'moral dilemma' will not be satisfactorily resolved by the straightforward application of a theory or principle. The application of ethics to practice demands an understanding of important ethical concepts (e.g. confidentiality); ethically important decision-making procedures (e.g. deciding when confidentiality should be maintained); the ability to apply such concepts and decision-making procedures to real-life cases; plus effective communication abilities (Gillon, 1996). In order that ethics may successfully contribute to practice, those involved in moral deliberation '... must be able to identify the morally relevant aspects of a situation and carefully consider the ethical concepts involved' (Chaloner, 1998, p. 28). In a study of ethical decision-making by health carers, it was found that a consistent and systematic pattern was not followed and that differences persisted between individuals' potential for moral thinking and their actual practice (Grundstein-Amado, 1993).

Identifying the 'rights' or 'wrongs' of a particular situation or issue can be the cause of dispute. Of course, simply defining 'right' or 'wrong' is an almost impossible task and requires some form of understanding between those involved before agreement can be reached. When attempting to respond effectively to a perceived ethical question it may be that each member of a clinical team has strongly held 'moral' views on a particular issue and that successful ethical deliberation is demanded in order that an 'ethical consensus' may be achieved which enables each team member to act in a manner which they can morally justify.

The process of deliberation may be assisted by reference to ethical theories and principles, by the application of professional codes and guidelines or by consideration of legal requirements although none of these provides a substitute for careful ethical reflection.

'Morality is not reducible to established laws, i.e. to examine what is legal, or what the law says on a particular matter, is not necessarily to discover what is morally right or wrong. On occasion, doing what is perceived to be right may require breaking the law. Therefore it is not possible simply to resolve moral dilemmas by resolving legal ones. The law itself may be subjected to moral scrutiny and the question of whether one is morally bound to obey an established law is always an open one' (Chaloner, 1997, p. 119).

The resolution of ethical dilemmas requires that a balance be achieved between the evaluative and objective components of decision-making. There must be an openness to consultation with others and a receptiveness to outside opinions in making ethical judgements. Central to this process should be the active development of therapeutic partnerships where there is equal power and participation in working towards mutual goals.

THE RELATIONSHIP BETWEEN ETHICS AND FORENSIC MENTAL HEALTH NURSING

Working within health care demands ethical sensitivity. An emphasis on patient-centred care strategies and an acknowledgement of individual autonomy requires that practitioners are able to see beyond the practical implications of their interventions.

For forensic mental health professionals who manage, treat and most importantly deliver *care* to individuals, many of whom have in effect contravened the moral rules of society, the requirements of ethical awareness may be claimed to be even more stringent than those of their non-forensic colleagues.

Forensic mental health care's associations with offending, criminality and deviance, in addition to the many and varied moral implications of mental disorder and its treatment, are the source of numerous ethical questions some of which are reflected in the sensationalist responses of the media to incidents related to forensic services (*The Mirror* 11 March 1997; *The Mail on Sunday* 8 June 1997).

Forensic mental health services are the subject of persistent public and professional curiosity. The perceived attitudes of nurses play a prominent role in inquiries into care management, and a comparatively small number of patients engender a large amount of negative social comment. The 'hidden world' of locked clinical facilities appears to be a particular focus for public and professional fascination and scrutiny (Kerr *et al.*, 1997; Gerrard, 1998).

Interestingly, despite their high profile, forensic mental health services do not appear to have devoted a great deal of time considering the moral basis for care. This is perhaps due to an acknowledgement of the morality of delivering 'care' to offender patients. The evident compassion displayed by the delivery of care and treatment (as opposed to imprisonment and punishment) may, for some, have offered sufficient moral justification for practice. Unfortunately, this may have led to the development of an 'inherent morality' – particularly within secure environments – providing some practitioners with an ethical defence for their role and possibly frustrating further moral scrutiny. A further obstacle to ethical inquiry may be that society as a whole has been unwilling to investigate the ethics of a 'difficult' and, to some degree, impenetrable health-care specialism.

Balancing the conflicting demands of the nurse's role is a constant source of debate. Nurses' clinical role demands an emphasis on therapeutic activity whilst a commitment to the wider needs of society requires that issues of safety and security are offered equal prominence (Burrow, 1993a).

An ethical conflict which arises as a result of this incongruity in role purpose relates to the ethical principle of 'respect for autonomy'. It is a principle which morally obliges us to respect another's autonomy, i.e. 'The capacity to think, decide and act on the basis of such thought and decision freely and independently' (Gillon, 1985, p. 60). In attempting to promote their patients' best interests within a treatment programme and, by so doing, acknowledging respect for autonomy, nurses may be frustrated by the limits to what they can and cannot agree to.

Obviously, an individual's autonomy may be diminished by the effects of a mental disorder or by measures imposed in response to their perceived risk of harm to others. However, it is possible that a fully autonomous patient may be unable to pursue a rehabilitative programme as a result of the many negative associations which forensic mental health services maintain. Therefore the ethical requirement to respect another's autonomy is frustrated, and considered reflection may be required on the moral nature and purpose of forensic mental health practice.

Traditionally, forensic mental health nursing was a professionally isolated undertaking. Within secure institutions nurses were able to exercise a great deal of control over their patients. Such control became an accepted aspect of 'care' and a means by which order could be successfully maintained. The freedom to exercise control within the comparative secrecy of secure environments may have led to the development of over-authoritative regimes in which other features of authority, such as punishment, became components of the nursing role. The essential need to maintain authority within such challenging environments may have deterred the questioning of these aspects of practice – at least from within these environments.

Nurses in secure institutions were frequently perceived as dominating and powerful figures (with regard to the physical control of their patients) and, as clinical areas developed a more open stance, such a negative image was exposed via a series of public inquiries: 'far from creating an atmosphere in which therapy can exist for the benefit of the patients, they seek to create a climate in which control and discipline – sometimes harsh and severe – are necessary instruments of a punitive approach' (Blom-Cooper *et al.*, 1992). A negative image of nursing in secure environments undoubtedly persists (Murphy, 1997; *The Times*, 7 June 1997) and this has implications for the way in which all who work within forensic services are regarded.

Close inspection of forensic services, particularly by the process of public inquiry, has encouraged the revision of 'traditional' practices, and attempts have been made to improve the image of the specialism. It is possible, however, that the need to demonstrate a positive approach to care, combined with an emphasis on respecting autonomy, can lead to misjudgements in care delivery leaving patients mismanaged and, ultimately, lacking care (Fallon *et al.*, 1999).

Although abuses of power cannot be ethically justified, many of the traditional aspects of forensic mental health practice – including the application of control and the considered use of power – were based on both practical and moral foundations. A contemporary shift away from paternalistic practice must be undertaken with consideration for the potentially damaging effects of healthcare professionals' withdrawal of control.

Fortunately, much of forensic mental health care is no longer practised within the comparative secrecy of the past. Political, media and public attention has compelled services to open their doors and to present an exposed and honest appraisal of their work, to develop both clinically and ethically in accordance with concomitant professional developments elsewhere and to cease to be practised 'in an ethical or clinical vacuum' (Rappeport, 1991).

CONTEMPORARY LITERATURE

Although there remains grounds for improvement, there has in recent years been an encouraging increase in the number and quality of papers attempting to examine the ethical nature of forensic mental health practice. Overviews of the ethical aspects of forensic psychiatry can be found within a number of dedicated book chapters (Gunn & Taylor, 1993; Faulk, 1994; Cope & Chiswick, 1995) and specific moral aspects of the forensic psychiatrist's role have been explored by, among others, Adshead & Mezey (1993) and Appelbaum (1990).

The majority of publications written by nurses which include an ethical perspective have focused on contentious practical aspects of the nurse's role such as physical control. The practice of seclusion remains a constant source of debate, much of which is concerned with the ethical propriety of placing a patient alone in a locked room as part of a supposedly therapeutic approach to care. Mason (1993) considered seclusion from a moral viewpoint, and in highlighting its accordance with ethical principles questioned its status as a 'benevolent or malevolent intervention'. Ethical issues relevant to other forms of physical restraint have also been addressed (Tarbuck, 1992; Hopton, 1995) and the practice of delivering care to dangerous individuals was examined by Chandley & Mason (1995). Chaloner (1998) addressed the various ethical issues relevant to nursing in secure environments.

There is some evidence available that nurses seek to examine the wider, contextual, ethical aspects of their specialism. Byrt (1993) provided one of the first ethical overviews of the forensic mental health nurse's role, and Burrow (1991, 1993a, 1994) outlined one of the debatable ethical aspects of practice when addressing the 'dilemma of therapeutic custody'. The role of the forensic mental health nurse within wider society was explored by Mason & Mercer (1996) who considered forensic nursing practice at the interface of medical and legal services and how nurses have moved into areas previously bereft of psychiatric intervention.

The influence on forensic mental health practice of international case law was considered by Mason (1998) in an overview of the US 'Tarasoff case' and its implications for practitioners' duty to third parties.

THE ETHICAL CONTEXT OF PRACTICE

The wide-ranging public and professional comment that forensic mental health services attract reflects the morally ambiguous status the specialism maintains for observers both within and beyond mental health practice. The positive moral basis for care receives little attention and, apart from defending their specialism at times of inspection, forensic mental health professionals tend not to participate in evaluations of the contextual morality of their role. An increasing amount of time is devoted to examining the practical aspects of care and their ethical implications (see below) but the ethical context in which forensic mental health services are delivered is less frequently addressed.

Forensic mental health services may be regarded as socially and professionally isolated (and isolating). Although there is now much more openness about care settings, the specialism retains many unique ethical features – the most pertinent of which, with regard to its 'contextual morality', is the requirement to treat and care for individuals who may be considered undeserving of social acceptability. Within the process of critical inspection, the aims and outcomes of practice may be contested and demands made for the closure of certain services (Snell, 1997).

As a result of the seriousness of their offences (despite the presence of mental disorder) it may be claimed that some mentally disordered offenders have forfeited a right to a compassion-based societal response. A supporting claim may be that the delivery of care and treatment to such individuals is both illogical and a waste of valuable resources and that society's only rational response to the extremes of offending behaviour should be punishment.

A degree of suspicion surrounds those who choose to work within the specialism. For those who question the therapeutic aims of forensic care the nurse's role may equate with that of a 'warder' or prison officer. This has obvious and unfortunate implications for the professional image of forensic mental health nursing and its aim to attract a well motivated and skilled workforce.

Negative attitudes towards forensic mental health services may reflect an instinctive association with immorality and deviance and the attention devoted to the negative aspects of practice may lead some practitioners to question the morality of their professional role. This of course is not necessarily an adverse reaction. It is essential that nurses investigate the morality of their work, and if public scepticism of various aspects of practice provides the impetus for moral appraisal this may be regarded as a positive response.

Within forensic mental health care arenas, to question the morality of providing care for mentally disordered offenders is perhaps regarded as an overly simplistic activity. But a considered reply to those who question the existence and moral foundations of forensic services requires an examination of a variety of issues relating to the moral context of care. Each has implications for the ethical context in which forensic mental health nursing is practised.

Patient contact

The practicalities of managing mentally disordered offenders remain a source of interest (and possible suspicion) for many. It may be assumed by uninformed observers that the extensive application of physical control is essential to managing such 'challenging' individuals. Such negative assumptions are assisted by the outcomes of some of the inquiries held into the working practices within high security settings (Blom-Cooper *et al.*, 1992; Fallou *et al.*, 1999). Claims that therapeutic activities remain at the head of the vast majority of practitioners' agendas may go unheard during public and professional debates which accompany such findings.

The need to combine therapeutic interventions with considerations of public and personal safety – 'the social control of a deviant group who are hospitalised for therapy; and the promotion of patients' interests while safeguarding the interests of the wider society' (Burrow, 1993a, p. 20) – raises specific difficulties for the nurse who seeks to provide an ethically justified balance to their role. It is undoubtedly one of the critical aspects of forensic mental health nursing and, it has been claimed, one which some nurses are unable to manage (Aiyegbusi, 1998).

Many mentally disordered offenders may become socially detached as a result of their mental disorder, the type of offences they may have committed or due to other antisocial behaviour displayed. Nurses must endeavour to deliver care to extremely challenging individuals who may consistently reject interventions and adopt aggressive and sometimes violent stances.

The ability to maintain a professionally non-judgemental approach is frequently claimed to be an essential requirement for this type of work. However, 'non-judgemental' suggests that the individual nurse should deny some of their essential skills of assessment, evaluation and personal inter-action – in other words 'judgement' – in order to effectively deliver care. This does not accord with the moral requirement that we should respect individual autonomy, and it is perhaps not therefore entirely applicable to ethical practice that a totally 'non-judgemental' approach is encouraged.

Power, control, coercion and paternalism

The application and potential abuse of the powerful position which foren-sic practitioners hold is an obvious cause of ethical concern and should be an issue for constant ethical inspection and analysis. The application of power and control may, to some extent, be required to maintain 'social order' within institutions but there are further areas for ethical concern with regard to the use of power in the wider aspects of forensic mental health care provision – for example, the contribution of forensic services to social control (Mason & Mercer, 1996). It may even be claimed that for-ensic services *are* used to deal with society's unwanted, and that in recent years some forms of offending behaviour have been 'medicalised' in order to deal with societal problems.

Could it be morally permissible to detain someone for what they might do rather than for what they have already done? 'The shortening of the periods of detention for treatment, deterrence or retribution have made a live issue of whether (or when) it is justifiable to detain violent and sexual offenders solely for the protection of others' (Walker, 1991; p. 755). Foren-sic mental health services are increasingly required to react to societal need for an effective response to dangerous individuals. The need for safe management of personality disordered individuals who have not necessarily committed an offence creates a dilemma to which forensic mental health professionals, and others, must respond.

Issues of power and control are as pertinent to those nurses working beyond the secure environment as to those within the locked ward:

'Nurses working in this specialist field should be concerned that their contribution to social policy may be as much associated with law enforcement as with health care, and that they are actively helping to prop up the inadequacies of community care' (Burrow, 1993b).

The concept of power and its use by mental health care teams was brought into the professional and public arena by the emergence of the Mental Health (Patients in the Community) Act 1995, and concern about the potential for abuse of such legislation has been expressed (Coffey, 1997).

The existence of a coercive element to the nursing role may not represent an ideal of practice but must surely be acknowledged:

'The imbalance in the carer/patient relationship suggests that the active participation in therapeutic programmes may be reliant on a degree of coercion, even if this is not intended. Patients may be motivated to co-operate with treatment and therapeutic programmes for pragmatic reasons – in relation to the prospect of earlier discharge or transfer from hospital for example' (Chaloner, 1998, p. 31).

The application of coercion does not accord with an 'ethical' approach to professional practice and, if intended, must presumably be morally justified by reference to consequentialist theories (see above) in which the perceived 'ends' may, in some circumstances, justify the 'means'.

Perhaps paternalism ('...intervention in another person's preferences, desires or actions with the intention of either avoiding harm to or benefiting the person' (Beauchamp & Childress, 1994, p. 274), which, in health care, is widely condemned as representing archaic practice) is also an essential contributor to forensic mental health nursing. It may possibly be ethically justified with regard to the need to create autonomy – prior to respecting it (Seedhouse, 1998). Creating autonomy and encouraging the autonomy of the individual may be one of the fundamental therapeutic activities in which all mental health professionals participate.

Treatment, care or punishment?

Whilst the justification for treating an individual's mental disorder may be unchallenged by the majority of people, as has been noted, the provision of 'care' to offender patients may be opposed by some who may regard it as an indication of a lenient approach to offending behaviour. It has been noted that the provision of 'care' is one of the moral foundations of forensic mental health practice: 'caring' for mentally disordered individuals who commit offences is perhaps a 'more moral' response than imprisonment or punishment. However, there may be some mentally disordered offenders – those who have committed the most grievous offences – for whom even this moral justification for care may be regarded as beyond acceptability. Such a denial of care for offenders may be even more vociferous with regard to personality disordered individuals who have traditionally offered intangible evidence of mental disorder:

'The peculiar individuals now known as psychopaths have so far presented an unsolved problem to the community afflicted with their presence, as well as to the doctors and lawyers who have to wrestle with their misdeeds, ... of old they were accounted as "moral imbeciles", for want of a more scientific word, indicating that their behaviour could not be judged by the normal moral code. But even nowadays it is uncertain who exactly these privileged beings are' (Partridge, 1953, p. 61).

The justification of a punitive response to mentally disordered offenders was encouraged by the publication of the Crime (Sentences) Act 1997 which introduced the provision of a combined hospital and prison direction (Eastman, 1997). This perhaps reflected an increasing trend in public opinion supportive of a more punitive legal disposal for some offenders. It undoubtedly raises interesting ethical questions. For example, how will nurses (and others) perceive the morality of their role which requires the delivery of care and treatment in order to prepare an individual for transfer to prison for completion of their 'hybrid' (hospital/prison) sentence (Eastman & Peay, 1998)?

Whilst it is arguable that societal retribution and, indeed, punishment are playing an increasingly prominent part in forensic mental health delivery, the restriction of a detained patient's liberty may be regarded as evidence in itself of a 'punitive' approach to care management. Of course, the identification of 'punitive' aspects of patient management may be dependent on individual perspectives.

Autonomy, rights, duties and responsibility

The restrictive aspects of forensic mental health practice – particularly with regard to legal detention – do not necessarily imply that all patients lack autonomy. Although many patients detained in hospital may be regarded as having restricted autonomy, an obligation to respect autonomy remains and is offered moral justification by both deontological and consequentialist ethical theories, i.e. it is both an 'ethical duty' and the respect for individual autonomy may be claimed to maximise overall welfare and bring about the 'best consequences'.

Do mentally disordered offenders have 'rights'? This may seem an unnecessary question – particularly with regard to their legal rights – but do such individuals also maintain moral rights, for example the right to be told the truth? In certain circumstances, may such rights be forfeited as a result of either the individual's innate character (Doyal, 1994) or their offending behaviour? The existence of moral rights may impose obligations on others to act in a certain way (Gillon, 1985, p. 57), i.e. such rights may create 'moral duties' in others and the identification of the focus of one's 'moral duties' is perhaps a key ethical aspect of forensic mental health nursing.

Perceptions of responsibility are central to the provision of forensic services and to the identification of those who may benefit from forensic mental health care. The assessment of culpable responsibility may be crucial to the determining of an individual's legal disposal, i.e. treatment or punishment. It may be proved that an individual 'did the act' but their perceived responsibility may be reduced as a result of an identifiable mental disorder. Moral responsibility, it may be claimed, is diminished by the presence of mental disorder and therefore treatment of the disorder is the logical and compassionate response. Once again, this may be supported by both deontological and consequentialist theories.

PRACTICE-BASED ETHICAL ISSUES

The most frequently considered ethical aspects of forensic mental health nursing are those that impact directly on daily practice and generate recognisable 'moral dilemmas'. The somewhat sparse literature pertaining to ethics and forensic mental health nursing tends to focus on such practical issues, many of which are a recurrent cause of professional and public concern. Nurses are required to identify and respond to ethical issues within their day-to-day role. Clear and informed ethical decisions are needed, particularly within the demanding schedule of clinical practice.

Assessing risk/danger

As is noted elsewhere in this book, recent years have seen a growing interest in the risks associated with people with mental disorder and the means by which such risks may be effectively assessed and managed. This has become a specialised aspect of mental health practice to which nurses have made a significant contribution (Allen, 1997).

Formal risk assessment and management require skilled intervention and, possibly, the application of specific measurement tools. Nurses are also involved, on a daily basis, with the less formal but equally meaningful kinds of risk assessment which take place, for example when a patient is to leave a clinical area for a short period within a constructive programme of rehabilitation.

The onerous responsibility for risk assessment may have both practical and moral implications for both the patient and others. It demands effective communication and close knowledge of the individual patient (Prins, 1996) and an understanding of the moral significance of making such important clinical appraisals. Identifying the focus of the risk, either to self and/or to others, may require that those who seek to implement risk management measures consider all the ethical implications of practice. For example, from a consequentialist perspective, a balance may be required between respecting the autonomy of the patient and achieving the best outcome, both for that individual and for others who may potentially be involved. It is perhaps ethically insufficient to simply declare that safety has been achieved by a process of effective assessment: the moral needs and concerns of all involved must be considered.

Physical interventions

The legal detention of mentally disordered offenders within secure environments implies some acceptance of the application of physical control measures. The need to physically control mentally disordered offenders and the methods employed to do so provide a source of ongoing commentary, much of which seeks to employ moral rationale to evaluate the application of physical measures (Mason, 1993; Hopton, 1995). But simple recourse to moral terminology does not necessarily provide either justification of a view nor evidence for the condemnation of practice.

Considerations of the principle of respect for autonomy appear to offer support to those who condemn the use of physical measures in the management of mentally disordered patients. The majority of papers concerning the use of seclusion in forensic mental health practice conclude that it is an inappropriate means of responding to physical disturbance and should have no place within a therapeutic programme. Such criticism focuses on a perceived need to respect the autonomy of the individual patient. Seclusion, it may be claimed, denies the individual the opportunity to exercise autonomy.

However, what is rarely considered within criticisms of seclusion as a means of managing disturbance is that the application of such an extreme measure of physical control may actually contribute to the creation of autonomy. By preventing disturbance and controlling behaviour in such a radical manner, nurses may be able to encourage the development of the patient's ability to exercise their autonomy. Such a moral justification may also support the considered application of other forms of physical restraint techniques.

Confidentiality

Nurses electing to work within forensic mental health care must acknowledge their obligation to maintain confidentiality within the confines of their professional role. The implications of such an obligation may, however, be somewhat ambiguous and the justification for disclosing confidential material should be made explicit.

Nurses may be exposed to a great deal of sensitive confidential information concerning their patients and others. On an individual basis, a deontological moral obligation to maintain confidentiality must be balanced against the needs of others to be aware of particular information. The claim that forensic mental health professionals may have a duty to warn third parties of the content of confidential exchanges has been highlighted (Mason, 1998).

The Access to Health Records Act 1990 gave patients the opportunity to acquire access to the majority of their written records and had particular implications for forensic mental health services: 'Psychiatric records are particularly sensitive because of the recording of opinions as well as facts, the nature of the diagnosis, the possible adverse response of the patient to disclosure, and the frequent inclusion of third party information' (Cope & Chiswick, 1995, p. 334). The need to ensure that patients are aware of their rights under the Act is accompanied by a requirement to maintain accurate records. The limitations to the patient's right of access to their records are particularly pertinent to forensic mental health practice (Box 14.1).

Box 14.1   Limitations to the Access to Health Records Act (Chiswick & Cope, 1995, p. 334)

Information can be withheld if:

(1)   Disclosure is 'likely to cause serious harm to the physical or mental health of the patient or any other individual'; or

(2)   The information is 'relating to, or provided by, an individual other than the patient, who could be identified by that information', unless the third party has consented.

Whether or not disclosure of confidential material is ever morally permissible remains a point for continuing debate and may ultimately rely on individual moral interpretation and justification.

Disclosure may be legally/professionally approved under certain specific circumstances, for example when the patient or their legal adviser gives written consent (General Medical Council, 1993).

W v. *Egdell* (1990) emphasised a judicial view in favour of disclosure in the public interest. The case concerned the communication of information contained within an independent 'confidential' report that Dr Egdell had prepared on patient 'W' who was detained in a secure hospital. The report, undertaken for a Mental Health Review Tribunal, opposed the patient's transfer to a medium secure facility and stated that, in Dr Egdell's opinion, W remained a danger. The patient's solicitors decided to withdraw the application for W's transfer and did not forward Dr Egdell's report to the Tribunal. To ensure that the contents of the report were not repressed, the doctor sent a copy both to W's hospital and to the Home Secretary. W's subsequent legal claim against Dr Egdell for damages for the breach of the duty of confidence was dismissed as was his subsequent appeal.

Acceptance and rejection of treatment

The concept of 'informed consent' is now an acknowledged aspect of health care practice and reflects a growing awareness of the need to both create and respect individual autonomy. The focus of obtaining consent has shifted from the doctor's responsibility to disclose information to a recognition of the patient's need to acquire and understand relevant information in order to make an informed decision. The central issue concerns self-determination and the perceived right of the individual to make an informed choice.

Requirements for obtaining consent to treatment of detained patients are outlined in Part IV of the Mental Health Act 1983. It should not automatically be assumed that a detained person will be unable or unwilling to offer informed consent to their treatment although the ability to offer such consent may be compromised by mental disorder. 'The fact that a person is suffering from a mental disorder, as defined in the Mental Health Act (1983) does not in itself preclude that person from giving a legally effective consent' (Skegg, 1988, p. 56). This also supports the right of such a patient to withdraw consent and reject treatment.

The rejection of many therapeutic interventions is a regular source of frustration for forensic practitioners: 'It is perhaps reasonable to suggest that compulsorily detained patients may be likely, at times, to reject treatment. Whilst individual autonomy should be acknowledged whenever possible [at least this is one moral view – see above], there may be occasions when autonomy has to be overridden in favour of perceived therapeutic benefit' (Chaloner, 1998, p. 32). An ethical challenge which nurses may frequently face is the requirement '... to confront the awkward question of how to respond to patients who reject treatment' (Clarke, 1998, p. 39). The overriding of autonomy demands ethical justification which may possibly be found within a consequentialist theory.

THE MORAL NATURE OF FORENSIC MENTAL HEALTH NURSES/NURSING

When one considers the many and varied ethical aspects of forensic mental health practice it is interesting to note that, within the body of literature relating to nursing, reference is rarely made to the character or attitudes of those who choose to care for mentally disordered offenders.

A consideration of the moral nature of those individuals who work within such a demanding health-care specialism must form an essential component of any examination of ethics and forensic mental health nursing. The specific nature of the nurse's role implies that a consideration of the moral nature of the individual practitioner could be of great value in identifying ethical foundations for practice. It may be argued that if it is not possible to determine the ethical intentions and characteristics of forensic mental health nurses, there is little point in trying to resolve the ethical dilemmas these individuals face in their day-to-day practice.

The 'action-based' ethical theories of deontology and consequentialism referred to above may be, in a sense, too simplistic to fully evaluate the morality of forensic nursing. Such theories are largely based on justifying decisions: you must always have an answer. A consideration of virtue ethics may allow a fuller exploration of the moral foundations of forensic practice. Virtue theorists may be somewhat sceptical about the moral claims of action-based theories: does there always have to be a 'right' answer? (Obviously in legal decisions there does, but legality and morality should not be confused: there is a particular risk of this within forensic mental health care). The most important aspect of virtue theories is that they define goodness and rightness (i.e. 'morality') not just in terms of the actions we perform but also how those actions came about (Scott, 1995). The virtue ethicist may consider that the morality of forensic nursing is best indicated by an assessment of the motives and intentions of the moral agent (the nurse) and perhaps a similar assessment of the motives and intentions of the profession?

Forensic mental health nursing is a demanding undertaking. The day-to-day association with mentally disordered offenders requires individuals who are able to cope effectively with the challenges of practice and respond appropriately to the diverse ethical nature of their role. The professional and public responsibilities of forensic mental health care are significant and the management of mentally disordered offenders requires careful consideration and a combination of rational and compassionate thinking.

FURTHER INQUIRY

The parameters of the forensic mental health nurse's role in caring for, treating and managing mentally disordered offenders have yet to be conclusively defined and the morality of care has yet to be exposed to a great deal of academic inspection. The indistinct nature of forensic mental health nursing which has led to what has been described as 'professional dysfunction' (Aiyegbusi, 1998) demands that the ethical aspects of practice receive as much attention as the more practical and visible issues which will undoubtedly continue to be exposed to increasing inspection.

The identification of the ethical basis for practice is needed. An examination of the practical ethical stances of those who deliver care to mentally disordered offenders will assist in this. Further investigation into the contribution of various ethical approaches – for example virtue ethics (see above), and the ethics of care (Beauchamp & Childress, 1994) – will offer a more comprehensive insight into the morality of both practice and practitioners.

CONCLUSION

Forensic mental health nursing requires a well developed moral awareness and the ability to identify and effectively respond to situations requiring ethical decisions. Moral dilemmas can frequently be anticipated and there is undoubtedly an acknowledged association between effective moral reasoning ability and skilled professional practice.

Forensic mental health nursing is, unfortunately but not surprisingly, closely associated with extremes of antisocial behaviour, physical control and custodial approaches to care. Such affiliations have generated a great deal of public, and possibly professional, misunderstanding about the true nature of forensic mental health care and certainly generated a substantial amount of moral concern regarding the 'rights' and 'wrongs' of this specialism.

Political, media and public attention has compelled forensic mental health services to develop more visible approaches to their work and to present open and honest appraisals of their services. Although forensic mental health establishments are no longer shrouded in the comparative 'secrecy' of the past, a number of misconceptions concerning the nature of practice remain.

There is an increasing need for an examination of the morality of all aspects of forensic mental health care. Such an examination may assist in the development of a considered ethical basis for practice and in formulating an informed response to the numerous and unusual ethical issues which this challenging specialism generates.

REFERENCES

Adshead, G. & Mezey, G. (1993) Ethical issues in the psychotherapeutic treatment of paedophiles: whose side are you on? *Journal of Forensic Psychiatry* 4(2), 361–8

Aiyegbusi, A. (1998) Forensic nursing is based on the flawed premise that care and custody can be combined (clinical review). *Nursing Times* 94(8), 51.

Allen, J. (1997) Assessing and managing risk of violence in the mentally disordered. *Journal of Psychiatric and Mental Health Nursing* 4, 369–78.

Appelbaum, P. S. (1990) The parable of the forensic psychiatrist: ethics and the problem of doing harm. *International Journal of Law and Psychiatry* 13(4), 249–59.

Beauchamp, T. & Childress, J. (1994) *Principles of Biomedical Ethics*. Oxford University Press, Oxford.

Blom-Cooper, L., Brown, M., Dolan, R. & Murphy, E. (1992) *Report of the Committee of Inquiry into Complaints about Ashworth Hospital*. HMSO, London.

Burrow, S. (1991) The Special Hospital Nurse and the dilemma of therapeutic custody. *Journal of Advances in Nursing and Health Care* 1(3), 21–38.

Burrow, S. (1993a) The role conflict of the forensic nurse ... facilitating the health-management of the mentally abnormal offender. *Senior Nurse* **13**(5), 20–25.

Burrow, S. (1993b) The contribution of secure hospitals to social control. *British Journal of Nursing* **2**(18), 891.

Burrow, S. (1994) Therapeutic security and the mentally disordered offender. *British Journal of Nursing* **3**(7), 314–15.

Byrt, R. (1993) Moral minefield. *Nursing Times* **89**(8), 63–6.

Chaloner, C. (1997) The legal and ethical context of mental health nursing. In *Stuart and Sundeen's Mental Health Nursing: Principles and Practice* (Thomas, B., Hardy, S. & Cutting, P., eds). Mosby, London.

Chaloner, C. (1998) Working in secure environments: ethical issues. *Mental Health Practice* **2**(2), 28–35.

Chandley, M. & Mason, T. (1995) Nursing chronically dangerous patients: ethical issues of behaviour management and patient health. *Psychiatric Care* **2**(1), 20–23.

Clarke, L. (1998) What's in a name? *Nursing Times* **94**(22), 38–9.

Coffey, M. (1997) Supervised discharge: concerns about the new powers for nurses. *British Journal of Nursing* **6**(4), 215–18.

Cope, R. & Chiswick, D. (eds) (1995) Ethical issues in forensic psychiatry. In *Seminars in Practical Forensic Psychiatry*. Royal College of Psychiatrists, London.

Doyal, L. (1994) Notes on the moral problems of diagnosing and treating psychopathic personality disorder. In *Report of the Department of Health and Home Office Working Group on Psychopathic Disorder*. Department of Health/Home Office, London.

Eastman, N. (1997) The Mental Health (Patients in the Community) Act 1995. *British Journal of Psychiatry* **170**, 492–6.

Eastman, N. & Peay, J. (1998) Sentencing psychopaths: is the 'Hospital and Limitation Direction' an ill-considered hybrid? *Criminal Law Review* February 93–108.

Fallon, P., Bluglass, R., Edwards, B. & Daniels, G. (1999) *The Report of the Committee of Inquiry into the Personality Disorder Unit, Ashworth Special Hospital*. HMSO, London.

Faulk, M. (1994) Ethics and forensic psychiatry. In *Basic Forensic Psychiatry*, 2nd edn (Faulk, M. ed.). Blackwell Science, Oxford.

General Medical Council (1993) *Professional Conduct and Discipline: Fitness to Practice*. GMC, London.

Gerrard, N. (1988) You must be mad to stay here. *The Observer*, 12 April.

Gillon, R. (1985) *Philosophical Medical Ethics*. Wiley, Chichester.

Gillon, R. (1996) Thinking about a medical school core curriculum for medical ethics and law. *Journal of Medical Ethics* **22**, 323–4.

Gillon, R. & Lloyd, A. (eds) (1994) *Principles of Health Care Ethics*. Wiley, Chichester.

Grundstein-Amado, R. (1993) Ethical decision-making processes used by health care providers. *Journal of Advanced Nursing* **18**, 1701–709.

Gunn, J. & Taylor, P. (eds) (1993) Ethics in forensic psychiatry. In *Forensic Psychiatry: Clinical, Legal and Ethical Issues*. Butterworth Heinemann, London.

Haslam, J. (1809) *Observations on Madness and Melancholy*. Callow, London.

Hopton, J. (1995) Control and restraint in contemporary psychiatric nursing: some ethical considerations. *Journal of Advanced Nursing* **22**, 110–15.

Kerr, G., Graley, R., Sandford, T. & Cresswell, J. (1997) What's so special? (Fish in a barrel/Taxing the councils/Behind closed doors/Trouble in the bins). *Open Mind* No. 86, 14–18.

Mason, T. (1993) Seclusion theory reviewed – a benevolent or malevolent intervention? *Medicine, Science and the Law* **33**(2), 95–102.

Mason, T. (1998) Tarasoff liability: its impact for working with patients who threaten others. *International Journal of Nursing Studies* **35**, 109–14.

Mason, T. & Mercer, D. (1996) Forensic psychiatric nursing: visions of social control. *Australia and New Zealand Journal of Mental Health Nursing* **5**(4), 153–62.

Murphy, E. (1997) The future of Britain's high security hospitals: the culture and values won't change until the Prison Officers' Association is ousted. *British Medical Journal* **314**, 1292–3.

Partridge, R. (1953) *Broadmoor. A History of Criminal Lunacy and Its Problems.* Chatto & Windus, London.

Prins, H. (1996) Taking chances: implications for decision makers. *Psychiatric Care* **3**(5), 181–7.

Rappeport, J. (1991) Ethics and forensic psychiatry. In *Psychiatric Ethics*, 2nd edn (Bloch, S. & Chodoff, P., eds). Oxford University Press, Oxford.

Scott, P. A. (1995) Aristotle, nursing and health care ethics. *Nursing Ethics* **2**(4), 279–85.

Seedhouse, D. (1998) *Ethics: the Heart of Health Care*, 2nd edn. Wiley, Chichester.

Singer, P. (1993) *Practical Ethics*, 2nd edn. Cambridge University Press, Cambridge.

Skegg, P. G. (1988) *Law, Ethics and Medicine.* Clarendon Press, Oxford.

Snell, J. (1997) 'I'd shut the bloody lot of them', Rowden tells Ashworth probe. *Health Service Journal* **107**, 584–8.

Tarbuck, P. (1992) Use and abuse of control and restraint. *Nursing Standard* **6**(52), 30–32.

Walker, N. (1991) Dangerous mistakes. *British Journal of Psychiatry* **158**, 752–7.

Chapter 15

History and Development

Stephan D. Kirby

INTRODUCTION

A number of authors have traced the history of mental health nursing, among them Barker (1990), Nolan (1993) and Nolan & Chung (1996), but very little has been written about the history and development of the forensic mental health nurse (FMHN).

The formal concept of mental health nursing emerged from under the skirts of the medical profession and was influenced by developments in psychology and sociology (Gijbels & Burnard, 1995). During the last 40 years, mental health nursing has been influenced by developments in psychopharmacology, changes in social policy – for example, the shift towards community-oriented services – and the emergence of other mental health professionals, such as social workers and occupational therapists. Major developments in mental health nurse education, the demise of local schools of nursing and the move towards a university-based pre- and post-registration educational system have all played a part in driving mental health nursing towards the millennium.

Nolan (1993) argues that nurses should feel empowered to disown the historical stereotypes with which they have been unfairly labelled and begin to reconstruct their past without fear. Similar thoughts are expressed by Hopton (1993) who supports this notion of a critical re-evaluation of the history of mental health nursing

Nolan (1993) states that a history confirms the legitimacy of the service one provides. Inclusion within the history of another group implies mere subordination, though the majority of historians have tended to see mental health nursing as an integral part of psychiatry, with no separate existence from it. This stereotypical image of the nurse–doctor relationship (Stein, 1968) is characterised by a perception of 'unquestioning obedience' and can be seen through rationalised bureaucratic dictate and by the historical socialisation process (Simpson, 1967; Davis, 1975) of the nurse into the hospital setting, with its emphasis on the medical model (Skevington, 1984) of organisational control. A review of the literature surrounding the history of British mental health nursing suggests that, at best, it has been considered an appendage of either general nursing or medicine and, at worst, an irrelevance meriting little or no acknowledgement in the history of care. This is a lamentable omission as the care of the mentally ill has a long and rich tradition and to tell its story should be of great significance to all mental health nurses (Nolan, 1993).

Care provision by mental health nurses is constantly changing and FMHNs are now exposed to a broad spectrum of care settings and patient groups. These include prison health-care settings (Gray, 1974; Saunders-Wilson, 1992); community-oriented services (Pederson, 1988; Chaloner & Kinsella, 1992; Evans, 1996); court diversion schemes (Kitchiner, 1996); plus forensic learning disability services, forensic adolescent services, and secure settings. The range of options within which FMHNs operate is comprehensive and continues to grow.

It is important to acknowledge that there is a cohort of patients within these services who are not offenders and are there as a result of behavioural management problems. The move to more community and less institutional provision implies that mentally disordered offenders will increasingly be cared for by nurses in mainstream mental health services, perhaps making those nurses 'forensic mental health nurses' by default.

The English National Board for Nursing, Midwifery and Health Visiting (ENB) describes forensic mental health nurses as registered nurses whose activities concern '... the employment of those skills necessary to address the needs of the ill individual who has offended, or is likely to offend, or who remains the subject of detention within the terms of legislation' (ENB, 1989).

THE PLACES AND THE PEOPLE

It may be claimed that, historically, mental hospitals were havens for the unwanted, antisocial, asocial and amoral. The goals of these institutions were to control such 'social misfits' and to protect society from their disruptive idiosyncrasies and themselves from society's rejection.

These goals were demanded of the institutions by society with its low tolerance to disruption and behaviour that was not the norm. Institutions were built away from the populace in large imposing bleak buildings with locked doors and a seemingly impenetrable brick wall surrounding this self-contained world, ostensibly to keep the inmates in.

If the asylums evolved because of society's intolerance towards 'misfits', a question could be raised: 'Which came first – the lunatic, the asylum or the people to care for the insane?'. It is commonly believed that the asylums were built because the immediate society was not prepared to put up with an individual's unusual behaviour, but, if society had been more tolerant and was prepared to look after its own 'oddities', would they have been built and would there have been the prevalence of 'labelled' mental illness on the scale it is now? It is a truism, after all, that a person only becomes a patient once he has been admitted to a hospital/asylum and not before. Perhaps if society had been more understanding, then the whole concept of community care would have taken on a new meaning (Kirby, 1985).

The history of the care and treatment of the mentally disordered is composed of many strands, distinct but interwoven: the growth of legislation to protect society from the insane and the insane from society; the development of institutional accommodation; the theorising of philosophers, politicians and men of law, as well as physicians about the nature and the cause of madness and the medical and psychological treatments in response to these theories.

Just as the emergence of medicine dominated the body, so the advent of psychiatry governed the mind (Mason & Mercer, 1996). The actual practice of care and the confinement of the insane stretches back more than 600 years in England. In fact, as far back as ninth century Britain the Celtic Church had a number of itinerant monks attached to each monastery. These were known as 'soul friends' who made mental health their particular concern. Their role was to befriend the disenchanted and melancholic and to form intimate spiritual relationships with them so as to 'steer them back into social harmony with kith and kin' (Clarke, 1975).

A select committee in 1807, studying the problem of lunatics in general, recommended that there should be one institution for 'His Majesty's Pleasure' (HMP) cases as well as 'county asylums' for ordinary pauper lunatics. The County Asylums Act (1808) and the ensuing Lunacy Act of 1845 heralded a new era in the care of the insane.

The emergence of the asylum system, however, simply reflected the increasing power of the state over the lives of individuals in the mid-nineteenth century. Although the asylums packaged their aims in medical rhetoric, as state-funded institutions their purpose was essentially social and lay in welfare administration (Nolan, 1993). Within a short period over 90% of the asylums' population were classified as paupers (Korman & Glennerster, 1990). The asylum programme in Britain effectively partitioned inmates from the rest of society. While there have always been bodies of people, either ecclesiastical or voluntary, who cared for the insane, it was the expansion of the asylum system and the opening of the County Asylums that allowed the role and responsibilities of the 'attendants' and 'warders' to be developed.

The equivalent institutional arrangements for the 'criminal lunatic' – altogether more modest – came with the statutory provisions of the Criminal Lunatic Act (1800) and the aforementioned County Asylums Act of 1808. These eventually led to the creation of the 'criminal lunatic asylum'.

In 1247 St. Mary Bethlem Priory opened in London's Bishopsgate, although it did not start caring for people who were mentally unwell until the latter half of the fourteenth century (McMillan, 1997). In 1624, visitors found the Hospital of St Mary at Bethlem overcrowded with 31 patients instead of 25, and so in 1776 the hospital moved to new buildings at Moorfields in London (McMillan, 1997). It was at this time that its name changed to The Bethlem Royal Hospital, which celebrated its 750th anniversary in 1997. Whilst the outside of the building was impressive, 'the inside was plainly a madhouse' (Russell, 1996). In the latter years of the seventeenth century, John Strype (1642–1737), an ecclesiastical historian writing about Bethlem Hospital, noted that there were three 'basket men' – possibly the predecessors of mental health nurses. Their title derived from the days when Bethlem was a monastery and monks with baskets went out to collect food and alms from the rich for the sick (Strype cited in Nolan, 1993).

In the early 1800s, while the Governors of Bethlem Hospital were negotiating for another hospital site in St. George's Fields, Southwark, they agreed that part of this venture would be a 'criminal lunatic asylum'. Two new buildings were put aside within the new hospital, one accommodating 45 male and the other 15 female prisoners. They were completed and occupied by October 1816. They were soon full, creating problems within the local county asylums, so much so that The Middlesex Asylum wrote to the Home Office objecting to taking criminal lunatics on the grounds that they did not have the security for that class of offender (Parker, 1985). During these early days of the asylum movement, the attendant's role was not clearly defined. There was no body of knowledge on which to base a coherent system of care and treatment. Their working day consisted primarily of cleaning, polishing, bed making, dressing patients and serving their meals (Hunter & Macalpine, 1974) – in short, attending to the inmates' basic needs; they also had to ensure that security was maintained.

Florence Nightingale observed that many of those who were employed to care for the sick would not have found work elsewhere because they were too old, alcoholic or simply too lazy. This image of an indolent, unmotivated workforce who were unable or unwilling to demonstrate compassion for patients and so unintelligent as to be totally dependent on rules and routines was rejected by Hunter (1956). This rejection was supported by Digby (1985) as it was felt that asylum keepers and attendants were the 'hidden dimension' of the asylum system whose work has been rarely described. It is now acknowledged that attendants were the backbone of the asylums, exercising considerable influence over the lives of patients. Russell (1996) noted that relationships between care staff and patients 'varied from brutality to the essence of kindness and consideration'.

In July 1835 the Home Office again wrote to the Governors of Bethlem, this time requesting that the male criminal department be enlarged to accommodate a further 30 occupants. This was agreed and the new wards were ready for occupation in 1838. Wide as its reach was, the 1845 Lunacy

Act was silent with regard to any further provision for criminal lunatics and the Bethlem criminal lunatic wings were soon overflowing into Fisherton House near Salisbury. The lunacy commissioners, returning regularly to the subject in their annual reports, continued to press for a separate asylum for criminal lunatics. They stated the opinion in 1855 (with particular reference to Bethlem) that it was 'highly objectionable' that such persons be detained in a 'general lunatic hospital'. In 1857 the commissioners triumphantly reported that the Government had agreed to provide a new state asylum for 600 criminal lunatics. This figure appears somewhat conservative as by this time there were already 581 criminal lunatics of whom 99 were in Bethlem (Parker, 1985).

It was during this time – the late eighteenth and early nineteenth centuries – that the term 'keeper' was regularly applied to those entrusted with the care of the mentally ill. 'Keeper' referred both to the owner of the house in which insane people were cared for, and to those employed to run such houses. With the emergence of the asylum system after 1845, Nolan (1993) reports that the term 'attendant' was preferred as it indicated a more humanitarian approach to care. The attendants 'attended' to the institution, keeping it clean and tidy, maintaining order by controlling inmates and ensuring there was sufficient farm and garden produce to render it viable. It is sad, however, that this period – one which has been deemed to be the start of the humanitarian era – has become renowned for '. . . the way in which people compared the mad to animals – that they could be violent, insensitive to heat and cold, and lacking in reason, that quality that distinguishes man from the beasts' (Russell, 1996).

At the same time as Bethlem was going through its radical changes and the way was being prepared for the building of an asylum for the criminally insane in England, the Irish were also taking this initiative. As a result of the Report on the District, Local and Private Lunatic Asylums in Ireland 1845, Dundrum Central Criminal Asylum was built and opened in 1850 (Forshaw & Rollin, 1990). This report noted that there were 84 criminal lunatics in asylums and 21 in gaols and the hospital opened with places for 80 males and 40 females. The staff of the hospital adopted a 'moral management' approach and the use of physical restraint was limited. Prior to its opening, the aforementioned report recommended that Dundrum, 'is not designed so that the building should partake of the character of a prison . . .'. Thus, where the Bethlem wings were overcrowded and oppressive, Dundrum was spacious and better suited to the moral management regimes.

In England, 'The Act for the Better Provision for the Custody and Care of Criminal Lunatics (1860)' allowed for the building of Broadmoor Criminal Lunatic Asylum which saw the closure of the criminal lunatic wings at Bethlem. It was decided that this institution would provide accommodation for only 400 men and 100 women, and would extend later if necessary (Parker, 1985). The building of Broadmoor began in March

1862. Ironically the workforce consisted of 254 convicts (together with their officers) who were transferred to the site from the public works prisons of Portland, Portsmouth and Chatham.

The new state asylum was completed in 1863. Within 12 months of opening, the Lunacy Commissioners reported that there was pressure for an immediate extension of Broadmoor, especially to the female wing. A new block for 50 women was opened in May 1867. It was again reported (in 1891), that Broadmoor was full and extensions were once more contemplated although the existing building had already been added to on several occasions. This situation reflected the shortage of provision generally for the insane. Throughout the last decade of the century Broadmoor operated to capacity and in the Lunacy Commissioners' report on their visit in May 1899 they commented:

'... the question of the provision of further accommodation for the criminal lunatics of the country is of pressing importance and is, we are informed, receiving consideration. Of the various proposals we have heard, the suggestion that another asylum should be built in the North of England is one which appears to us to have some special advantages' (Parker, 1985).

To alleviate the situation while a new state asylum was being built, an outbuilding of Parkhurst Prison was converted into Parkhurst Criminal Lunatic Asylum in 1900 (Faulk, 1994). Initially the reports were favourable but after a few years this picture had changed. There was an over-use of seclusion; no remuneration or tobacco allowance as at Broadmoor; the patients wore convict uniform; and there was only a limited area for exercise. In short the asylum was more like a prison.

About this time there was one of the earliest attempts to provide attendants with some form of training through a series of one-off lectures (Weir, 1992). Nolan & Chung (1996) argue that the introduction of formal training did not lead to greater control for these attendants, but resulted in further subservience towards the medical profession. They claim that the positivistic tradition of the day has been a perverted force in its influence on the history of mental health care in this country and subsequently mental health nursing training and practice (Gijbels & Burnard, 1995).

The term 'nurse' was first used around this period, but it referred solely to females while the men were still called 'attendants'; however, by the end of the century 'nurse' had become a neutral term for both male and female carers. From this time onwards there was a steady increase in admissions to mental hospitals. In 1890 there had been 86 067 people detained under the Lunacy Laws; by 1920 that number had increased to 120 344 and in 1930 there were an estimated 142 000 mental patients in hospitals in Britain (Ramon, 1985).

Rampton Criminal Lunatic Asylum was opened in October 1912 and within 8 months 88 men and 40 women were transferred in from Broadmoor leaving space for the Parkhurst patients to move before it was closed in 1913. The transferred patients were carefully selected as 'non-refractory' and preference was given to North Country people whose homes or friends were in the general vicinity of the asylum. In 1914, the Board of Control purchased Moss Side Institution in Merseyside – previously an epileptic colony – for the same sort of patients as were in Rampton. In 1919, Moss Side opened for 'dangerous male and female defectives' with 33 residents, though these were, over the next two years, transferred back to Rampton when it became the 'state institution for mental defectives'.

On the completion of extra accommodation, women were transferred to Rampton in 1922. By the early 1930s, however, both Rampton and Broadmoor were full, having reached their limit of expansion, and this was alleviated by Moss Side coming back into the possession of the Board of Control for the third time. It reopened in 1933, again as a state institution for 'dangerous and violent mental defectives', and 50 men and 51 women were transferred there in October.

By 1927 psychiatry was employing new terms: 'hospital' was being preferred to 'asylum'; and 'mental illness' and 'psychiatrist' to 'insanity' and 'asylum doctor'. The term 'nurse' began to be used for both male and female carers (Nolan, 1993), a usage which followed the setting up, in 1923, of the Supplementary Register for Mental Nurses under the General Nursing Council (GNC) where the title 'mental nurse' became 'official'.

In 1930, Rampton opened a juvenile section for children who could not be satisfactorily dealt with elsewhere. Consisting of two houses, one for boys and one for girls, each accommodating 36 children – and a school, it was set some distance from the main institution. This provision for children within Rampton was discontinued in 1956, with nobody under the age of 13 admitted to a high security hospital since 1980.

In Scotland, work began in 1936 to construct a State Institution for Mental Defectives at Carstairs. The State Hospital was completed in 1939 though during the Second World War the hospital was used by the British Army to treat military personnel who were suffering from 'mental breakdown as a result of their wartime experiences'. This ended in 1948 when the hospital became a secure institution for 'mental defectives'.

The use of the phrase 'psychiatric nurse' was first noted in the 1940s. This was based on the psychoanalytical model of mental illness, which was being adopted in certain hospitals, as it was felt to be different from the treatment provided in traditional mental hospitals.

The ownership of Rampton and Moss Side passed to the Minister of Health under Section 49(4) of the National Health Act 1946 with Broadmoor also being vested in the Ministry of Health, in accordance with Section 62 of the Criminal Justice Act 1948. At this time Broadmoor dropped the title 'Criminal Lunatic Asylum' and was named 'Broadmoor Institution', while Rampton and Moss Side became 'hospitals'. The Mental Health Act 1959 changed the name of the institutions to that of 'Special Hospitals' – on the basis that special security was needed to contain those who had shown a capacity to cause harm to others, in contrast to the remaining relatively harmless psychiatric population (Burrow, 1993a).

From the 1950s onwards, there was a dramatic move to revolutionise care within general psychiatric hospitals. To a large extent psychiatric care owes a debt of thanks to the high-security hospitals (Hamilton, 1985). If it had not been for their existence, then Dr George Bell at Dingleton Hospital, Melrose, would not have been able to pioneer the 'open door' policy. The special hospitals took the dangerous and difficult patients and those who needed to be cared for in conditions of security, thereby allowing this 'revolution' to develop and spread. The achievements of Dr Bell and his contemporaries were all the more commendable as they pre-dated the use of tranquillisers. Supported by the legislation of the 1959 Mental Health Act, which allowed patients to be admitted to hospital on a voluntary basis and encouraged their return to the community, terms such as 'open-door policy', 'therapeutic community' and 'community care' entered the psychiatric vocabulary.

In 1961 the then Minister of Health, Enoch Powell, appointed a working party to consider the provision of security in psychiatric hospitals and the future of the Special Hospitals (Ministry of Health, 1961). Its authors clearly recognised the consequences of this 'therapeutic community, open door' policy and observed that:

(1) security precautions cannot be disposed of for all psychiatric patients
(2) security precautions are a necessary part of treatment for the sake of the patient as well as the public
(3) the maximum security provided by Special Hospitals should not be used if suitable facilities can be made available locally
(4) patients should be treated near their homes, in so far as this is possible, to maintain links with the local community

Emery *et al.* (Ministry of Health, 1961) succinctly highlighted the need for the introduction of local secure facilities, not necessarily high secure, but certainly something between that and the open ward. The seeds for Regional Secure Units were sown. Despite the notion of regional medium secure provision being conceived in the early 1960s, the reality did not transpire until after the publication of both the Glancy Report (DHSS, 1974) and the final Butler Report (Home Office/Department of Health and Social Security, 1975) reports. Both envisaged a regional network of medium secure units (MSUs) as essential to the resolution of problems relating to the management and the placement of the 'mentally abnormal offender' as these patients had now become known.

Following plans in 1962 to update and extend Broadmoor again, it was decided to build a new hospital rather than modernise. A site next to Moss Side was chosen and while the two hospitals were to be separate entities they would share administrative facilities. In October 1974 an advance unit of the new hospital – Park Lane – was opened in buildings previously owned by Moss Side with the official opening of the entire new hospital in September 1984 (Hamilton, 1985). Also, in 1974, while these changes were occurring within high secure provision, the Secretary of State for Social Services announced the Government's acceptance of the Butler proposals for the establishment of Regional Secure Units. It was decided that, initially, 1000 secure places be provided as a matter of urgency. Meanwhile interim secure arrangements were being made in NHS psychiatric hospitals until the new units were built (Snowden, 1990).

The Butler Report (Home Office/Department of Health and Social Security, 1975) and the Glancy Report (Department of Health and Social Security, 1974) provided the general principles, but each region found it necessary to create its own concept of medium secure provision. Those Regional Health Authorities who already had a resident forensic psychiatrist took account of existing facilities, population density and the size of the region before deciding on a service model and the site for a permanent unit. The solution of these regional, medium secure units was an attempt to escape the dichotomies of prison versus hospital and criminal versus sick person.

In its report on the future of the Special Hospitals the Royal College of Psychiatrists (1980) said, '. . . it is clear that Regional Secure Units will only be able to function effectively with patients who do not need treatment in conditions of maximum security. For other patients Special Hospitals will still be required and they have advantages of providing a range of facilities appropriate for patients requiring more than a short range of stay in hospital'.

The first purpose-built Regional Secure Unit to be officially opened was the Hutton Unit (now the Hutton Centre), at St. Luke's Hospital, Middlesbrough, in November 1980. This period was the most influential in the creation and future development of the FMHN. Up to the mid-1980s all staff within the Special Hospitals were employed by the Department of Health and Social Security (DHSS). Therefore all staff were regarded as civil servants and required to sign the Official Secrets Act. With the development of the MSU movement, within NHS establishments and organisation, the staff were employed by the NHS and no Home Office or DHSS requirements were placed upon them. For the first time nurses working within secure environments were able to seek representation by nursing unions rather than the Prison Officers Association (POA) which had been the case in the Special Hospitals. It could be suggested that this was the turning point in the history of the FMHN. It was here that the specialism came of age and started to emerge from its (partly self-imposed, partly bureaucratically imposed) veil of secrecy.

Park Lane and Moss Side Hospitals amalgamated in 1989 to form Ashworth Hospital. The impetus for the amalgamation of the two Merseyside hospitals coincided with the management of all the English Special Hospitals transferring from the Department of Health to the newly established Special Hospital Services Authority (SHSA). The SHSA took over the running of the Special Hospitals on 1 October 1989. The immediate task of the authority was to get a firm grip on its management responsibilities whilst at the same time launching initiatives which would help shape medium- to long-term strategies by testing fresh approaches to care and providing new information. At the time that the SHSA was set up the Government set them six objectives (see Box 15.1)

Box 15.1   Objectives of the Special Hospitals Service Authority (SHSA, 1995a)

- To ensure the continuing safety of the public
- To provide appropriate treatment for patients
- To ensure a good quality of life for both patients and staff
- To develop the hospitals as centres of excellence for training of staff of all disciplines in forensic and other branches of psychiatric care and treatment
- To develop closer links with local and regional NHS psychiatric services
- To promote research into fields related to forensic psychiatry

---

Towards the end of 1995, when the SHSA was preparing for its metamorphosis into the High Security Psychiatric Services Commissioning Board (HSPSCB), it produced five strategies which, commenced by the SHSA, would be completed by the HSPSCB (Box 15.2). Some of the MSUs also saw these strategies as viable areas for service development. An example was the Hutton Centre's opening the first medium-secure long-stay ward (within the NHS) in 1996, not long after this range of strategies was announced.

Box 15.2   Strategies for high security services (SHSA, 1995b)

- Patients with learning disabilities
- Long-term medium security
- Patients with mental illness
- Patients with personality disorder
- Women requiring secure psychiatric services

Dramatic changes resulted not only from the influence of both the SHSA and the HSPSCB but also, and probably more directly, from the ever changing need of staff, patients, the public, and purchasers of secure services as well as in response to the changing face and direction of forensic mental health practice in general.

In April 1996 the HSPSCB set about integrating the high security services much more closely with mainstream NHS services. This was designed to be carried out through the following points (Bowis, 1995):

- separation of responsibility for commissioning and provision of high security services
- local management for the three Special Hospitals
- integration of high security services with other parts of the mental health services
- direct involvement of local NHS health purchasers in commissioning high security services

ADDITIONAL CARE SCENARIOS

Forensic mental health nursing is practised in a large number of care environments. The 'controlled' environment is an integral but not exclusive part of the health care process. Over the past few years there has been a rapid development in community care for the mentally disordered offender, while at the other end of the security spectrum there has been a growing awareness of the needs of mentally ill individuals in prison. This has resulted in an increase in the number of qualified nurses working within the prison health-care service and more inter-agency collaboration between the NHS and the Prison Service.

Prisons

Kirby & Maguire (1997) point out that, considering that a large percentage of the overall prison population is drawn from the socially disadvantaged, unemployed, unemployable, and restless quarters of society, it is perhaps unsurprising to find that large numbers of this population have a psychiatric disorder classifiable in terms of ICD-10 (World Health Organisation, 1992). No prison, or part of a prison, is recognised as a hospital. Under the purposes of the Mental Health Act 1983, prisoners cannot, except in cases of life-threatening emergencies, be treated without their consent. This obviously poses serious problems for the severely psychotic or paranoid patient who lacks insight or fears the persecution of vendettas and poisoning and therefore refuses treatment. These difficulties are compounded further if there is a delay in transferring the prisoner to a secure hospital setting under a section of the Mental Health Act 1983.

A number of variations in approaches to mental health care of prisoners have been developed. One example is that the 'local' forensic service employs the nursing staff and holds the contract that provides mental health care to the prison population. Another example is the prison which 'buys in' forensic health care from contracted forensic mental health services on a sessional basis.

Diversion schemes

Kitchiner (1996) points out that it became government policy to highlight and encourage local initiatives between health and social services and other appropriate professionals, with a view to improving arrangements for the identification and treatment of mentally disordered offenders. This was highlighted in Circulars 66/90 (Home Office, 1990) and 12/95 (Home Office, 1995) and resulted in the introduction of diversion schemes at many magistrates courts in England and Wales. Forensic community mental health nurses, forensic psychiatrists, approved social workers and probation officers are now available to offer these courts an 'on the spot' brief mental state assessment and, where possible, recommendations of support or treatment as an alternative to being remanded to custody (Joseph, 1990, 1991; James & Hamilton, 1991; Exworthy & Parrot, 1993; Hillis, 1993; Joseph & Potter, 1993; Kitchiner, 1995; Kitchiner & Davies, in press).

Kitchiner (1996) goes on to state that there is no definition that adequately describes a court diversion scheme. There are differences between schemes depending upon the membership of the team; the particular parent forensic service; the resources available; and the particular court framework. However, a court diversion/liaison scheme is a system which gives non-health-care staff who come into contact with perceived mentally disordered offenders the opportunity of referring them to health-care professionals with psychiatric assessment and diagnostic skills. The aim of this referral is to provide the court with a mental health assessment that will suggest alternatives to custody via treatment and/or support in the least secure environment appropriate to their needs.

FROM 'PSYCHIATRIC' TO 'FORENSIC MENTAL HEALTH' NURSE

The concept of the FMHN appears not to have been initiated and cultivated until the late 1970s and early 1980s, coinciding with the birth and rapid growth of the MSU movement. It would be a fair assumption to say that, prior to this time, nurses working within secure environments had rested in an air of complacency, safe in the knowledge that their practice and environments would not change. At this time the high secure hospitals dominated the field of forensic mental health nursing.

Most mental health professionals are familiar with the term 'forensic psychiatry' but they are perhaps less likely to have a clear conception of the forensic mental health nurse. Unlike many specialities there is little understanding of what forensic nursing represents (Burrow, 1993b).

Forensic clients fall into the well established diagnostic categories, but within these broad classifications there is a mosaic of subtle divisioning, including medico-legal and criminal issues. In addition to this 'judicial' element, conventional psychiatric hospitals and units often hand over to the secure environments responsibility for clients who display persistent challenging and disruptive behaviour. Such patients have often committed some serious assault or a series of dangerous acts in a hospital setting, but have not had formal contact with the criminal justice system.

One major argument against the establishment and furtherment of the specialised secure units is the perceived de-skilling of staff within conventional psychiatric services. Following the 'open door' revolution it became evident, within a decade or so, that staff were finding it increasingly difficult to deal with the types of patients and behaviours which historically they had always cared for within the conventional locked environment.

This revolution in the delivery of care also included the advent of psychotropic drugs and less restrictive regimes, and culminated in a gradual erosion of the traditional skills of both nursing and medical staff in dealing with difficult and dangerous patients (Snowden, 1985). This had the effect that a large number of 'conventional' psychiatric services were (and perhaps, remain) unwilling and/or unable to accept such patients, preferring to refer and subsequently transfer these patients to the specialist forensic/ secure services.

The forensic mental health nursing role has had to incorporate both legal and physical boundaries of therapeutic yet custodial detention. As Burrow (1991) pointed out, herein lies the essential paradox of the forensic treatment process and the nursing role, owing to the incompatibilities of therapeutic custody. Therapy and security have become inextricably linked. The therapy versus custody debate is about whether it is possible to provide individualised, patient-centred, health-promoting care while detaining patients, often for many years, to ensure the protection of the general public (Burrow, 1993b).

The therapeutic balance of security and therapy is an issue which has long been debated and appears to be no nearer resolution or even a satisfactory compromise. Invariably there are cases where security is sacrificed in favour of therapeutic activity and unnecessary and unfortunate incidents occur, or the need for security outweighs the therapeutic value of an intervention or action and the patient makes no clinical progress.

SKILLS AND COMPETENCIES

Tarbuck (1994) and Tarbuck & Rooney (1997) produced a discussion document which identified the skills and competencies of the FMHN which would be seen as attractive to external purchasers seeking to bring in these specialist nursing skills. These competencies (combined with those put forward by Kirby & Maguire in 1997) include the following (Box 15.3):

Box: 15.3   Competencies required by the forensic mental health nurse

- maintaining a safe and secure environment
- the assessment and management of dangerousness
- risk assessment and management
- psychodynamic psychotherapies
- assessment and treatment of offending behaviours
- management of personality disorders with associated offending behaviour
- understanding associated ethical issues in the management of the mentally disordered offender

---

THE EMERGENCE OF THE FORENSIC COMMUNITY MENTAL HEALTH NURSE

'In the 19th Century, mental patients were locked in and in the 20th Century they are locked out' (Wallace, 1985). The history of forensic mental health nursing in the community is incomplete, though Pederson (1988) reported some activity during the late 1970s, when nurses from secure units were providing a follow-up service to discharged MSU in-patients. What started as an after-care service for discharged in-patients now encompasses the wider needs of mentally disordered offenders in the community (Chaloner & Kinsella, 1992) and other non-hospital settings, i.e. within the prison setting. This group of patients has always been in existence though, as Pederson (1988) points out, it was not until the mid to late 1980s that the provision of specialist staff was recognised as a resource priority and forensic community mental health nurses (FCMHNs) were being recruited.

Evidence suggests that the forensic patient in the community requires an extended area of expertise. The role of the FCMHN was expanded upon by Moon (1993) to include such areas as the assessment of risk relating to violence, criminal offending, criminal or other antisocial behaviour and liaison with police, probationary services and forensic resources. Evans

(1996) expands this role by stating that they provide care for patients both inside and outside the secure environment, based upon individual patients' needs. Also they are the main link between the patient, the forensic clinical team and, crucially, the patient's family. The particular needs of relatives and the isolation and stigma associated with offending behaviour all require the skill of an experienced FCMHN who is able to interact effectively with a family to enable them, initially, to deal with their own needs as preparation for supporting their relative upon discharge.

Despite the specific circumstances of much forensic work, the actual practice of FCMHNs is similar to that carried out by generic community nurses (Chaloner & Kinsella, 1992); they have, however, been described as ambassadors for forensic psychiatry (Pederson, 1988). Pederson (1988) states that effective liaison between them and related agencies is vital owing to the professionally isolated nature of some establishments and the guarded way in which mentally disordered offenders are viewed by society.

CONCLUSION

The overall function of forensic mental health nursing could be described as primarily providing health care (as opposed to secondary issues of custody) for mentally disordered offenders within, on occasions, conditions of special security which is required for their dangerous, violent or criminal propensities. Although a somewhat simplistic view, it captures the essence of the forensic mental health nurse's function.

Being required to deliver health care to people who have a mental illness whilst being agents of social control for their deviant and antisocial behaviours demonstrates how the nurse's role is caught up within a web of contradictory issues. It is very important for nurses to show faith, trust and respect for their patients despite past and present behaviours. Forensic mental health nurses have a responsibility to take an active role in promoting this unique patient group to the rest of society by consciously raising the status of the patient to someone deserving of appropriate health facilities and treatments.

Over the years forensic mental health nursing has built a firm foundation of specialist knowledge and skills which are disseminated throughout general and forensic mental health arenas. It is necessary that nurses build on this foundation in order to take the care and treatment of the mentally disordered offender into the next century with a continued positive, dynamic and united approach.

The research, academic skills and knowledge base are increasing and nurses are in a position to demonstrate to their peers and colleagues from all professions that they have the determination and ability to meet these challenges head on and will continue to provide the best forensic mental health care that their patients require. It is time to take the nursing care of the mentally disordered offender into the new century.

REFERENCES

Barker, P. J. (1990) The conceptual basis of mental health nursing. *Nurse Education Today* 10, 339–48.

Bowis, J. (1995) High Security Psychiatric Services: Changes in Funding and Organisation. Announcement by Parliamentary Under-Secretary of State for Health. NHS Executive, London.

Burrow, S. (1991) The special hospital nurse and the dilemma of therapeutic custody. *Journal of Advanced Nursing and Health Care* 1(3), 21–38.

Burrow, S. (1993a) Inside the walls. *Nursing Times* 89(37), 38–40.

Burrow, S. (1993b) An outline of the forensic nursing role. *British Journal of Nursing* 2(18), 899–904.

Chaloner, C. & Kinsella, C. (1992) Care with conviction. *Nursing Times* 88(17), 50–52.

Clarke, B. (1975) *Mental Disorder in Early Britain*. University of Wales Press, Cardiff.

Davis, F. (1975) Professional socialisation as subjective experiences: the process of doctrinal conversion among student nurses. In *A Sociology of Medical Practice* (Cox, C. & Mead, A., eds). Collier-Macmillan, London.

Department of Health and Social Security (1974) *Revised Report of the Working Party on Security in National Health Service Hospitals (Glancy Report)*. HMSO, London.

Digby, A. (1985) *Madness, Morality and Medicine – A Study of the York Retreat*. Cambridge University Press, Cambridge.

English National Board for Nursing, Midwifery and Health Visiting (1989) Nursing in Controlled Environments: Course No. 770 Curriculum, ENB, London.

Evans, N. (1996) Defining the role of the forensic community mental health nurse. *Nursing Standard* 10(49), 35–7.

Exworthy, T. & Parrot, J. M. (1993) Evaluation of a diversion from custody scheme at magistrates' courts. *Journal of Forensic Psychiatry* 4, 497–505.

Faulk, M. (1994) *Basic Forensic Psychiatry*, 2nd edn. Blackwell Science, Oxford.

Forshaw, D. & Rollin, H. (1990) The history of forensic psychiatry in England. In *Principles and Practice of Forensic Psychiatry* (Bluglass, R. & Bowden, P., eds). Churchill Walker, Edinburgh.

Gijbels, H. & Burnard, P. (1995) *Exploring the Skills of Mental Health Nurses*. Avebury, Aldershot.

Gray, W. J. (1974) Grendon Prison. *British Journal of Hospital Medicine* 12, 299–308.

Hamilton, J. R. (1985) The special hospitals. In *Secure Provision* (Gostin, L., ed.). Tavistock Publications, London.

Hillis, G. (1993) Birmingham Diversion Services. Reaside Clinic, Birmingham (unpublished).

Home Office (1990) Circular 66/90 Provision for the Mentally Disordered. HMSO, London.

Home Office (1995) Circular 12/95 Progress Report on the Implications of Circular 66/90. HMSO, London.

Home Office/Department of Health and Social Security (1975) Report of the Committee on Abnormal Offenders (Butler Report). Cmnd 6244. HMSO, London.

Hopton, J. (1993) The contradictions of mental health nursing. *Nursing Standard* 8(11), 37–9.

Hunter, R. (1956) The rise and fall of mental nursing. *The Lancet* 1, 98–9.

Hunter, R. & Macalpine, I. (1974) *Psychiatry for the Poor*. Dawsons of Pall Mall, London.

James, D. V. & Hamilton, L. W. (1991) The Clerkenwell Scheme: assessing efficacy and cost of a psychiatric liaison service to a magistrates' court. *British Medical Journal* 303, 282–5.

Joseph, P. L. A. (1990) Mentally disordered offenders: diversion from the criminal justice system. *Journal of Forensic Psychiatry* 1(2), 133–7.

Joseph, P. L. A. (1991) *Psychiatric Assessment at the Magistrates' Court*. Home Office Research Planning Unit. HMSO, London.

Joseph, P. L. A. & Potter, M. (1993) Diversion from custody. 1. Psychiatric assessments at the magistrates' court. *British Journal of Psychiatry* 162, 325–30.

Kirby, S. D. (1985) The development of an existential, behavioural and social model of care for the rehabilitation of mentally ill people. ENB 945 Course Project, Central Hospital, Warwick (unpublished).

Kirby, S. D. & Maguire, N. A. (1997) Forensic psychiatric nursing. In *Stuart & Sundeen's Mental Health Nursing: Principles and Practice – UK Version* (Thomas, B., Hardy, S. & Cutting, P., eds). Mosby, London.

Kitchiner, N. J. (1995) A court diversion scheme for the mentally disordered offender. MSc (Nursing), University of Wales, College of Health, Cardiff (unpublished).

Kitchiner, N. J. (1996) Forensic community mental health nurses and court diversion schemes. *Psychiatric Care* 3(2), 65–9.

Kitchiner, N. J. & Davies, A. (In press) The development of a mental health assessment and diversion scheme for the mentally disordered offender in two magistrates courts in South Wales. In *Issues in Forensic Mental Health Nursing* (Tarbuck, P., Topping-Morris, B. & Burnard, P., eds). Whurr Publishers, London.

Korman, N. & Glennerster, N. (1990) *Hospital Closure*. Open University Press, Milton Keynes.

McMillan, I. (1997) Insight into Bedlam: one hospital's history. *Journal of Psychosocial Nursing* 35(6), 28–34.

Mason, T. & Mercer, D. (1996) Forensic psychiatric nursing: visions of social control. *Australian and New Zealand Journal of Mental Health Nursing* 5, 153–62.

Ministry of Health (1961) *Special Hospitals: Report of a Working Party* (Emery Report). HMSO, London.

Moon, W. (1993) The expanding role of the forensic community psychiatric nurse. *Journal for Nurses and Other Professionals in Forensic Psychiatry* 3, 12–13.

Nolan, P. (1993) *A History of Mental Health Nursing*. Chapman & Hall, London.

Nolan, P. & Chung, C. (1996) Science and early development of mental health nursing. *Nursing Standard* **10**(48), 44–7.

Parker, E. (1985) The development of secure provision. In *Secure Provision* (Gostin, L., ed.). Tavistock, London.

Pederson, P. (1988) The role of community psychiatric nurses in forensic psychiatry. *Community Psychiatric Nursing Journal* 8(3), 12–17.

Ramon, S. (1985) *Psychiatry in Britain – Meaning and Policy*. Croom Helm, London.

Royal College of Psychiatrists (1980) *Secure Facilities for Psychiatric Patients: A Comprehensive Policy*. Royal College of Psychiatrists, London.

Russell, D. (1996) *Scenes from Bedlam: A History of Caring for the Mentally Disordered at Bethlem Royal Hospital and the Maudsley*. Baillière Tindall, London.

Saunders-Wilson, D. (1992) Her Majesty's Prison Grendon: A maverick prison. *Journal of Forensic Psychiatry* 2(2), 179–83.

SHSA (1995a) *Special Hospitals Service Authority Review 1995*. Special Hospitals Service Authority, London

SHSA (1995b) *Service Strategies for Secure Care*. Special Hospitals Service Authority, London.

Simpson, I. H. (1967) Patterns of socialisation into professions: the case of student nurses. *Sociological Inquiry* 37, 47–54.

Skevington, S. (ed.) (1984) *Understanding Nurses: the Social Psychology of Nursing*. Wiley, Chichester.

Snowden, P. (1985) A survey of the Regional Secure Unit Programme. *British Journal of Psychiatry* **147**, 499–507.

Snowden, P. (1990) Regional Secure Units and forensic services in England and Wales. In *Principles and Practice of Forensic Psychiatry* (Bluglass, R. & Bowden, P., eds). Churchill Walker, Edinburgh.

Stein, L. I. (1968) The doctor/nurse game. *American Journal of Nursing* 68, 101–105.

Tarbuck, P. (1994) *Buying Forensic Mental Health Nursing: A Guide for Purchasers*. RCN, London.

Tarbuck, P. & Rooney, J. (1997) *Buying Forensic Mental Health Nursing*. RCN, London.

Wallace, M. (1985) When freedom is a life sentence. *The Times*, 16 December.

Weir, R. (1992) An experimental course of lectures on moral treatment for mentally ill people. *Journal of Advanced Nursing* 17, 390–95.

World Health Organisation (1992) *The ICD-10: Classification of Mental and Behavioural Disorders*. WHO, Geneva.

Postscript

Forensic mental health nursing can be both challenging and rewarding. It requires a range of professional and personal qualities and offers practitioners the potential for professional development and role satisfaction. The evolution of the specialism owes much to those who have highlighted the nurse's role and its general contribution to the treatment, care and management of mentally disordered offenders. Its development is ongoing and the future for nurses working within this unique area of mental health care offers much in relation to both personal and professional attainment.

Although forensic mental health nursing has yet to completely define its skills and knowledge base, the establishment of the specialism is confirmed and the foundations that have been laid offer an exciting future for those currently working within forensic mental health services and for nurses considering this area as a means to professional growth and challenge.

The contents of this book provide evidence of the significant advances made by forensic mental health nurses in recent years and demonstrate that the role has progressed significantly from that of 'asylum attendant' to one which is more consistent with the 'health' focus implied in the title.

As we look forward to the continued emergence of the forensic mental health nurse it is important that we do not lose sight of the origins of the specialism. The foundations for the role lie within in-patient secure environments and this is where the majority of forensic mental health nurses continue to practise. The emergence of discrete roles for nurses, within community mental health teams for example, is but one overt indicator of the progress which has been made. However, there is increasing evidence available of the many developments made by ward-based nurses working within medium and high secure services, and it should be noted that the 'specialist' aspect of the forensic mental health nursing role does not refer purely to practice undertaken within specific roles. The in-patient role has equal specialist validity to that of community-based practice.

How will the specialism develop? The development of a generic forensic mental health nursing programme is a possible means by which progress may be made. Further integration with the prison health care service and the development of long-term medium secure provision should widen and further enhance the scope of the forensic mental health nurse's role. Potential changes in mental health legislation together with increased interdisciplinary and multi-professional collaboration may lead to greater professional autonomy for some nurses. Another indication of nurses' expanding their role is in the area of work with relatives and families of patients.

Broadening nurses' understanding of risk assessment to include exploitation and iatrogenic factors may be required so that the sole focus of nursing interactions with patients is not centred on the negative aspects of their personalities. The regional nature of forensic community services may need to be reviewed to enable the provision of tenable comprehensive services. Nurses should participate in multi-disciplinary creative thinking with regard to the development of services, for example with regard to considerations regarding the integration of community forensic mental health teams with generic mental health services. This may allow realistic responses to patient-identified needs such as out-of-hours and crisis work.

With regard to clinical practice, it would appear prudent for forensic mental health nurses to review their practice in order to ensure interventions have demonstrable benefits to their patient group. Some of these, such as psychosocial interventions, have been addressed within this book and many other possibilities exist and are ripe for exploration. Practically this means using the evidence which currently exists to offer effective interventions within both hospital and community settings. For example, although the evidence accrued from case management is varied and often related to research-funded services, the core principles can be assimilated into practice. This will require a sense of vision and creativity in the application of resources but the potential benefits support the case for the adoption of these principles.

Of course, there should be little preventing forensic mental health nurses from collecting 'hard evidence' for the effectiveness of their interventions. Passively waiting for relevant findings from others' research is not representative of a professional specialism. For forensic mental health services, the incorporation of an evaluative framework into practice to enable the identification and collection of evidence-based outcomes will hopefully form an essential component of service delivery.

The humanistic principles on which much of mental health nursing is founded should not be offloaded in the rush to embrace newer ideologies. Efforts to promote the individual autonomy of forensic mental health patients may be hindered by, for example, the walls of a high secure hospital or indeed the confines of a legal detention order, but even within such parameters there exists the potential for the development of empathic relationships.

Of course, in approaching their patients effectively it is vital that nurses do not ignore their own needs for support and the prevention of the potentially negative effects of stress and 'burnout'. As evidence emerges of the stressful nature of forensic mental health nursing, it would be prudent for both nurses and their managers to develop supportive mechanisms to address these issues.

CONCLUSION

We hope that the discussion contained within this book has been both useful and informative. We have endeavoured to balance the exposure of current knowledge with indications towards future developments, and we hope that much of what has been written will stimulate ideas for individual practice and professional development.

Forensic mental health services represent one of the fastest developing areas of mental health care, and the many and varied influences on the delivery of these services and the persistently high public and professional profile they maintain require that all forensic mental health professionals work towards developing their specialist role and their skills and knowledge. Nurses must ensure that their contribution to forensic mental health services contributes to the process of development whilst consolidating the achievements made so far.

Chris Chaloner
Michael Coffey

Index